Nicholas Culepper

The English physician

enlarged with 369 medicines made of English herbs

Nicholas Culepper

The English physician
enlarged with 369 medicines made of English herbs

ISBN/EAN: 9783742840349

Manufactured in Europe, USA, Canada, Australia, Japa

Cover: Foto ©Lupo / pixelio.de

Manufactured and distributed by brebook publishing software
(www.brebook.com)

Nicholas Culepper

The English physician

THE

ENGLISH PHYSICIAN ENLARGED,

With Three Hundred and Sixty-Nine

MEDICINES,

MADE OF

ENGLISH HERBS,

That were not in any IMPRESSION until THIS.

BEING

An Astrologo-Physical discourse of the Vulgar Herbs of this Nation, containing a complete Method of Physic, whereby a Man may preserve his Body in Health, or cure himself, being Sick, for Three-pence Charge, with such Things only as grow in England, they being most fit for English Bodies.

Herein is also shewed these Seven Things, viz. 1. The Way of Making Plaisters, Ointments, Oils, Poultices, Syrups, Decoctions, Juleps, or Waters, of all Sorts of Physical Herbs, that you may have them ready for your Use at all times of the Year. 2. What Planet governeth every Herb or Tree (used in Physic) that groweth in England. 3. The time of gathering all Herbs, both Vulgarly and Astrologically. 4. The Way of drying and keeping the Herbs all the Year. 5. The way of keeping their Juice ready for Use at all Times. 6. The Way of making and keeping all kinds of useful Compounds made of Herbs. 7. The Way of mixing Medicines according to the Cause and Mixture of the Disease and Part of the Body afflicted.

BY *NICH. CULPEPPER*, GENT.

STUDENT IN PHYSIC AND ASTROLOGY.

LONDON:

Printed for P. M'QUEEN, J. LAIKINGTON, J. MATHEWS; WILSON and SPENCE, York; J. BINNS, Leeds; JO. CLARKE and Co. Manchester; JO. MOZLEY, Gainsborough; and W. COKE, Leith.

M.DCC.LXXXVIII.

An Alphabetical TABLE *of all the* HERBS *and* PLANTS *in this* BOOK; *as alſo what* PLANET *governeth every one of them.*

Clowns

Liver-

English

wall-

The CONTENTS of the DIRECTIONS for making *Syrups, Conferves, Oils, Ointments, Plaifters,* &c. of *Herbs, Roots, Flowers,* &c. whereby you may have them ready for ufe all the year long.

SECT. I.

The way of gathering, drying, and preferving Simples, and their Juices.

SECT. II.

The way of making and keeping all neceffary compounds.

THE ENGLISH PHYSICIAN ENLARGED.

AMARA DULCIS.

CONSIDERING divers ſhires in this nation give divers names to one and the ſame herb, and that the common name which it bears in one county, is not known in another, I ſhall take the pains to ſet down all the names that I know of each herb: Pardon me for ſetting that name firſt which is common to myſelf. Beſides Amara Dulcis, ſome call it Mortal, others Bitter-ſweet; ſome Woody Night-ſhade, and others Félon-wort.

Deſcript.] It grows up with woody ſtalks even to a man's height, and ſometimes higher. The leaves fall off at the approach of Winter, and ſpring out of the ſame ſtalk at Spring-time: The branch is compaſſed about with a whitiſh bark, and hath a pith in the middle of it: The main branch brancheth itſelf into many ſmall ones with claſpers, laying hold on what is next to them, as vines do: It bears many leaves, they grow in no order at all, at leaſt in no regular order: The leaves are longiſh, though ſomewhat broad, and pointed at the ends; many of them have two little leaves growing at the end of their foot-ſtalk; ſome have but one, and ſome none. The leaves are of a pale green colour; the flowers are of a purple colour, or of a perfect blue like to violets, and they ſtand many of them together in knots; the berries are green at firſt, but when they are ripe they are very red; if you taſte them, you ſhall find them juſt as the crabs which we in Suſſex call bitter-ſweets, *viz.* ſweet at firſt, and bitter afterwards.

Place.] They grow commonly almoſt throughout England, eſpecially in moiſt and ſhady places.

Time.] The leaves ſhoot out about the end of March, if the temperature of the air be ordinary; it flowereth in July, and the ſeeds are ripe ſoon after, uſually in the next month.

Government and Virtues.] It is under the planet Mercury, and a notable herb of his alſo, if it be rightly gathered under his influence. It is excellent good to remove witchcraft both in men and beaſts, as alſo all ſudden diſeaſes whatſoever. Being tied round about the neck, is one of the admirableſt remedies for the vertigo or dizzineſs in the head that is; and that is the reaſon (as Tragus ſaith) the people in Germany commonly hang it about their cattles necks, when they fear any ſuch evil hath betided them: Country people commonly uſe to take the berries of it, and having bruiſed them, they apply them to felons, and thereby ſoon rid their fingers of ſuch troubleſome gueſts.

We have now ſhewed you the external uſe of the herb; we ſhall ſpeak a word or two of the internal, and ſo conclude. Take notice, it is a Mercurial herb, and therefore of very ſubtle parts, as indeed all mercurial plants are; therefore take a pound of the wood and leaves together, bruiſe the wood (which you may eaſily do, for it is not ſo hard as oak) then put it in a pot, and put to it three pints of white wine, put on the pot-lid and ſhut it cloſe; and let it infuſe hot over a gentle fire twelve hours, then ſtrain it out, ſo have you a moſt excellent drink to open obſtructions of the liver and ſpleen, to help difficulty of breath, bruiſes and falls, and congealed blood in any part of the body, it helps the yellow jaundice, the dropſy and black-jaundice, and to cleanſe women newly brought to bed. You may drink a quarter of a pint of the infuſion every morning. It purgeth the body very gently, and not churliſhly, as ſome hold. And when you find good by this remember me.

They that think the uſe of theſe medicines is too brief, it is only for the cheapneſs of the book; let them read thoſe books of mine, of the laſt edition, *viz. Riverius, Veſlingus, Riolunus, Johnſon, Sennertus*, and *Phyſic for the Poor.*

All-heal.

IT is called All-heal, Hercules's All-heal, and Hercules's Wound-wort, becauſe it is ſuppoſed that Hercules learned the herb and its virtues from Chiron, when he learned phyſic of him. Some call it Panay, and others Opopane-wort.

Deſcript.

Descript.] Its root is long, thick, and exceeding full of juice, of a hot and biting taste, the leaves are great and large, and winged almost like ash-tree leaves, but that they are something hairy, each leaf consisting of five or six pair of such wings set one against the other upon foot-stalks, broad below, but narrow towards the end; one of the leaves is a little deeper at the bottom than the other, of a fair yellowish, fresh green colour; they are of a bitterish taste, being chewedi n the mouth. From among these ariseth up a stalk, green in colour, round in form, great and strong in magnitude, five or six feet high in altitude, with many joints, and some leaves thereat: Towards the top come forth umbels of small yellow flowers, after which are passed away, you may find whitish, yellow, short, flat seeds, bitter also in taste.

Place.] Having given you the description of the herb from the bottom to the top, give me leave to tell you, that there are other herbs called by this name; but because they are strangers in England, I give only the description of this, which is easily to be had in the gardens of divers places.

Time.] Although Gerrard saith, That they flower from the beginning of May to the end of December, experience teacheth them that keep it in their gardens, that it flowers not till the latter end of the Summer, and sheds its seed presently after.

Government and Virtues.] It is under the dominion of Mars, hot, biting, and cholerick; and remedies what evils Mars afflicts the body of man with, by sympathy, as vipers flesh attracts poison, and the loadstone iron. It kills the worms, helps the gout, cramp, and convulsions, provokes urine, and helps all joint-aches. It helps all cold griefs of the head, the vertigo, falling-sickness, the lethargy, the wind-cholick, obstructions of the liver and speen, stone in the kidneys and bladder. It provokes the terms, expels the dead birth: It is excellent good for the griefs of the sinews, itch, stone, and took-ach, the biting of mad-dogs and venomous beasts, and purgeth choler very gently.

ALKANET.

BESIDES the common name, it is called Orchanet, and Spanish Bugloss, and by apothecaries, Enchusa.

Descript.] Of the many sorts of this herb, there is but one known to grow commonly in this nation; of which one take this description: It hath a great and thick root, of a reddish colour, long, narrow, hairy leaves, green like the leaves of Buglofs, which lie very thick upon the ground; the stalks rise up compassed round about, thick with leaves, which are lesser and narrower than the former; they are tender, and slender, the flowers are hollow, small, and of a reddish colour.

Place.] It grows in Kent near Rochester, and in many places in the West Country, both in Devonshire and Cornwall.

Time.] They flower in July, and the beginning of August, and the seed is ripe soon after, but the root is in its prime, as carrots and parsnips are, before the herb runs up to stalk.

Government and Virtues.] It is an herb under the dominion of Venus, and indeed one of her darlings, though somewhat hard to come by. It helps old ulcers, hot inflammations, burnings by common fire, and St Anthony's fire, by antipathy to Mars; for these uses, your best way is to make it into an ointment; also, if you make a vinegar of it, as you make vinegar of roses, it helps the morphew and leprosy; if you apply the herb to the privities, it draws forth the dead child. It helps the yellow-jaundice, spleen, and gravel in the kidneys. Dioscorides saith, it helps such as are bitten by a venomous beast, whether it be taken inwardly, or applied to the wound; nay, he saith further, if any one that hath newly eaten it, do but spit into the mouth of a serpent, the serpent instantly dies. It stays the flux of the belly, kills worms, helps the fits of the mother. Its decoction made in wine, and drank, strengthens the back, and easeth the pains thereof: It helps bruises and falls, and is as gallant a remedy to drive out the small pox and measles as any is; an ointment made of it, is excellent for green wounds, pricks or thrusts.

ADDER'S TONGUE, or SERPENT'S TONGUE.

Descript.] THIS herb hath but one leaf, which grows with the stalk a finger's length above the ground, being flat and of a fresh green colour; broad like Water Plantane, but less, without any rib in it; from the bottom of which leaf, on the inside, riseth up (ordinarily) one,

one, ſometimes two or three ſlender ſtalks, the upper half whereof is ſomewhat bigger, and dented with ſmall dents of a yellowiſh green colour, like the tongue of an adder ſerpent (only this is as uſeful as they are formidable.) The roots continue all the year.

Place.] It grows in moiſt meadows, and ſuch like places.

Time.] It is to be found in May or April, for it quickly periſheth with a little heat.

Government and Virtues.] It is an herb under the dominion of the Moon and Cancer, and therefore if the weakneſs of the retentive faculty be cauſed by an evil influence of Saturn in any part of the body governed by the Moon, or under the dominion of Cancer, this herb cures it by ſympathy: It cures theſe diſeaſes after ſpecified, in any part of the body under the influence of Saturn, by antipathy.

It is temperate in reſpect of heat, but dry in the ſecond degree. The juice of the leaves drank with the diſtilled water of Horſe-tail, is a ſingular remedy for all manner of wounds in the breaſts, bowels, or other parts of the body, and is given with good ſucceſs unto thoſe that are troubled with caſting, vomiting, or bleeding at the mouth or noſe, or otherwiſe downwards. The ſaid juice given in the diſtilled water of Oaken-buds, is very good for women who have their uſual courſes, or the whites flowing down too abundantly. It helps ſore eyes. Of the leaves infuſed or boiled in oil, omphacine, or unripe olives, ſet in the ſun for certain days, or the green leaves ſufficiently boiled in the ſaid oil, is made an exellent green balſam, not only for green and freſh wounds, but alſo for old and inveterate ulcers, eſpecially if a little fine clear turpentine be diſſolved therein. It alſo ſtayeth and refreſheth all inflammations that ariſe upon pains by hurts and wounds.

What parts of the body are under each planet and ſign, and alſo what diſeaſe, may be found in my aſtrological judgment of diſeaſes; and for the internal work of nature in the body of man; as vital, animal, natural, and procreative ſpirits of man; the apprehenſion, judgment, and memory; the external ſenſes, *viz.* Seeing, hearing, ſmelling, taſting and feeling; the virtues attractive, retentive, digeſtive, expulſive, &c. under the dominion of what planets they are, may be found in my *Ephemeris* for the year 1651. In both which you ſhall find the chaff of authors blown away by the fame of Dr Reaſon, and nothing but rational truths left for the ingenious to feed upon.

Laſtly, To avoid blotting paper with one thing many times, and alſo to eaſe your purſes in the price of the book, and withal to make you ſtudious in phyſic; you have at the latter end of the book, the way of preſerving all herbs either in juice, conſerve, oil, ointment or plaiſter, electuary, pills or troches.

AGRIMONY.

Deſcript.] THIS hath divers long leaves (ſome greater ſome ſmaller) ſet upon a ſtalk, all of them dented about the edges, green above, and greyiſh underneath, and a little hairy withal. Among which ariſeth up uſually but one ſtrong, round, hairy, brown ſtalk, two or three feet high, with ſmaller leaves ſet here and there upon it At the top hereof grow many ſmall yellow flowers, one above another, in long ſpikes; after which come rough heads of ſeed, hanging downwards, which will cleave to and ſtick upon garments, or any thing that ſhall rub againſt them. The knot is black, long, and ſomewhat woody, abiding many years, and ſhooting afreſh every Spring; which root, though ſmall, hath a reaſonable good ſcent.

Place.] It groweth upon banks, near the ſides of hedges.

Time.] It flowereth in July and Auguſt, the ſeed being ripe ſhortly after.

Government and Virtues.] It is an herb under Jupiter, and the ſign Cancer; and ſtrengthens thoſe parts under the planet and ſign, and removes diſeaſes in them by ſympathy, and thoſe under Saturn, Mars, and Mercury by antipathy, if they happen in any part of the body governed by Jupiter, or under the ſigns Cancer, Sagittary, or Piſces, and therefore muſt needs be good for the gout, either uſed outwardly in oil or ointment, or inwardly in an electuary, or ſyrup, or concerted juice; for which ſee the latter end of this book.

It is of a cleanſing and cutting faculty, without any manifeſt heat, moderately drying and binding. It openeth and cleanſeth the liver, helpeth the jaundice, and is very beneficial to the bowels, healing all inward wounds, bruiſes,

hurts,

hurts, and other distempers. The decoction of the herb made with wine, and drank, is good against the biting and stinging of serpents, and helps them that make foul, troubled, or bloody water, and make them piss clear speedily. It also helpeth the cholick, cleanseth the breast, and rids away the cough. A draught of the decoction taken warm before the fit, first removes, and in time rids away the tertian or quartan agues. The leaves and seeds taken in wine, stays the bloody flux; outwardly applied, being stamped with old swines grease, it helpeth old sores, cancers, and inveterate ulcers, and draweth forth thorns, and splinters of wood, nails, or any other such things gotten in the flesh. It helpeth to strengthen the members that be out of joint; and being bruised and applied, or the juice dropped in it, helpeth foul and imposthumed ears.

The distilled water of the herb is good to all the said purposes, either inward or outward, but a great deal weaker.

It is a most admirable remedy for such whose lives are annoyed either by heat or cold. The liver is the former of blood, and blood the nourisher of the body, and Agrimony a strengthener of the liver.

I cannot stand to give you a reason in every herb, why it cureth such diseases; but if you please to peruse my judgment in the herb Wormwood, you shall find them there, and it will be well worth your while to consider it in every herb, you shall find them true throughout the book.

WATER AGRIMONY.

IT is called, in some countries, Water Hemp, Bastard Hemp, and Bastard Agrimony, Eupatorium, and Hepatorium, because it strengthens the liver.

Descript.] The root continues a long time, having many long slender strings. The stalk grows up about two feet high, sometimes higher. They are of a dark purple colour: The branches are many, growing at distances the one from the other, the one from the one side of the stalk, the other from the opposite point. The leaves are winged, and much indented at the edges. The flowers grow at the top of the branches, of a brown yellow colour, spotted with black spots, having a substance within the midst of them like that of a Daisy: If you rub them between your

your fingers, they ſmell like roſin or cedar when it is burnt. The ſeeds are long, and eaſily ſtick to any woollen thing they touch.

Place.] They delight not in heat, and therefore they are not ſo frequently found in the ſouthern parts of England, as in the northern, where they grow frequently: You may look for them in cold grounds, by ponds and ditches ſides, as alſo by running waters; ſometimes you ſhall find them grow in the midſt of the waters.

Time.] They all flower in July or Auguſt, and the ſeed is ripe preſently after.

Government and Virtues.] It is a plant of Jupiter, as well as the other Agrimony, only this belongs to the celeſtial ſign Cancer. It healeth and drieth, cutteth and cleanſeth thick and tough humours of the breaſt, and for this I hold it inferior to but few herbs that grow. It helps the cachexia or evil diſpoſition of the body, the dropſy and yellow jaundice. It opens obſtructions of the liver, mollifies the hardneſs of the ſpleen, being applied outwardly. It breaks impoſthumes taken inwardly: It is an excellent remedy for the third day ague. It provokes urine and the terms; it kills worms, and cleanſeth the body of ſharp humours, which are the cauſe of itch and ſcabs; the herb being burnt, the ſmoke thereof drives away flies, waſps, &c. It ſtrengthens the lungs exceedingly. Country people give it to their cattle when they are troubled with the cough, or broken-winded.

ALEHOOF, or GROUND-IVY.

SEVERAL counties give it ſeveral names, ſo that there is ſcarce an herb growing of that bigneſs that has got ſo many: It is called Cats-foot, Ground-ivy, Gill-go-by-ground, and Gill-creep-by-ground, Turnhoof, Haymaids, and Alehoof.

Deſcript.] This well known herb lieth, ſpreadeth, and creepeth upon the ground, ſhooteth forth roots, at the corners of tender jointed ſtalks, ſet with two round leaves at every joint ſomewhat hairy, crumpled, and unevenly dented about the edges with round dents; at the joints likewiſe, with the leaves towards the end of the branches, come forth hollow, long flowers, of a blueiſh purple co-

lour,

lour, with small white spots upon the lips that hang down. The root is small with strings.

Place.] It is commonly found under hedges, and on the sides of ditches, under houses, or in shadowed lanes, and other waste grounds, in almost every part of this land.

Time.] They flower somewhat early, and abide a great while; the leaves continue green until Winter, and sometimes abide, except the Winter be very sharp and cold.

Government and Virtues.] It is an herb of Venus, and therefore cures the diseases she causes by sympathy, and those of Mars by antipathy; you may usually find it all the year long, except the year be extremely frosty; it is quick, sharp, and bitter in taste, and is thereby found to be hot and dry; a singular herb for all inward wounds, exulcerated lungs, or other parts, either by itself, or boiled with other the like herbs; and being drank, in a short time it easeth all griping pains, windy and cholerick humours in the stomach, spleen or belly; helps the yellow jaundice, by opening the stoppings of the gall and liver, and melancholy, by opening the stoppings of the spleen; expelleth venom or poison, and also the plague; it provokes urine and womens courses; the decoction of it in wine drank for sometime together, procureth ease unto them that are troubled with the sciatica, or hip-gout; as also the gout in hands, knees, or feet; if you put to the decoction some honey and a little burnt alum, it is excellent good to gargle any sore mouth or throat, and to wash the sores and ulcers in the privy parts of man or woman; it speedily helpeth green wounds, being bruised and bound thereto. The juice of it boiled with a little honey and verdigrease, both wonderfully cleanse fistulas, ulcers, and stayeth the spreading or eating of cancers and ulcers; it helpeth the itch, scabs, wheals, and other breakings out in any part of the body. The juice of Celandine, Field-daisies, and Ground-ivy clarified, and a little fine sugar dissolved therein, and dropped into the eyes, is a sovereign remedy for all pains, redness, and watering of them; as also for the pin and web, skins and films growing over the sight; it helpeth beasts as well as men. The juice dropped into the ears, doth wonderfully help the noise and singing of them, and helpeth the hearing which is decayed. It is good to tun up with new drink, for it will clarify it in a night, that it will be the fitter to be drank the next morning; or if any drink be thick with removing, or any other accident, it will do the like in a few hours.

ALEXANDER.

IT is alſo called Aliſander, Horſe-parſley, and Wild-parſley, and the Black Pot-herb; the ſeed of it is that which is uſually ſold in apothecaries ſhops for Macedonian Parſley-ſeed.

Deſcript.] It is uſually ſown in all the gardens in Europe, and ſo well known that it needs no farther deſcription.

Time.] It flowereth in June and July; the ſeed is ripe in Auguſt.

Government and Virtues.] It is an herb of Jupiter, and therefore friendly to nature, for it warmeth a cold ſtomach, and openeth a ſtoppage of the liver and ſpleen; it is good to move womens courſes, to expel the after-birth, to break wind, to provoke urine, and helpeth the ſtrangury; and theſe things the ſeeds will do likewiſe. If either of them be boiled in wine, or being bruiſed and taken in wine, is alſo effectual againſt the biting of ſerpents. And you know what Alexander Pottage is good for, that you may no longer eat it out of ignorance, but out of knowledge.

The Black ALDER-TREE.

Deſcript.] THIS tree ſeldom groweth to any great bigneſs, but for the moſt part abideth like a hedge-buſh, or a tree ſpreading its branches, the woods of the body being white, and a dark red cole, or heart; the outward bark is of a blackiſh colour, with many whitiſh ſpots therein; but the inner bark next the wood is yellow, which being chewed, will turn the ſpittle near into a ſaffron colour. The leaves are ſomewhat like thoſe of an ordinary Alder-tree, or the Female Cornet, or Dogberry-tree, called in Suſſex Dog-wood, but blacker, and not ſo long. The flowers are white, coming forth with the leaves at the joints, which turn into ſmall round berries, firſt green, afterwards red, but blackiſh when they are thorough ripe, divided as it were, into two parts, wherein is contained two ſmall round and flat ſeeds. The root runneth

not

not deep into the ground, but spreads rather under the upper crust of the earth.

Place.] This tree or shrub may be found plentifully in St John's wood by Hornsey, and the woods upon Hamstead-heath; as also a wood called the Old Park in Barcomb in Essex, near the brooks sides.

Time.] It flowereth in May, and the berries are ripe in September.

Government and Virtues.] It is a tree of Venus, and perhaps under the celestial sign Cancer. The inner yellow bark hereof purgeth downwards both choler and phlegm, and the watery humours of such that have the dropsy, and strengthens the inward parts again by binding. If the bark hereof be boiled with Agrimony, Woormwood, Dodder, Hops, and some Fennel, with Smallage, Endive, and Succory roots, and a reasonable draught taken every morning for some time together, it is very effectual against the jaundice, dropsy, and the evil disposition of the body, especially if some suitable purging medicines have been taken before, to void the grosser excrements: It purgeth and strengtheneth the liver and spleen, cleansing them from such evil humours and hardness as they are afflicted with. It is to be understood that these things are performed by the dried bark; for the fresh green bark taken inwardly provokes strong vomitings, pains in the stomach, and gripings in the belly; yet if the decoction may stand and settle two or three days, until the yellow colour be changed black, it will not work so strongly as before, but will strengthen the stomach, and procure an appetite to meat. The outward bark contrariwise doth bind the body, and is helpful for all lasks and fluxes thereof, but this also must be dried first, whereby it will work the better. The inner bark thereof boiled in vinegar is an approved remedy to kill lice, to cure the itch, and take away scabs, by drying them up in a short time. It is singular good to wash the teeth, to take away the pains, to fasten those that are loose, to cleanse them, and keep them sound. The leaves are good fodder for kine, to make them give more milk.

If in the Spring-time you use the herbs before-mentioned, and will take but a handful of each of them, and to them add an handful of Elder buds, and having bruised

them

them all, boil them in a gallon of ordinary beer, when it is new; and having boiled them half an hour, add to this three gallons more, and let them work together, and drink a draught of it every morning, half a pint, or thereabouts, it is an excellent purge for the Spring, to consume the phlegmatic quality the Winter hath left behind it, and withal to keep your body in health, and consume those evil humours which the heat of Summer will readily stir up. Esteem it as a jewel.

The common ALDER-TREE,

Descript.] GROWETH to a reasonable hight, and spreads much if it like the place. It is so generally well known unto country people, that I conceive it needless to tell that which is no news.

Place and Time.] It delighteth to grow in moist woods and watry places; flowering in April or May, and yielding ripe seed in September.

Government and Use.] It is a tree under the dominion of Venus, and of some watry sign or other, I suppose Pisces; and therefore the decoction, or distilled water of the leaves, is excellent against burnings and inflammations, either with wounds or without, to bathe the place grieved with, and especially for that inflammation in the breast, which the vulgar call an ague.

If you cannot get the leaves (as in Winter 'tis impossible) make use of the bark in the same manner.

The leaves and bark of the Alder-tree are cooling, drying, and binding. The fresh leaves laid upon swellings dissolve them, and stay the inflammations. The leaves put under the bare feet galled with travelling, are a great refreshing to them. The said leaves gathered while the morning dew is on them, and brought into a chamber troubled with fleas, will gather them thereunto, which being suddenly cast out, will rid the chamber of those troublesome bed-fellows.

ANGELICA.

TO write a description of that which is so well known to be growing almost in every garden, I suppose is altogether needless; yet for its virtues it is of admirable use.

In

In time of Heathenism, when men had found out any excellent herb, they dedicated it to their gods; as the Bay-tree to Apollo, the Oak to Jupiter, the Vine to Bacchus, the Poplar to Hercules. These the Papists following as the Patriarchs, they dedicate to their Saints; as our Lady's Thistle to the Blessed Virgin, St John's Wort to St John, and another Wort to St Peter, *&c.* Our physicians must imitate like apes (though they cannot come off half so cleverly) for they blasphemously call Phansies or Hearts-ease, *an herb of the Trinity*, because it is of three colours: And a certain ointment, *an ointment of the Apostles*, because it consists of twelve ingredients: Alas, I am sorry for their folly, and grieved at their blasphemy; God send them wisdom the rest of their age, for they have their share of ignorance already. Oh! Why must ours be blasphemous, because the Heathens and Papists were idolatrous? Certainly they have read so much in old rusty authors, that they have lost all their divinity; for unless it were amongst the Ranters, I never read or heard of such blasphemy. The Heathens and Papists were bad, and ours worse; the Papists giving idolatrous names to herbs for their virtues sake, not for their fair looks; and therefore some called this an herb of the *Holy Ghost*; others more moderate called it Angelica, because of its angelical virtues, and that name it retains still, and all nations follow it so near as their dialect will permit.

Government and Virtues.] It is an herb of the Sun in Leo; let it be gathered when he is there, the Moon applying to his good aspect; let it be gathered either in his hour, or in the hour of Jupiter, let Sol be angular; observe the like in gathering the herbs of other planets, and you may happen to do wonders. In all epidemical diseases caused by Saturn, that is as good a preservative as grows: It resists poison, by defending and comforting the heart, blood, and spirits; it doth the like against the plague and all epidemical diseases, if the root be taken in powder to the weight of half a dram at a time, with some good treacle in Carduus water, and the party thereupon laid to sweat in his bed; if treacle be not to be had, take it alone in Carduus or Angelica-water. The stalks or roots candied and eaten fasting, are good preservatives in time of infection; and at other times to warm and comfort a cold ſtomach. The root alſo ſteeped in vinegar, and a little of that vinegar taken ſometimes faſting, and the root ſmelled unto, is good for the ſame purpoſe. A water diſtilled from the root ſimply, as ſteeped in wine, and diſtilled in a glaſs, is much more effectual than the water of the leaves; and this water, drank two or three ſpoonfuls at a time, eaſeth all pains and torments coming of cold and wind, ſo that the body be not bound; and taken with ſome of the root in powder, at the beginning, helpeth the pleuriſy as alſo all other diſeaſes of the lungs and breaſt, as coughs, phthyſick, and ſhortneſs of breath; and a ſyrup of the ſtalks do the like. It helps pains of the colick, the ſtrangury and ſtoppage of the urine, procureth womens courſes, and expelleth the after-birth, openeth the ſtoppings of the liver and ſpleen, and briefly eaſeth and diſcuſſeth all windineſs and inward ſwellings. The decoction drunk before the ſit of an ague, that they may ſweat (if poſſible) before the fit comes, will, in two or three times taking, rid it quite away; it helps digeſtion, and is a remedy for a ſurfeit. The juice, or the water, being dropped into the eyes or ears, helps dimneſs of ſight and deafneſs; the juice put into the hollow teeth, eaſeth their pains. The root in powder, made up into a plaiſter with a little pitch, and laid on the biting of mad dogs, or any other venomous creature, doth wonderfully help. The juice or the water dropped, or tents wet therein, and put into filthy dead ulcers, or the powder of the root (in want of either) doth cleanſe and cauſe them to heal quickly, by covering the naked bones with fleſh; the diſtilled water applied to places pained with the gout, or ſciatica, doth give a great deal of eaſe.

The wild Angelica is not ſo effectual as the garden; although it may be ſafely uſed to all the purpoſes aforeſaid.

AMARANTHUS.

BESIDES its common name, by which it is beſt known by the floriſts of our days, it is called Flower Gentle, Flower Velure, Floramor, and Velvet Flower.

Deſcript.] It being a garden flower, and well known to every one that keeps it, I might forbear the deſcription; yet, notwithſtanding, becauſe ſome deſire it, I ſhall give it. It runneth up with a ſtalk a cubit high, ſtreaked, and ſomewhat reddiſh toward the root, but very ſmooth, divided towards the top with ſmall branches, among which ſtand long broad leaves of a reddiſh green colour, ſlippery; the flowers are not properly flowers, but tuſts, very beautiful to behold, but of no ſmell, of reddiſh colour; if you bruiſe them, they yield juice of the ſame colour; being gathered, they keep their beauty a long time; the ſeed is of a ſhining black colour.

Time.] They continue in flower from Auguſt till the time the froſt nip them.

Government and Virtues.] It is under the dominion of Saturn, and is an excellent qualifier of the unruly actions and paſſions of Venus, though Mars alſo ſhould join with her. The flowers dried and beaten into powder, ſtop the terms in women, and ſo do almoſt all other red things. And by the icon, or image of every herb, the ancients at firſt found out their virtues. Modern writers laugh at them for it; but I wonder in my heart, how the virtues of herbs came at firſt to be known, if not by their ſignatures; the moderns have them from the writings of the ancients; the ancients had no writings to have them from: But to proceed. The flowers ſtop all fluxes of blood; whether in man or woman bleeding either at the noſe or wound. There is alſo a ſort of Amaranthus that bears a white flower, which ſtops the whites in women, and the running of the reins in men, and is a moſt gallant antivenereal, and a ſingular remedy for the French pox.

Anemone.

Called alſo Wind Flower, becauſe they ſay the flowers never open but when the wind bloweth. Pliny is my author; if it be not ſo, blame him. The ſeed alſo (if it bears any at all) flies away with the wind.

Place and Time.] They are ſown uſually in the gardens of the curious, and flower in the Spring-time. As for deſcription I ſhall paſs it, being well known to all thoſe that ſow them.

Government and Virtues.] It is under the dominion of Mars, being ſuppoſed to be a kind of Crow-foot. The leaves provoke the terms mightily, being boiled, and the decoction drunk. The body being bathed with the decoction of them, cures the leprosy. The leaves being stamped, and the juice snuffed up in the nose, purgeth the head mightily; so doth the root, being chewed in the mouth, for it procureth much spitting, and bringeth away many watery and phlegmatic humours, and is therefore excellent for the lethargy. And when all is done, let physicians prate what they please, all the pills in the dispensatory purge not the head like to hot things held in the mouth. Being made into an ointment, and the eyelids anointed with it, it helps inflammations of the eyes, whereby it is palpable, that every stronger draweth its weaker like. The same ointment is excellent good to cleanse malignant and corroding ulcers.

GARDEN ARRACH.

CALLED also Orach, and Arage.

Descript.] It is so commonly known to every housewife, it were labour lost to discribe it.

Time.] It flowereth and seedeth from June to the end of August.

Government and Virtues.] It is under the government of the Moon; in quality cold and moist like unto her. It softeneth and loosenerh the body of man being eaten, and fortifieth the expulsive faculty in him. The herb, whether it be bruised and applied to the throat; or boiled, and in like manner applied, it matters not much, it is excellent good for swellings in the throat; the best way, I suppose, is to boil it, and having drunk the decoction inwardly, apply the herb outwardly: The decoction of it besides, is an excellent remedy for the yellow jaundice.

ARRACH, wild and stinking.

CALLED also Vulvaria, from that part of the body, upon which the operation is most; also Dogs Arrach, Goats Arrach, and Stinking Motherwort.

Descript.] This hath small and almost round leaves, yet a little pointed and without dent or cut, of a dusky mealy colour, growing on the slender stalks and branches that spread on the ground, with small flowers in clusters set with the leaves, and small seeds succeeding like the rest,

rest, perishing yearly, and rising again with its own sowing. It smells like rotten fish, or something worse.

Place.] It grows usually upon dunghills.

Time.] They flower in June and July, and their seed is ripe quickly after.

Government and Virtues.] Stinking Arrach is used as a remedy to help women pained, and almost strangled with the mother, by smelling to it; but inwardly taken there is no better remedy under the moon for that disease. I would be large in commendation of this herb, were I but eloquent. It is an herb under the dominion of Venus, and under the sign Scorpio; it is common almost upon every dunghill. The works of God are given freely to man, his medicines are common and cheap, and easy to be found: ('Tis the medicines of the College of Physicians that are so dear and scarce to find) I commend it for an universal medicine for the womb, and such a medicine as will easily, safely, and speedily cure any disease thereof, as the fits of the mother, dislocation, or falling out thereof; it cools the womb being over-heated. And let me tell you this, and I will tell you the truth, heat of the womb is one of the greatest causes of hard labour in child-birth. It makes barren women fruitful. It cleanseth the womb if it be foul, and strengthens it exceedingly; it provokes the terms if they be stopped, and stops them if they flow immoderately; you can desire no good to your womb, but this herb will effect it; therefore if you love children, if you love health, if you love ease, keep a syrup always by you, made of the juice of this herb, and sugar, (or honey, if it be to cleanse the womb) and let such as be rich keep it for their poor neighbours; and bestow it as freely as I bestow my studies upon them, or else let them look to answer it another day, when the Lord shall come to make inquisition of blood.

ARCHANGEL.

TO put a gloss upon their practice, the physicians call an herb (which country people vulgarly know by the name of Dead Nettle) Archangel; whether they savour more of superstition or folly, I leave to the judicious reader. There is more curiosity than courtesy to my countrymen used by others in the explanation as well of the names, as description of this so well known herb; which, that I may not also be guilty of, take this short description, first of the Red Archangel.

Descript.] This has divers square stalks, some what hairy, at the joints whereof grow two sad green leaves dented about the edges, opposite to one another to the lowermost upon long foot stalks, but without any toward the tops, which are somewhat round, yet pointed, and a little crumpled and hairy; round about the upper joints, where the leaves grow thick, are sundry gaping flowers of a pale reddish colour; after which come the seeds three or four in a husk. The root is smaller and thready, perishing every year; the whole plant hath a strong scent, but not stinking.

White Archangel hath divers square stalks, none standing straight upward, but bending downward, whereon stand two leaves at a joint, larger and more pointed than the other, dented about the edges, and greener also, more like unto Nettle leaves, but not stinking, yet hairy. At the joints with the leaves stand larger and more open gaping white flowers, husks round about the stalks, but not with such a bush of leaves as flowers set in the top, as is on the other wherein stand small roundish black seeds; the root is white, with many strings at it, not growing downward, but lying under the upper crust of the earth, and abideth many years increasing; this hath not so strong a scent as the former.

Yellow Archangel is like the White in the stalks and leaves; but that the stalks are more straight and upright, and the joints with leaves are farther asunder, having longer leaves than the former, and the flowers a little larger and more gaping, of a fair yellow colour in most, in some paler. The roots are like white, only they creep not so much under the ground.

Place.] They grow almost every way (unless it be in the middle of the street) the yellow most usually in the wet grounds of woods, and sometimes in the drier, in divers counties of this nation.

Time.] They flower from the beginning of the Spring all the Summer long.

Virtues

Virtues and Use.] The Archangels are somewhat hot and drier than the stinging Nettles, and used with better success for the stopping and hardness of the spleen, than they, by using the decoction of the herb in wine, and afterwards applying the herb hot unto the region of the spleen as a plaister, or the decoction with spunges. Flowers of the White Archangel are preserved or conserved to be used to stay the whites, and the flowers of the red to stay the reds in women. It makes the heart merry, drives away melancholy, quickens the spirits, is good against quartan agues, stancheth bleeding at mouth and nose, if it be stamped and applied to the nape of the neck; the herb also bruised, and with some salt and vinegar and hogs-grease, laid upon an hard tumour or swelling, or that vulgarly called the king's evil, do help to dissolve or discuss them; and being in like manner applied, doth much allay the pains, and give ease to the gout, sciatica, and other pains of the joints and sinews. It is also very effectual to heal green wounds, and old ulcers; also to stay their fretting, gnawing and spreading. It draweth forth splinters, and such like things gotten into the flesh, and is very good against bruises and burnings. But the yellow Archangel is most commended for old, filthy, corrupt sores and ulcers, yea although they grow to be hollow; and to dissolve tumours. The chief use of them is for women, it being a herb of Venus, and may be found in my *Guide for Women.*

ARSSMART.

THE hot Arssmart is called also Water-pepper, or Culrage. The mild Arssmart is called dead Arssmart Percicaria, or Peach-wort, because the leaves are so like the leaves of a peach-tree; it is also called Plumbago.

Description of the Mild.] This hath broad leaves set at the great red joint of the stalks; with semi-circular blackish marks on them, usually either bluish or whitish, with such like seed following. The root is long, with many strings thereat, perishing yearly; this hath no sharp taste (as another sort hath, which is quick and biting) but rather sour like sorrel, or else a little drying, or without taste.

Place.] It grows in watry places, ditches, and the like, which

which for the most part are dry in Summer.

Time.] It flowereth in June, and the seed is ripe in August.

Government and Virtues.] As the virtue of both these is various, so is also their government; for that which is hot and biting, is under the dominion of Mars, but Saturn challengeth the other, as appears by that leaden coloured spot he hath placed upon the leaf.

It is of a cooling and drying quality, and very effectual for putrified ulcers in man or beast, to kill worms, and cleanse the putrefied places. The juice thereof dropped in, or otherwise applied, consumeth all cold swellings, and dissolveth the congealed blood of bruises by strokes, falls, &c. A piece of the root, or some of the seeds bruised, and held to an aching tooth, taketh away the pain. The leaves bruised and laid to the joint that hath a felon thereon taketh it away. The juice destroyeth worms in the ears, being dropped into them; if the hot Arssmart be strewed in a chamber, it will soon kill all the fleas; and the herb or juice of the cold Arssmart, put to a horse, or other cattle's sores, will drive away the fly in the hottest time of Summer; a good handful of the hot biting Arssmart put under a horse's saddle, will make him travel the better, although he were half tired before. The mild Arssmart is good against all imposthumes and inflammations at the beginning, and to heal green wounds.

All authors chop the virtues of both sorts of Arssmart together, as men chop herbs to the pot, when both of them are of clean contrary qualities. The hot Arssmart groweth not so high or tall as the mild doth, but hath many leaves of the colour of peach leaves, very seldom or never spotted; in other particulars it is like the former, but may easily be known from it, if you will but be pleased to break a leaf of it cross your tongue, for the hot will make your tongue to smart, so will not the cold. If you see them both together, you may easily distinguish them, because the mild hath far broader leaves: And our College of Physicians, out of the learned care of the publick good, *Anglice*, their own gain, mistake the one for the other in their *New Master-piece*, whereby they discover, 1. Their ignorance. 2. Their carelessness; and he

that

that hath but half an eye, may see their pride without a pair of spectacles. I have done what I could to distinguish them in the virtues, and when you find not the contrary named, use the cold. The truth is, I have not yet spoken with Dr Reason, nor his brother Dr Experience concerning either of them.

ASARABACCA.

Descript.] ASARABACCA hath many heads rising from the roots, from whence come many smooth leaves, every one upon his own foot-stalks, which are rounder and bigger than Violet leaves, thicker also, and of a dark green shining colour on the upper side, and of a pale yellow green underneath, little or nothing dented about the edges, from among which rise small, round, hollow, brown green husks, upon short stalks, about an inch long, divided at the brims into five divisions, very like the cups or heads of the Henbane seed, but that they are smaller: and these be all the flowers it carrieth, which are somewhat sweet, being smelled unto, and wherein, when they are ripe, is contained small cornered rough seeds, very like the kernels or stones of grapes or raisins. The roots are small and whitish, spreading divers ways in the ground, increasing into divers heads; but not running or creeping under the ground, as some other creeping herbs do. They are somewhat sweet in smell, resembling Nardus, but more when they are dry than green; and of a sharp but not unpleasant taste.

Place.] It groweth frequently in gardens.

Time.] They keep their leaves green all Winter; but shoot forth new in the Spring, and with them come forth those heads or flowers which give ripe seed about Midsummer, or somewhat after.

Government and Virtues.] 'Tis a plant under the dominion of Mars, and therefore inimical to nature, This herb being drank not only provoketh vomiting, but purgeth downward, and by urine also, purgeth both choler and phlegm: If you add to it some spikenard, with the whey of goat's milk, or honeyed water, it is made more strong, but it purgeth phlegm more manifestly than choler, and therefore doth much help pains in the hips, and other parts;

parts; being boiled in whey, they wonderfully help the obſtructions of the liver and ſpleen, and therefore profitable for the dropſy and jaundice; being ſteeped in wine and drank, it helps thoſe continual agues that come by the plenty of ſtubborn humours; an oil made thereof by ſetting in the ſun, with ſome laudanum added to it, provoketh ſweating, (the ridge of the back being anointed therewith) and thereby driveth away the ſhaking fits of the ague. It will not abide any long boiling, for it looſeth its cheif ſtrength thereby; nor much beating, for the finer powder doth provoke vomits and urine, and the coarſer purgeth downwards.

The common uſe hereof is, to take the juice of five or ſeven leaves in a little drink to cauſe vomiting; the roots have alſo the ſame virtue, though they do not operate ſo forcibly; they are very effectual againſt the biting of ſerpents, and therefore are put as an ingredient both into Mithridate and Venice treacle. The leaves and roots being boiled in lee, and the head often waſhed therewith while it was warm, comforteth the head and brain that is ill affected by taking cold, and helpeth the memory.

I ſhall deſire ignorant people to forbear the uſe of the leaves; the roots purge more gently, and may prove beneficial in ſuch as have cancers, or old putrified ulcers, or fiſtulas upon their bodies, to take a dram of them in powder in a quarter of a pint of white wine in the morning. The truth is, I fancy purging and vomiting medicines as little as any man breathing doth, for they weaken nature, nor ſhall ever adviſe them to be uſed, unleſs upon urgent neceſſity. If a phyſician be nature's ſervant, it is his duty to ſtrengthen his miſtreſs as much as he can, and weaken her as little as may be.

ASPARAGUS, SPARAGUS, or SPERAGE.

Deſcript.] IT riſeth up at firſt with divers whit and green ſcaly heads, very brittle or eaſy to break while they are young, which afterwards riſe up in very long and ſlender green ſtalks, of the bigneſs of an ordinary riding wand, at the bottom of moſt, or bigger or leſſer, as the roots are of growth; on which are ſet divers branches of green leaves ſhorter and ſmaller than fennel

to

to the top; at the joints whereof come forth small yellowish flowers, which turn into round berries, green at first, and of an excellent red colour when they are ripe, shewing like bead or coral, wherein are contained exceeding hard black seeds, the roots are dispersed from a spongeous head into many long, thick, and round strings, wherein is sucked much nourishment out of the ground, and increaseth plentifully thereby.

Prickly ASPARAGUS, or SPERAGE.

Descript.] IT groweth usually in gardens, and some of it grows wild in Appleton meadows, in Gloucestershire, where the poor people do gather the buds of young shoots, and sell them cheaper than our garden Asparagus is sold at London.

Time.] They do for the most part flower, and bear their berries late in the year, or not at all, although they are housed in Winter.

Government and Virtues.] They are both under the dominion of Jupiter. The young buds or branches boiled in ordinary broth, make the belly soluble and open, and boiled in white wine, provoke urine, being stopped, and is good against the stranguary or difficulty of making water; it expelleth the gravel and stone out of the kidneys, and helpeth pains in the reins. And boiled in white wine or vinegar, it is prevalent for them that have their arteries loosened, or are troubled with the hip-gout or sciatica. The decoction of the roots boiled in wine and taken, is good to clear the sight, and being held in the mouth easeth the tooth-ach; and being taken fasting several mornings together, stirreth up bodily lust in man or woman (whatever some have written to the contrary.) The garden Asparagus nourisheth more than the wild, yet hath it the same effects in all the afore-mentioned diseases: The decoction of the roots in white wine, and the back and belly bathed therewith, or kneeling or lying down in the same, or sitting therein as a bath, hath been found effectual against pains of the reins and bladder, pains of the mother and colick, and generally against all pains that happen to the lower parts of the body, and no less effectual against stiff and benumbed sinews, or those that are shrunk by cramps and convulsions, and helpeth the sciatica.

ASH

Ash Tree.

THIS is so well known, that time will be mispent in writing a description of it; and therefore I shall only insist upon the virtues of it.

Government and Virtues.] It is governed by the sun; and the young tender tops, with the leaves taken inwardly, and some of them outwardly applied, are singular good against the biting of viper, adder, or any other venomous beast; and the water distilled therefrom being taken a small quantity every morning fasting, is a singular medicine for those that are subject to dropsy, or to abate the greatness of those that are too gross or fat. The decoction of the leaves in white wine helpeth to break the stone, and expel it, and cureth the jaundice. The ashes of the bark of the Ash made into lee, and those heads bathed therewith, which are leprous, scabby, or scald, they are thereby cured. The kernels within the husks, commonly called Ashen Keys, prevail against stiches and pains in the sides, proceeding of wind, and voideth away the stone by provoking urine.

I can justly except against none of all this, save only the first, *viz.* That Ash-tree tops and leaves are good against the bitings of serpents and vipers. I suppose this had its rise from Gerard or Pliny, both which hold, That there is such an antipathy between an adder and an Ash-tree, that if an adder be encompassed round with Ash-tree leaves, she will sooner run through the fire than through the leaves: The contrary to which is the truth, as both my eyes are witness. The rest are virtues something likely, only if it be in winter when ye cannot get the leaves, you may safely use the bark instead of them. The keys you may easily keep all the year, gathering them when they are ripe.

Avens, called also Colewort, and Herb Bonet.

Descript.] THE ordinary Avens hath many long, rough, dark green winged leaves, rising from the root, every one made of many leaves set on each side of the middle rib, the largest three whereof grow at the end, and are snipped or dented round about the edges; the other being small pieces, sometimes two and sometimes four.

four, standing on each side of the middle rib underneath them. Among which do rise up divers rough or hairy stalks about two feet high, branching forth with leaves at every joint, not so long as those below, but almost as much cut in on the edges, some into three parts, some into more. On the tops of the branches stand small, pale, yellow flowers, consisting of five leaves, like the flowers of Cinquefoil, but large, in the middle whereof standeth a small green herb, which, when the flower is fallen, groweth to be round, being made of many long greenish purple seeds (like grains) which will stick upon your clothes. The root consists of many brownish strings or fibres, smelling somewhat like unto cloves, especially those which grow in the higher, hoter, and drier grounds, and in free and clear air.

Place.] They grow wild in many places under hedges sides, and by the path-ways in fields; yet they rather delight to grow in shadowy than sunny places.

Time.] They flower in May and June for the most part, and their seed is ripe in July at the farthest.

Government and Virtues.] It is governed by Jupiter, and that gives hopes of a wholesome healthful herb. It is good for the diseases of the chest or breast, for pains, and stitches in the side, and to expel crude and raw humours from the belly and stomach, by the sweet savour and warming quality. It dissolves the inward congealed blood happening by falls or bruises, and the spitting of blood, if the roots, either green or dry, be boiled in wine and drank; as also all manner of inward wounds or outward, if washed or bathed therewith. The decoction also being drank, comforts the heart, and strengtheneth the stomach and a cold brain, and therefore is good in the Spring-time to open obstructions of the liver, and helpeth the wind colick; it also helps those that have fluxes, or are bursten, or have a rupture; it taketh away spots or marks in the face, being washed therewith. The juice of the fresh root, or powder of the dried root, hath the same effect with the decoction. The root in the Spring-time steeped in wine, doth give it a delicate savour and taste, and being drank fasting every morning, comforteth the heart, and is a good preservative against the plague, or any other poison. It helpeth digestion, and warmeth a cold stomach, and openeth obstructions of the liver and spleen.

It is very safe; you need have no dose prescribed; and is very fit to be kept in every body's house.

BALM.

THIS herb is so well known to be an inhabitant almost in every garden, that I shall not need to write any description thereof, although the virtues thereof, which are many, may not be omitted.

Government and Virtues.] It is an herb of Jupiter, and under Cancer, and strengthens nature much in all its actions. Let a syrup made with the juice of it and sugar (as you shall be taught at the latter end of the book) be kept in every gentlewoman's house, to relieve the weak stomachs and sick bodies of their poor sickly neighbours; as also the herb kept dry in the house, that so with other convenient simples, you may make it into an electuary with honey, according as the disease is, you shall be taught at the latter end of my book. The Arabian physicians have extolled the virtues thereof to the skies; although the Greeks thought it not worth mentioning. Seraphio saith, it causeth the mind and heart to become merry, and reviveth the heart, faintings and swoonings, especially of such who are overtaken in sleep, and driveth away all troublesome cares and thoughts out of the mind, arising from melancholy or black choler; which Avicen also confirmeth. It is very good to help digestion, and open obstructions of the brain, and hath so much purging quality in it (saith Avicen) as to expel those melancholy vapours from the spirits and blood which are in the heart and arteries, although it cannot do so in other parts of the body. Dioscorides saith, That the leaves steeped in wine, and the wine drank, and the leaves externally applied, is a remedy against the stings of a scorpion, and the bitings of mad dogs; and commendeth the decoction thereof for women to bathe or sit in to procure their courses; it is good to wash aching teeth therewith, and profitable for those that have the bloody-flux. The leaves also with a little nitre taken in drink, are good against the

the surfeit of mushrooms, helps the griping pains of the belly; and being made into an electuary, it is good for them that cannot fetch their breath: Used with salt, it takes away wens, kernels, or hard swellings in the flesh or throat; it cleanseth foul sores, and easeth pains of the gout. It is good for the liver and spleen. A tansy or caudle made with eggs, and juice thereof while it is young, putting to it some sugar and rose-water, is good for a woman in child-bed, when the after-birth is not thoroughly voided, and for their faintings upon or in their sore travel. The herb bruised and boiled in a little wine and oil, and laid warm on a boil, will ripen it, and break it.

BARBERRY.

THE shrub is so well known by every boy and girl that hath but attained to the age of seven years, that it needs no description.

Government and Virtues.] Mars owns the shrub, and presents it to the use of my countrymen to purge their bodies of choler. The inner rind of the Barberry-tree boiled in white wine, and a quarter of a pint drank each morning, is an excellent remedy to cleanse the body of cholerick humours, and free it from such diseases as choler causeth, such as scabs, itch, tetters, ringworms, yellow jaundice, boils, &c. It is excellent for hot agues, burnings, scaldings, heat of the blood, heat of the liver, bloody flux; for the berries are as good as the bark, and more pleasing; they get a man a good stomach to his victuals, by strengthening the attractive faculty which is under Mars, as you may see more at large at the latter end of my EPHEMERIS for the year 1651: The hair washed with the lee made of ashes of the tree and water, will make it turn yellow, viz. of Mars' own colour. The fruit and rind of the shrub, the flowers of broom and of heath, or furz, cleanse the body of choler by sympathy, as the flowers, leaves, and bark of the peach-tree do by antipathy; because these are under Mars, that under Venus.

BARLEY.

THE continual usefulness hereof hath made all in general so acquainted herewith, that it is altogether needless to describe it, several kinds hereof plentifully growing, being yearly sown in this land. The virtues thereof take as followeth.

Government and Virtues.] It is a notable plant of Saturn; if you view diligently its effects by sympathy and antipathy, you may easily perceive a reason of them; as also why barley-bread is so unwholesome for melancholy people. Barley in all the parts and composions thereof (except malt) is more cooling than wheat, and a little cleansing: And all the preparations thereof, as barley-water and other things made thereof, do give great nourishment to persons troubled with fevers, agues, and heats in the stomach. A poultice made of barley meal or flour boiled in vinegar and honey, and a few dry figs put into them, dissolveth all hard imposthumes, and assuageth inflammations, being thereto applied. And being boiled with melilot and camomile-flowers, and some linseed, fenugreek and rue in powder, and applied warm, it easeth pains in side and stomach, and windiness of the spleen. The meal of barley and fleawort boiled in water, and made a poultice with honey and oil of lilies applied warm, cureth swellings under the ears, throat, neck, and such like; and a plaister made thereof with tar, wax, and oil, helpeth the king's evil in the throat; boiled with sharp vinegar into a poultice, and laid on hot, helpeth the leprosy; being boiled in red wine with pomgranate rinds, and myrtles, stayeth the lask or other flux of the belly; boiled with vinegar and quince, it easeth the pains of the gout; barley-flour, white salt, honey, and vinegar mingled together, taketh away the itch speedily and certainly. The water distilled from the green barley in the end of May, is very good for those that have defluctions of humours fallen into their eyes, and easeth the pain being dropped into them; or white bread steeped therein, and bound on the eyes, doth the same.

GARDEN BAZIL, or SWEET BAZIL.

Descript.] THE greater or ordinary Bazil riseth up usually with one upright stalk diversely branching forth on all sides, with two leaves at every joint, which are somewhat broad and round, yet pointed, of a pale green colour, but fresh; a little snipped about the edges, and of a strong healthy scent. The flowers are small and white, and standing at the tops of the branches, with two small leaves at the joints, in some places green, in others brown, after which come black seed. The root perisheth at the approach of Winter, and therefore must be new sown every year.

Place.] It groweth in gardens.

Time.] It must be sowed late, and flowers in the heart of Summer, being a very tender plant.

Government and Virtues.] This is the herb which all authors are together by the ears about, and rail at one another (like lawyers.) Galen and Dioscorides hold it not fitting to be taken inwardly; and Chrysippus rails at it, with downright Billinsgate rhetoric; Pliny, and the Arabian physicians, defend it.

For mine own part, I presently found that speech true;

Non nostrum inter nos tantas componere lites.

And away to Dr Reason went I, who told me it was an herb of Mars, and under the Scorpion, and perhaps therefore called Basilicon, and it is no marvel if it carry a kind of virulent quality with it. Being applied to the place bitten by venomous beasts, or stung by a wasp or hornet, it speedily draws the poison to it; *Every like draws his like.* Mizaldus affirms, that, being laid to rot in horse-dung, it will breed venomous beasts. Hilarius, a French physician, affirms upon his own knowledge, that an acquaintance of his, by common smelling to it, had a Scorpion bred in his brain. Something is the matter, this herb and rue will not grow together, no, nor near one another; and we know rue is as great an enemy to poison as any that grows.

To conclude: It expelleth both birth and after-birth; and as it helps the deficiency of Venus in one kind, so it spoils all her actions in another. I dare write no more of it.

The BAY TREE.

THIS is so well known that it needs no description; I shall therefore only write the virtues thereof, which are many.

Government and Virtues.] I shall but only add a word or two to what my friend hath written, viz. That it is a tree of the sun, and under the celestial sign Leo, and resisteth witchcraft very potently, as also all the evils old Saturn can do to the body of man, and they are not a few; for it is the speech of one, and I am mistaken if it were not Mizaldus, that neither witch nor devil, thunder nor lightening, will hurt a man in the place where a Bay-tree is. Galen said, That the leaves or bark do dry and heal very much, and the berries more than the leaves; the bark of the root is less sharp and hot, but more bitter, and hath some astriction withal, whereby it is effectual to break the stone, and good to open obstructions of the liver, spleen, and other inward parts, which bring the jaundice, dropsy, &c. The berries are very effectual against all poison of venomous creatures, and the sting of wasps and bees; as also against the pestilence, or other infectious diseases, and therefore put into sundry treacles for that purpose: They likewise procure womens courses; and seven of them given to a woman in sore travel of child-birth, do cause a speedy delivery, and expel the after-birth, and therefore not to be taken by such as have not gone out their time, lest they procure abortion, or cause labour too soon. They wonderfully help all cold and rheumatic distillations from the brain to the eyes, lungs, or other parts; and being made into an electuary with honey, do help the consumption, old coughs, shortness of breath, and thin rheums; as also the megrim. They mightily expel the wind, and provoke urine; help the mother, and kill the worms. The leaves also work the like effects. A bath of the decoction of the leaves and berries, is singular good for women to sit in, that are troubled with the mother, or the diseases thereof, or the stoppings of their courses, or for the diseases of the bladder, pains in the bowels by wind and stopping of urine. A decoction likewise of equal parts of Bay-berries, cummin-feed, hyssop, origanum, and euphorbium, with some honey, and the head bathed therewith, doth wonderfully help distillations and rheums, and settleth the palate of the mouth into its place. The oil made of the berries is very comfortable in all cold griefs of the joints, nerves, arteries, stomach, belly, or womb, and helpeth palsies, convulsions, cramp, aches, tremblings and numbness in any part, weariness also, and pains that come by sore travelling. All griefs and pains proceeding from wind, either in the head, stomach, back, belly, or womb, by anointing the parts affected therewith: And pains in the ears are also cured by dropping in some of the oil, or by receiving into the ears the fume of the decoction of the berries through a funnel. The oil takes away the marks of the skin and flesh by bruises, falls, &c. and dissolveth the congealed blood in them: It helpeth also the itch, scabs, and weals in the skin.

BEANS.

BOTH the garden and field beans are so well known that it saveth me the labour of writing any description of them. Their virtues follow:

Government and Virtues.] They are plants of Venus, and the distilled water of the flower of garden beans is good to clean the face and skin from spots and wrinkles, and the meal or flour of them, or the small beans doth the same. The water distilled from the green husks, is held to be very effectual against the stone, and to provoke urine. Bean flour is used in poultices to assuage inflammations rising upon wounds, and the swelling of womens breasts, caused by the curdling of their milk, and represseth their milk: Flour of beans and fenugreek mixed with honey, and applied to felons, boils, bruises, or blue marks by blows, or the imposthumes in the kernels of the ears, helpeth them all; and with rose leaves, frankinscense, and the white of an egg, being applied to the eyes, helpeth them that are swollen or do water, or have received any blow upon them, if used with wine. If a Bean be parted in two, the skin being taken away, and laid on the place where the leech hath been set that bleedeth too much, stayeth the bleeding. Bean flour boiled

to

to a poultice with wine and vinegar, and ſome oil put thereto, eaſeth both pains and ſwellings of the cods. The huſks boiled in water to the conſumption of a third part thereof, ſtayeth a laſk: And the aſhes of the huſks, made up with old hog's greaſe, helpeth the old pains, contuſions, and wounds of the ſinews, the ſciatica and gout. The field Beans have all the afrementioned virtues as the garden Beans.

Beans eaten are extreme windy meat; but if after the Dutch faſhion, when they are half boiled you huſk them, and then ſtew them (I cannot tell you how, for I never was cook in all my life) they are wholeſome food.

French Beans.

Deſcript.] THIS French or Kidney-Bean ariſeth at firſt but with one ſtalk, which afterwards divides itſelf into many arms or branches, but all ſo weak that if they be not ſuſtained with ſticks or poles, they will be fruitleſs upon the ground. At ſeveral places of theſe branches grow foot ſtalks, each with three broad, round and pointed green leaves at the end of them; towards the top come forth divers flowers made like unto peaſe bloſſoms, of the ſame colour for the moſt part that the fruit will be of; that is to ſay, white, yellow, red, blackiſh, or of a deeper purple, but white is the moſt uſual; after which come long and ſlender flat cods, ſome crooked, ſome ſtraight, with a ſtring running down the back thereof, wherein is flattiſh round fruit made like a kidney; the root long, ſpreadeth with many ſtrings annexed to it, and periſheth every year.

There is another ſort of French Beans commonly growing with us in this land, which is called the Scarlet flowered Bean.

This ariſeth with ſundry branches as the other, but runs higher, to the length of hop-poles, about which they grow twining, but turning contrary to the ſun, having foot-ſtalks with three leaves on each, as on the other; the flowers alſo are like the other, and of a moſt orient ſcarlet colour. The Beans are larger than the ordinary kind, of a dead purple colour turning black when ripe and dry: The root periſheth in Winter.

Government

Government and Virtues.] These also belong to Dame Venus, and being dried and beat to powder, are as great strengtheners of the kidneys as any are; neither is there a better remedy than it; a dram at a time taken in white wine, to prevent the stone, or to cleanse the kidneys of gravel or stoppage. The ordinary French Beans are of an easy digestion; they move the belly, provoke urine, enlarge the breast that is straitened with shortness of breath, engender sperm, and incite to venery. And the scarlet coloured Beans, in regard of the glorious beauty of their colour, being set near a quickset hedge, will bravely adorn the same by climbing up thereon, so that they may be discerned a great way, not without admiration of the beholders at a distance. But they will go near to kill the quicksets by cloathing them in scarlet.

LADIES BED-STRAW.

BESIDES the common name above written, it is called Cheese-Rennet, because it performs the same office; as also Gallion, Pettimugget, and Maid-Hair; and by some Wild Rosemary.

Descript.] This riseth up with divers small, brown and square upright stalks a yard high or more; sometimes branches forth into divers parts, full of joints, and with divers very fine small leaves at every one of them, little or nothing rough at all; at the tops of the branches grow many long tufts or branches of yellow flowers very thick set together, from the several joints which consist of four leaves a piece, which smell somewhat strong, but not unpleasant. The seed is small and black like poppy seed, two for the most part joined together; The root is reddish, with many small threads fastened unto it, which take strong hold of the ground, and creepeth a little; and the branches leaning a little down to the ground, take root at the joints thereof, whereby it is easily encreased.

There is another sort of Ladies Bed-straw growing frequently in England which beareth white flowers as the other doth yellow; but the branches of this are so weak that unless it be sustained by the hedges, or other things near which it groweth, it will lie down to the ground: The leaves a little bigger than the former, and the flow-

ers

ers not so plentiful as these; and the root hereof is also thready and abiding.

Place.] They grow in meadows and pastures both wet and dry, and by the hedges.

Time.] They flower in May for the most part, and the seed is ripe in July and August.

Government and Virtues.] They are both herbs of Venus, and therefore strengthening the parts both internal and external, which she rules. The decoction of the former of those being drank, is good to fret and break the stone, provoke urine, stayeth inward bleeding, and healeth inward wounds. The herb or flour bruised and put up into the nostrils, stayeth their bleeding likewise: The flowers and herbs being made into an oil, by being set in the sun, and changed after it hath stood ten or twelve days; or into an ointment being boiled in *Axunga*, or sallet oil, with some wax melted therein, after it is strained; either the oil made thereof, or the ointment, do help burnings with fire, or scaldings with water: The same also, or the decoction of the herb and flower, is good to bathe the feet of travellers and lacquies, whose long running causeth weariness and stiffness in their sinews and joints. If the decoction be used warm, and the joints afterwards anointed with ointment, it helpeth the dry scab, and the itch in children; and the herb with the white flower is also very good for the sinews, arteries, and joints, to comfort and strengthen them after travel, cold, and pains.

BEETS.

OF Beets there are two sorts, which are best known generally, and whereof I shall principally treat at this time, *viz.* the white and red Beets, and their virtues.

Descript.] The common white Beet hath many great leaves next the ground, somewhat large, and of a whitish green colour. The stalk is great, strong, and ribbed, bearing great store of leaves upon it, almost to the very top of it: The flowers grow in very long tufts, small at the end, and turning down their heads, which are small, pale, greenish, yellow buds, giving cornered prickly seed. The

The root is great, long, and hard, and when it hath given feed, is of no ufe at all.

The common red Beet differeth not from the white, but only it is leffer, and the leaves and the roots are fomewhat red: The leaves are differently red, fome only with red ftalks or veins; fome of a frefh red, and others of a dark red. The root thereof is red, fpungy, and not ufed to be eaten.

Government and Virtues.] The government of thefe two forts of Beets are far different; the red Beet being under Saturn, and the white under Jupiter; therefore take the virtues of them apart, each by itfelf: The white Beet doth much loofen the belly, and is of a cleanfing, digefting quality, and provoketh urine. The juice of it openeth obftructions both of the liver and fpleen, and is good for the head-ach and fwimmings therein, and turnings of the brain; and is effectual alfo againft all venomous creatures; and applied unto the temples, ftayeth inflammations in the eyes; it helpeth burnings, being ufed without oil, and with a little alum put to it; is good for St Anthony's fire. It is good for all wheals, pufhes, blifters, and blains in the fkin: The herb boiled and laid upon chilblains or kibes, helpeth them. The decoction thereof in water and fome vinegar, healeth the itch, if bathed therewith, and cleanfeth the head of dandruff, fcurf, and dry fcabs, and doth much good for fretting and running fores, ulcers, and cankers in the head, legs, or other parts, and is much commended againft baldnefs and fhedding the hair

The red Beet is good to ftay the bloody-flux, womens courfes, and the whites, and to help the yellow jaundice: The juice of the root put into the noftrils, purgeth the head, helpeth the noife in the ears, and the tooth-ach; the juice fnuffed up the nofe, helps a ftinking breath, if the caufe lies in the nofe, as many times it doth, if any bruife hath been there; as alfo want of fmell coming that way.

WATER BETONY.

CALLED alfo Brown-wort, and in Yorkfhire, Bifhops-leaves.

Defcript.] Firft, of the Water Betony, which rifeth up with-

with square, hard, greenish stalks, sometimes brown, set with broad dark green leaves dented about the edges with notches somewhat resembling the leaves of the Wood Betony, but much larger too, for the most part set at a joint. The flowers are many, set at the tops of the stalks and branches, being round bellied and opened at the brims, and divided into two parts, the uppermost being like a hood, and the lowermost like a hip hanging down, of a dark red colour, which passing, there comes in their places small round heads with small points at the ends, wherein lie small and brownish seeds: the root is a thick bush of strings and shreds growing from the head.

Place.] It groweth by the ditch-side, brooks, and other water-courses, generally through this land, and is seldom found far from the water-side.

Time.] It flowereth about July, and the seed is ripe in August.

Government and Virtues.] Water Betony is an herb of Jupiter in Cancer, and is appropriated more to wounds and hurts in the breasts than Wood Betony, which follows: It is an excellent remedy for sick hogs. It is of a cleansing quality: The leaves bruised and applied are effectual for all old and filthy ulcers; and especially if the juice of the leaves be boiled with a little honey, and dipped therein, and the sores dressed therewith: as also for bruises or hurts, whether inward or outward: The distilled water of the leaves is used for the same purpose; as also to bathe the face and hands spotted or blemished, or discoloured by sun-burning.

I confess I do not much fancy distilled waters, I mean such waters as are distilled cold; some virtues of the herb they may happily have (it were a strange thing else;) but this I am confident of, that being distilled in a pewter still, as the vulgar and apish fashion is, both chymical oil and salt is left behind, unless you burn them, and then all is spoiled, water and all, which was good for as little as can be by such a distillation in my translation of the London Dispensatory.

WOOD BETONY.

Descrip.] COMMON or Wood Betony hath many leaves rising from the root, which are some-

ſomewhat broad and round at the end, roundly dented about the edges, ſtanding upon long foot ſtalks, from among which ariſe up ſmall, ſquare, ſlender, but upright hairy ſtalks, with ſome leaves thereon to a piece at the joints, ſmaller than the lower, whereon are ſet ſeveral ſpiked heads of flowers like lavender, but thicker and ſhorter for the moſt part, and of a reddiſh or purple colour, ſpotted with white ſpots both in the upper and lower part. The ſeeds being contained within the huſks that hold the flowers, are blackiſh, ſomewhat long and uneven. The roots are many white thready ſtrings; the ſtalk periſheth, but the roots, with ſome leaves thereon, abide all the Winter. The whole plant is ſomething ſmall.

Place.] It groweth frequently in woods, and delighteth in ſhady places.

Time.] And it flowereth in July; after which the ſeed is quickly ripe, yet in its prime in May.

Government and Virtues.] The herb is appropriated to the planet Jupiter, and the ſign Aries. Antonius Muſa, phyſician to the Emperor Auguſtus Cæſar, wrote a peculiar book of the virtues of this herb; and among other virtues, ſaith of it, that it preſerveth the liver and bodies of men from the danger of epidemical diſeaſes, and from witchcrafts alſo; it helpeth thoſe that loath or cannot digeſt their meat, thoſe that have weak ſtomachs, or ſour belchings, or continual riſing in their ſtomach, uſing it familiarly either green or dry; either the herb or root, or the flowers in broth, drink, or meat, or made into conſerve, ſyrup, water, electuary, or powder, as every one may beſt frame themſelves unto, or as the time or ſeaſon requireth; taken any of the aforeſaid ways, it helpeth the jaundice, falling-ſickneſs, the palſy, convulſions, or ſhrinking of the ſinews, the gout, and thoſe that are inclined to dropſy, thoſe that have continual pains in their heads, although it turn to phrenſy. The powder mixed with pure honey, is no leſs available for all ſorts of coughs or colds, wheeſing, or ſhortneſs of breath, diſtillations of thin rheum upon the lungs, which cauſeth conſumptions. The decoction made with mead, and a little penny-royal, is good for thoſe that are troubled with putrid agues, whether quotidian, tertian, or quartan, and to draw down and evacuate the blood and humours, that by falling into the eyes, do hinder the ſight; the decoction thereof made in wine, and taken, killeth the worms in the belly, openeth obſtructions both of the ſpleen and liver; cureth ſtitches, and the pains in the back or ſides, the torments and griping pains of the bowels, and the wind-colick; and mixed with honey purgeth the belly, helpeth to bring down womens courſes, and is of ſpecial uſe for thoſe that are troubled with the falling down of the mother, and pains thereof, and cauſeth an eaſy and ſpeedy delivery of women in child-birth. It helpeth alſo to break and expel the ſtone, either in the bladder or kidneys. The decoction with wine gargled in the mouth, eaſeth the tooth-ach. It is commended againſt the ſtinging or biting of venomous ſerpents, or mad dogs, being uſed inwardly and applied outwardly to the place. A dram of the powder of Betony, taken with a little honey in ſome vinegar, doth wonderfully refreſh thoſe that are over wearied by travel. It ſtayeth bleeding at the mouth or noſe, and helpeth thoſe that piſs or ſpit blood, and thoſe that are burſten or have a rupture, and is good for ſuch as are bruiſed by any fall or otherwiſe. The green herb bruiſed, or the juice applied to any inward hurt, or outward green wound in the head or body, will quickly heal and cloſe it up; as alſo any veins or ſinews that are cut; and will draw forth any broken bone or ſplinter, thorn or other things got into the fleſh. It is no leſs profitable for old ſores or filthy ulcers; yea, though they be fiſtulous and hollow. But ſome do adviſe to put a little ſalt to this purpoſe, being applied with a little hog's lard, it helpeth a plague ſore, and other boils and puſhes. The fumes of the decoction while it is warm, received by a funnel into the ears, eaſeth the pains of them, deſtroyeth the worms and cureth the running ſores in them. The juice dropped into them doth the ſame. The root of Betony is diſpleaſing both to the taſte and ſtomach, whereas, the leaves and flowers, by their ſweet and ſpicy taſte, are comfortable both to meat and medicine.

Theſe are ſome of the many virtues Antony Muſe, an expert phyſician (for it was not the practice of Octavius Cæſar

Cæſar to keep fools about him) appropriates to Betony; it is a very precious herb, that is certain, and moſt fitting to be kept in a man's houſe, both in ſyrup, conſerve, oil, ointment, and plaiſter. The flowers are uſually conſerved.

The BEECH TREE.

IN treating of this tree, you muſt underſtand that I mean the green Maſt-beech, which is, by way of diſtinction from that other ſmall rough ſort, called in Suſſex the ſmaller Beech, but in Eſſex Horn-bean.

I ſuppoſe it is needleſs to deſcribe it, being already too well known to my countrymen.

Place.] It groweth in woods amongſt oaks and other trees, and in parks, foreſts, and chaſes, to feed deer; and in other places to fatten ſwine.

Time.] It bloometh in the end of April, or beginning of May, for the moſt part, and the fruit is ripe in September.

Government and Virtues.] It is a plant of Saturn, and therefore performs his qualities and proportion in theſe operations: The leaves of the Beech tree are cooling and binding, and therefore good to be applied to hot ſwellings to diſcuſs them; the nuts do much nouriſh ſuch beaſts as feed thereon. The water that is found in the hollow places of decaying Beeches will cure both man and beaſt of any ſcurf, ſcab, or running tetters, if they be waſhed therewith; you may boil the leaves into a poultice, or make an ointment of them when time of year ſerves.

BILBERRIES, *called by ſome* WHORTS, *and* WHORTLE-BERRIES.

Deſcript.] OF theſe I ſhall only ſpeak of two ſorts which are common in England, viz. The black and red berries. And firſt of the black.

The ſmall buſh creepeth along upon the ground, ſcarce riſing half a yard high, with divers ſmall dark green leaves ſet in the green branches, not always one againſt the other, and a little dented about the edges: At the foot of the leaves come forth ſmall, hollow, pale, bluiſh coloured flowers, the brims ending in five points, with a reddish thread in the middle, which pass into small round berries of the bigness and colour of juniper berries, but of a purple, sweetish, sharp taste; the juice of them giveth a purplish colour in their hands and lips that eat and handle them, especially if they break them. The root groweth aslope under ground, shooting forth in sundry places as it creepeth. This loseth its leaves in Winter.

The Red Bilberry, or Wortle-Bush, riseth up like the former, having sundry hard leaves, like the Box-tree leaves, green and round pointed, standing on the several branches, at the top whereof only, and not from the sides, as in the former, come forth divers round, reddish, sappy berries, when they are ripe, of a sharp taste. The root runneth in the ground, as in the former, but the leaves of this abide all the Winter.

Place.] The first groweth in forests, on the heaths, and such like barren places: The red grows in the north parts of this land, as Lancashire, Yorkshire, &c.

Time.] They flower in March and April, and the fruit of the black is ripe in July and August.

Government and Virtues.] They are under the dominion of Jupiter. It is a pity they are used no more in physick than they are. The Black Bilberries are good in hot agues, and to cool the heat of the liver and stomach; they do somewhat bind the belly, and stay vomitings and loathings; the juice of the berries made in a syrup, or the pulp made into a conserve with sugar, is good for the purposes aforesaid, as also for an old cough, or an ulcer in the lungs, or other diseases therein. The Red Worts are more binding, and stop womens courses, spitting of blood, or any other flux of blood or humours, being used as well outwardly as inwardly.

BIFOIL, OR TWABLADE.

Descript.] THIS small herb, from a root somewhat sweet, shooting downwards many long strings, riseth up a round green stalk, bare or naked next the ground for an inch, two or three to the middle thereof, as it is in age or growth; as also from the middle upward to the flowers, having only two broad plantain-like leaves (but whiter) set at the middle of the stalk one against

gainst another, compasseth it round at the bottom of them.

Place.] It is an usual inhabitant in woods, copses, and in many other places in this land.

There is another sort groweth in wet grounds and marshes, which is somewhat different from the former. It is a smaller plant, and greener, having sometimes three leaves; the spike of the flowers is less than the former, and the roots of this do run or creep in the ground.

They are much and often used by many to good purpose for wounds, both green and old, and to consolidate or knit ruptures; and well it may, being a plant of Saturn.

The Birch Tree.

Descript.] THIS groweth a goodly tall straight tree, fraught with many boughs, and slender branches bending downward; the old being covered with a discoloured chapped bark, and the younger being browner by much. The leaves at the first breaking out are crumpled, and afterwards like the beech leaves, but smaller and greener, and dented about the edges. It beareth small short cat-skins, somewhat like those of the hazel nut-tree, which abide on the branches a long time, until growing ripe, they fall on the ground, and their seed with them.

Place.] It usually groweth in woods.

Government and Virtues.] It is a tree of Venus; the juice of the leaves, while they are young, or the distilled water of them, or the water that comes from the tree being bored with an auger, and distilled afterwards; any of these being drank for some days together, is available to break the stone in the kidneys and bladder, and is good also to wash sore mouths.

Bird's Foot.

THIS small herb groweth not above a span high, with many branches spread upon the ground, set with many wings of small leaves. The flowers grow upon the branches, many small ones of a pale yellow colour being set a-head together, which afterwards turneth into small jointed cods, well resembling the claws of small birds, whence it took its name.

There is another ſort of Bird's-foot in all things like the former, but a little larger; the flower of a pale whitiſh red colour, and the cods diſtinct by joints like the other, but a little more crooked; and the roots do carry many ſmall white knots or kernels amongſt the ſtrings.

Place.] Theſe grow on heaths, and many open untilled places of this land.

Time.] They flower and ſeed in the end of Summer.

Government and Virtues.] They belong to Saturn, and are of a drying, binding quality, and thereby very good to be uſed in wound drinks; as alſo to apply outwardly for the ſame purpoſe. But the latter Bird's-foot is found by experience to break the ſtone in the back or kidneys, and drives them forth, if the decoction thereof be taken; and it wonderfully helpeth the rupture, being taken inwardly, and outwardly applied to the place.

All ſalts have beſt operation upon the ſtone, as ointments and plaiſters have upon wounds; and therefore you may make a ſalt of this for the ſtone; the way how to do ſo may be found in my tranſlation of the London Diſpenſatory; and it may be I may give you it again in plainer terms at the latter end of this book.

BISHOPS-WEED.

BESIDES the common name Biſhop-weed, it is uſually known by the Greek name *Ammi* and *Ammios*; ſome call it Æthiopian Cummin-ſeed, and others Cummin-royal, as alſo Herb William, and Bull-wort.

Deſcript.] Common Biſhops-weed riſeth up with a round ſtraight ſtalk, ſometimes as high as a man, but uſually three or four feet high, beſet with divers ſmall, long, and ſomewhat broad leaves, cut in ſome places, and dented about the edges, growing one againſt another, of a dark green colour, having ſundry branches on them, and at the top ſmall umbels of white flowers, which turn into ſmall round ſeeds, little bigger than parſley-ſeeds, of a quick hot ſcent and taſte: the root is white and ſtringy, periſhing yearly, and uſually riſeth again on its own ſowing.

Place.] It groweth wild in many places in England and Wales, as between Greenhith and Graveſend.

Government and Virtues.] It is hot and dry in the third

degree of a bitter taste, and somewhat sharp withal; it provokes lust to purpose: I suppose Venus owns it. It digesteth humours, provoketh urine and womens courses, dissolveth wind, and being taken in wine it easeth pain and griping in the bowels, and is good against the biting of serpents; it is used to good effects in those medicines which are given to hinder the poisonous operation of Cantharides upon the passage of the urine; being mixed with honey and applied to black and blue marks, coming of blows or bruises, it takes them away; and being drank or outwardly applied, it abateth an high colour, and makes it pale; and the fumes thereof taken with rosin or raisins, cleanseth the mother.

BISTORT, or SNAKEWEED.

IT is called Snakeweed, English Serpentary, Dragonwort, Osterick, and Passions.

Descript.] This hath a thick short knobbed root, blackish without, and somewhat reddish within, a little crooked or turned together, of a hard astringent taste, with divers black threads hanging there, from whence spring up every year divers leaves standing upon long foot-stalks, being somewhat broad and long like a dock leaf, and a little pointed at the ends, but that it is of a blueish green colour on the upper side, and of an ash-colour grey, and a little purplish underneath, with divers veins therein, from among which rise up divers small and slender stalks, two feet high, and almost naked and without leaves, or with a very few, and narrow, bearing a spikey bush of pale-coloured flowers; which being past, there abideth small seed, like unto sorrel-seed, but greater.

There are other sorts of Bistort growing in this land, but smaller, both in height, root, and stalks, and especially in the leaves. The root blackish without, and somewhat whitish within; of an austere binding taste, as the former.

Place.] They grow in shadowy moist woods, and at the foot of hills, but are chiefly nourished up in gardens. The narrow leafed Bistort groweth in the north, in Lancashire, Yorkshire, and Cumberland.

Time.

Time.] They flower about the end of May, and the feed is ripe about the beginning of July.

Government and Virtues.] It belongs to Saturn, and is in operation cold and dry; both the leaves and roots have a powerful faculty to resist all poison. The root in powder taken in drink expelleth the venom of the plague, the small-pox, measles, purples, or any other infectious disease, driving it out by sweating. The root in powder, the decoction thereof in wine being drank, stayeth all manner of inward bleeding, or spitting of blood, and any fluxes in the body of either man or woman, or vomiting. It is also very available against ruptures, or burstings, or all bruises of falls, dissolving the congealed blood, and easing the pains that happen thereupon; it also helpeth the jaundice.

The water distilled from both leaves and roots, is a singular remedy to wash any place bitten or stung by any venomous creature; as also for any of the purposes before spoken of, and is very good to wash any running sores or ulcers. The decoction of the root in wine being drank, hindereth abortion or miscarriage in child-bearing. The leaves also kill the worms in children, and is a great help to them that cannot keep their water; if the juice of plantain be added thereto, and outwardly applied, much helpeth the gonorrhea, or running of the reins. A dram of the powder of the root taken in water thereof, wherein some red hot iron or steel hath been quenched, is also an admireable help thereto, so as the body be first prepared and purged from the offensive humours. The leaves, seed, or roots, are all very good in decoctions, drinks, or lotions, for inward or outward wounds, or other sores. And the powder strewed upon any cut or wound in a vein, stayeth the immoderate bleeding thereof. The decoction of the root in water, whereunto some pomegranate peels and flowers are added, injected into the matrix, stayeth the immoderate flux of the courses. The root thereof with pellitory of Spain, and burnt alum, of each a little quantity, beaten small and made into paste, with some honey, and a little piece thereof put into an hollow tooth, or held between the teeth, if there be no hollowness in them, stayeth the defluction of rheum upon on them, which causeth pains, and helps to cleanse the head, and void much offensive water. The distilled water is very effectual to wash sores or cankers in the nose, or any other part; if the powder of the root be applied thereunto afterwards. It is good also to fasten the gums, and to take away the heat and inflammations that happen in the jaws, almonds of the throat, or mouth, if the decoction of the leaves, roots, or seeds bruised, or the juice of them be applied; but the roots are most effectual to the purposes aforesaid.

One Blade.

Descript.] THIS small plant never beareth more than one leaf, but only when it riseth up with its stalk, which thereon beareth another, and seldom more, which are of a blueish green colour, broad at the bottom, and pointed with many ribs or veins like plantain; at the top of the stalk grow many small flowers star-fashion, smelling somewhat sweet; after which cometh small reddish berries when they are ripe: The root small of the bigness of a rush, lying aud creeping under the upper crust of the earth, shooting forth in divers places.

Place.] It grows in moist, shadowy, grassy places of woods, in many places of this realm.

Time.] It flowereth about May, and the berries be ripe in June, and then quickly perisheth, until the next year it springeth from the same again.

Government and Virtues.] It is an herb of the sun, and therefore cordial; half a dram, or a dram at most, of the roots hereof in powder, taken in wine and vinegar, of each a like quantity, and the party presently laid to sweat, is held to be a sovereign remedy for those that are infected with the plague, and have a sore upon them, by expelling the poison, and defending the heart and spirits from danger. It is also accounted a singular good wound herb, and therefore used with other herbs in making such balms as are necessary for curing of wounds, either green or old, and especially if the nerves be hurt.

The BRAMBLE, or BLACK-BERRY BUSH.

IT is ſo well known that it needeth no deſcription. The virtues thereof are as followeth.

Government and Virtues.] It is a plant of Venus in Aries. You ſhall have ſome directions at the latter end of the book for the gathering of all herbs and plants, &c. If any aſk the reaſon why Venus is ſo prickly? Tell them 'tis becauſe ſhe is in the houſe of Mars. The buds, leaves, and branches, while they are green, are of a good uſe in the ulcers and putrid ſores of the mouth and throat, and of the quinſey, and likewiſe to heal other freſh wounds and ſores; but the flowers and fruits unripe are very binding, and ſo profitable for the bloody-flux, laſks, and are a fit remedy for ſpitting of blood. Either the decoction or powder of the root being taken, is good to break or drive forth gravel and the ſtone in the reins and kidneys. The leaves of brambles, as well green as dry, are excellent good lotions for ſores in the mouth, or ſecret parts. The decoction of them, and of the dryed branches, do much bind the belly, and are good for too much flowing of womens courſes; the berries of the flowers are a powerful remedy againſt the poiſon of the moſt venomous ſerpents; as well drank as outwardly applied, helpeth the ſores of the fundament, and the piles; the juice of the berries mixed with the juice of mulberries, do bind more effectually, and help all fretting and eating ſores and ulcers wheresoever. The diſtilled water of the branches, leaves, and flowers, or the fruit, is very pleaſant in taſte, and very effectual in fevers, and hot diſtempers of the body, head, eyes, and other parts, and for the purpoſes aforeſaid. The leaves boiled in lee, and the head waſhed therewith, healeth the itch, and the running ſores thereof, and maketh the hair black. The powder of the leaves ſtrewed on cankers and running ulcers, wonderfully helps to heal them. Some uſe to condenſate the juice of the leaves, and ſome the juice of the berries, to keep for their uſe all the year, for the purpoſes aforeſaid.

BLITES.

BLITES.

Descript.] OF these there are two sorts commonly known, viz. White and red. The White hath leaves somewhat like unto beets, but smaller, rounder, and of a whitish green colour, every one standing upon a small long foot-stalk; the stalk rises up two or three feet high, with such like leaves thereon; the flowers grow at the top in long round tufts or clusters, wherein are contained small and round seeds; the root is very full of threads or strings.

The Red Blite is in all things like the White, but that his leaves and tufted heads are exceeding red at first, and after turn more purplish.

There are other kinds of Blites which grow differing from the two former sorts but little, but only the wild are smaller in every part.

Place.] They grow in gardens, and wild in many places in this land.

Time.] They seed in August and September.

Government and Virtues.] They are all of them cooling, drying, and binding, serving to restrain the fluxes of blood in either man or woman, especially the Red; which also stayeth the over-flowing of the womens reds, as the white Blites stayeth the whites in women: It is an excellent secret; you cannot well fail in the use: They are all under the dominion of Venus.

There is another sort of wild Blites like the other wild kinds, but have long and spikey heads of greenish seeds, seeming by the thick setting together to be all seed.

This sort the fishers are delighted with, and it is a good and usual bait; for fishes will bite fast enough at them, if you have but wit enough to catch them when they bite.

BORAGE and BUGLOSS.

THESE are so well known to be inhabitants in every garden, that I hold it needless to describe them.

To these I may add a third sort, which is not so common, nor yet so well known, and therefore I shall give you its name and description.

It is called *Langue de Beuf;* but why then should they call

call one herb by the name Buglofs, and another by the name *Langue de Beuf*? It is fome queftion to me, feeing one fignifies Ox-tongue in Greek, and the other fignifies the fame in French.

Defcript.] The leaves whereof are fmaller than thofe of Buglofs, but much rougher; the ftalks arifing up about a foot and a half high, and is moft commonly of a red colour; the flowers ftand in fcaly rough heads, being compofed of many fmall yellow flowers, not much unlike to thofe of Dandelions, and the feed flieth away in down, as that doth; you may eafily know the flowers by their tafte, for they are very bitter.

Place.] It groweth wild in many places of this land, and may be plentifully found near London, as between Rotherhith and Deptford, by the ditch-fide. Its virtues are held to be the fame with Borage and Buglofs, only this is fomewhat hotter.

Time.] They flower in June and July, and the feed is ripe fhortly after.

Government and Virtues.] They are all three herbs of Jupiter, and under Leo, all great cordials, and great ftrengtheners of nature. The leaves and roots are to very good purpofe ufed in putrid and peftilential fevers, to defend the heart, and help to refift and expel the poifon, or the venom of other creatures; the feed is of the like effects; and the feed and leaves are good to increafe milk in womens breafts; the leaves, flowers, and feed, all or any of them, are good to expel penfivenefs and melancholy; it helpeth to clarify the blood, and mitigate heat in fevers. The juice made into a fyrup, prevaileth much to all the purpofes aforefaid, and is put with other cooling, opening and cleanfing herbs to open obftructions, and help the yellow jaundice, and mixed with fumitory, to cool, cleanfe, and temper the blood thereby; it helpeth the itch, ringworms, and tetters, or other fpreading fcabs or fores. The flowers candied or made into a conferve, are helpful in the former cafes, but are chiefly ufed as a cordial, and are good for thofe that are weak in long ficknefs, and to comfort the heart and fpirits of thofe that are in a confumption, or troubled with often fwoonings, or paffions of the heart; The diftilled water is is no less effectual to all the purposes aforesaid, and helpeth the redness and inflammations of the eyes, being washed therewith; the dried herb is never used, but the green; yet the ashes thereof, boiled in mead, or honied water, is available against the inflammations and ulcers in the mouth or throat to gargle it therewith; the roots of Bugloss are effectual, being made into a licking electuary for the cough, and to condensate thick phlegm, and the rheumatick distillations upon the lungs.

BLUE-BOTTLE.

IT is called Syanus, I suppose from the colour of it; Hurtsickle, because it turns the edge of the sickles that reap the corn; Blue-blow, Corn-flower, and Blue-bottle.

Descript.] I shall only describe that which is commonest, and in my opinion most useful; its leaves spread upon the ground, being of a whitish green colour, somewhat on the edges like those of cornscabions, amongst which ariseth up a stalk divided into divers branches, beset with long leaves of a greenish colour, either but very little indented, or not at all; the flowers are of a blue colour, from whence it took its name, consisting of an innumerable company of small flowers set in a scaly head, not much unlike those of knap-weed; the seed is smooth, bright and shining, wrapped up in a woolly mantle; the root perisheth every year.

Place.] They grow in corn-fields, amongst all sorts of corn (pease, beans, and tares excepted.) If you please to take them up from thence, and transplant them in your garden, especially towards the full of the moon, they will grow more double than they are, and many times change colour.

Time.] They flower from the beginning of May to the end of harvest.

Government and Virtues.] As they are naturally cold, dry, and binding, so they are under the dominion of Saturn. The powder or dried leaves of the Blue-bottle, or Corn-flower, is given with good success to those that are bruised by a fall, or have broken a vein inwardly, and void much blood at the mouth; being taken in the water of plantain, horsetail, or the greater comfrey, it is a remedy against the poison of the scorpion, and resisteth all venoms and poison. The seed or leaves taken in wine, is very good against the plague, and all infectious diseases, and is very good in pestilential fevers. The juice put into fresh or green wounds, doth quickly solder up the lips of them together, and is very effectual to heal all ulcers and sores in the mouth. The juice dropped into the eyes takes away the heat and inflammation of them. The distilled water of this herb, hath the same properties, and may be used for the effects aforesaid.

BRANK URSINE.

BESIDE the common name Brank Ursine, it is also called Bears-breech, and Acanthus, though I think our English names to be more proper; for the Greek word *Acanthus*, signifies any thistle whatsoever.

Descript.] This thistle shooteth forth very many large, thick, sad green smooth leaves upon the ground, with a very thick and juicy middle rib; the leaves are parted with sundry deep gashes on the edges; the leaves remain a long time before any stalk appears, afterwards riseth up a reasonable big stalk, three or four feet high, and bravely decked with flowers from the middle of the stalk upwards; for on the lower part of the stalk there is neither branches nor leaf. The flowers are hooded and gaping, being white in colour, and standing in brownish husks, with a long small undivided leaf under each leaf; they seldom seed in our country. Its roots are many, great, and thick, blackish without, and whitish within, full of a clammy sap; a piece of them, if you set in the garden, and defend it from the first Winter cold, will grow and flourish.

Place.] They are only nursed up in the gardens in England, where they will grow very well.

Time.] It flowereth in June and July.

Government and Virtues.] It is an excellent plant under the dominion of the Moon: I could wish such as are studious, would labour to keep it in the gardens. The leaves being boiled and used in clisters, are excellent good to mollify the belly, and make the passage slippery. The decoction

decoction drank inwardly, is excellent and good for the bloody-flux. The leaves being bruised, or rather boiled and applied like a poultice, are excellent good to unite broken bones, and strengthen joints that have been put out. The decoction of either leaves or roots being drank, and the decoction of leaves applied to the place, is excellent good for the king's evil that is broken and runneth; for by the influence of the Moon, it reviveth the ends of the veins which are relaxed: There is scarce a better remedy to be applied to such places as are burnt with fire than this is, for it fetches out the fire, and heals it without a scar. This is an excellent remedy for such as are bursten, being either taken inwardly or applied to the place. In like manner used, it helps the cramp and the gout. It is excellent good in hectic fevers, and restores radical moisture to such as are in consumptions.

BRIONY, or WILD VINE.

IT is called Wild, and Wood Vine, Tamus or Ladies Seal. The white is called White Vine by some; and the black, Black Vine.

Descript.] The common White Briony groweth ramping upon the hedges, sending forth many long, rough, very tender branches at the beginning, with many very rough, and broad leaves thereon, cut (for the most part) into five partitions, in form very like a vine leaf, but smaller, rough, and of a whitish hoary green colour, spreading very far, spreading and twining with his small claspers (that come forth at the joints with the leaves) very far on whatsoever standeth next to it. At the several joints also (especially towards the top of the branches) cometh forth a long stalk bearing many whitish flowers together on a long tuft, consisting of five small leaves apiece, laid open like a star, after which come the berries separated one from the other, more than a cluster of grapes, green at the first, and very red when they are thorough ripe, of no good scent, but of a most loathsome taste, provoking vomit. The root groweth to be exceeding great, with many long twines or branches going from it, of a pale whitish colour on the outside, and more white within, and of a sharp, bitter, loathsome taste.

 Place,

Place.] It groweth on banks, or under hedges, through this country.

Time.] It flowereth in July and August, some earlier, and some later than the other.

Government and Virtues.] They are furious martial plants. The root of Briony purges the belly with great violence, troubling the stomach and burning the liver, and therefore not rashly to be taken: but being corrected, is very profitable for the diseases of the head, as falling-sickness, giddiness and swimmings, by drawing away much phlegm and rheumatick humours that oppress the head, as also the joints and sinews; and is therefore good for palsies, convulsions, cramps, and stitches in the sides, and the dropsy, and in provoking urine; it cleanseth the reins and kidneys from gravel and stone, by opening the obstructions of the spleen, and consumeth the hardness and swelling thereof. The decoction of the root in wine, drunk once a week at going to bed, cleanseth the mother, and helpeth the rising thereof, expelleth the dead child; a dram of the root in powder taken in white wine, bringeth down their courses. An electuary made of the roots and honey, doth mightily cleanse the chest of rotten phlegm, and wonderfully help any old strong cough, to those that are troubled with shortness of breath, and is very good for them that are bruised inwardly, to help to expel the clotted or congealed blood. The leaves, fruit and root do cleanse old and filthy sores, are good against all fretting and running cankers, gangrenes, and tetters, and therefore the berries are by some country people called tetter-berries. The root cleanseth the skin wonderfully from all black and blue spots, freckles, morphew, leprosy, foul scars, or other deformity whatsoever; also all running scabs and manginess are healed by the powder of the dried root, or the juice thereof, but especially by the fine white hardened juice. The distilled water of the root worketh the same effects, but more weakly; the root bruised and applied of itself to any place where the bones are broken, helpeth to draw them forth, as also splinters and thorns in the flesh; and being applied with a little wine mixed therewith, it breaketh boils, and helpeth whitelows on the joints.—For all these latter,

beginning

beginning at sores, cancers, &c. apply it outwardly, and take my advice in my translation of the London Dispensatory, among the preparations at the latter end, where you have a medicine called *Fæcula Brionia*, which take and use, mixing it with a little hog's grease, or other convenient ointment.

As for the former diseases where it must be taken inwardly, it purgeth very violently, and needs an abler hand to correct it than most country people have; therefore it is a better way for them in my opinion to let the simple alone, and take the compound water of it mentioned in my Dispensatory, and that is far more safe, being wisely corrected.

BROOK-LIME, or WATER-PIMPERNEL.

Descript.] THIS sendeth forth from a creeping root that shooteth forth strings at every joint, as it runneth, divers and sundry green stalks, round and sappy, with some branches on them, somewhat broad, round, deep green, and thick leaves set by couples thereon; from the bottom whereof shoot forth long foot-stalks, with sundry small blue flowers on them, that consist of five small round pointed leaves a-piece.

There is another sort nothing differing from the former, but that it is greater, and the flowers of a paler green colour.

Place.] They grow in small standing waters, and usually near water cresses.

Time.] And flowers in June and July, giving seed the next month after.

Government and Virtues.] It is a hot and biting martial plant. Brook-lime and water-cresses are generally used together in diet-drink, with other things serving to purge the blood and body from all ill humours that would destroy health, and are helpful to the scurvy. They do all provoke urine, and help to break the stone, and pass it away; they procure womens courses, and expel the dead child. Being fried with butter and vinegar, and applied warm, it helpeth all manner of tumours, swellings, and inflammations.

Such drinks ought to be made of sundry herbs, according to the malady. I ſhall give a plain and eaſy rule at the latter end of this book.

Butchers Broom.

IT is called Ruſcus, and Bruſcus, Kneeholm, Kneeholy, Kneehulver, and Pettigree.

Deſcript.] The firſt ſhoots that ſprout from the root of Butchers Broom, are thick, whitiſh, and ſhort, ſomewhat like thoſe of aſparagus, but greater, they riſing up to be a foot and a half high, are ſpread into divers branches, green, and ſomewhat creſſed with the roundneſs, tough and flexible, whereon are ſet ſomewhat broad and almoſt round hard leaves, and prickly, pointed at the end, of a dark green colour, two for the moſt part ſet at a place, very cloſe and near together; about the middle of the leaf, on the back and lower ſide from the middle rib, breaketh forth a ſmall whitiſh green flower, conſiſting of four ſmall round pointed leaves, ſtanding upon little or no foot-ſtalk, and in the place whereof cometh a ſmall round berry, green at the firſt, and red when it is ripe, wherein are two or three white, hard, round ſeeds contained. The root is thick, white, and great at the head, and from thence ſendeth forth divers thick, white, long, tough ſtrings.

Place.] It groweth in copſes, and upon heaths and waſte grounds, and oftentimes under or near the holly buſhes.

Time.] It ſhooteth forth its young buds in the Spring, and the berries are ripe about September, the branches of the leaves abiding green all the Winter.

Government and Virtues.] 'Tis a plant of Mars, being of a gallant cleanſing and opening quality. The decoction of the root made with wine openeth obſtruction, provoketh urine, helpeth to expel gravel and the ſtone, the ſtranguary and womens courſes, alſo the yellow jaundice and the head-ach: And with ſome honey or ſugar put thereunto, cleanſeth the breaſt of phlegm, and the cheſt of ſuch clammy humours gathered therein. The decoction of the root drank, and a poultice made of the berries and leaves being applied, are effectual in kniting and conſolidating broken bones or parts out of joint. The common way of uſing it, is to boil the root of it, and parſley

and

and fennel, and ſmallage in white wine, and drink the decoction, adding the like quantity of graſs-root to them: The more of the root you boil, the ſtronger will the decoction be; it works no ill effects, yet I hope you have wit enough to give the ſtrongeſt decoction to the ſtrongeſt bodies.

BROOM, and BROOM-RAPE.

TO ſpend time in writing a deſcription hereof is altogether needleſs, it being ſo generally uſed by all the good houſewives almoſt through this land to ſweep their houſes with, and therefore very well known to all ſorts of people.

The Broom-rape ſpringeth up on many places from the roots of the broom (but more often in fields, as by hedge-ſides and on heaths.) The ſtalk whereof is of the bigneſs of a finger or thumb, above two feet high, having a ſhew of leaves on them, and many flowers at the top, of a reddiſh yellow colour, as alſo the ſtalks and leaves are.

Place.] They grow in many places of this land commonly, and as commonly ſpoil all the land they grow in.

Time.] And flower in the Summer months, and give their ſeed before Winter.

Government and Virtues.] The juice or decoction of the young branches, or ſeed, or the powder of the ſeed taken in drink, purgeth downwards, and draweth phlegmatick and watry humours from the joints, whereby it helpeth the dropſy, gout, ſciatica, and pains of the hips and joints; it alſo provoketh ſtrong vomits, and helpeth the pains of the ſides, and ſwelling of the ſpleen, cleanſeth alſo the reins or kidneys and bladder of the ſtone, provoketh urine abundantly, and hindereth the growing again of the ſtone in the body. The continual uſe of the powder of the leaves and ſeed doth cure the black jaundice. The diſtilled water of the flowers is profitable for all the ſame purpoſes; it alſo helpeth ſurfeits, and altereth the fits of agues, if three or four ounces thereof, with as much of the water of the leſſer centaury, and a little ſugar put therein, be taken a little before the fit cometh, and the party be laid down to ſweat in his bed. The oil or water that is drawn from the end of the green ſticks heated ed in the fire, helpeth the tooth-ach. The juice of young branches made into an ointment of old hog's greafe, and anointed, or the young branches bruifed and heated in oil or hog's greafe, and laid to the fides pained by wind, as in ftitches, or the fpleen, eafeth them in once or twice ufing it. The fame boiled in oil is the fafeft and fureft medicine to kill lice in the head or body of any; and is an efpecial remedy for joint-aches, and fwollen knees, that come by the falling down of humours.

The BROOM-RAPE *alfo is not without its Virtues.*

The decoction thereof in wine, is thought to be as effectual to void the ftone in the kidneys and bladder, and to provoke urine, as the Broom itfelf. The juice thereof is a fingular good help to cure as well green wounds, as old and filthy fores and malignant ulcers. The infolate oil, wherein there hath been three or four repititions of infufion of the top ftalks, with flowers ftrained and cleared, cleanfeth the fkin from all manner of fpots, marks, and freckles that rife either by the heat of the fun, or the malignity of humours. As for the Broom and Broom-rape, Mars owns them, and is exceeding prejudicial to the liver; I fuppofe by reafon of the antipathy between Jupiter and Mars, therefore if the liver be difaffected, minifter none of it.

BUCKS-HORN PLANTAIN.

Defcript.] THIS being fown of feed, rifeth up at firft with fmall, long, narrow, hairy, dark green leaves like grafs, without any divifion or gafh in them, but thofe that follow are gafhed in on both fides the leaves into three or four gafhes, and pointed at the ends, refembling the knags of buck's horn, (whereof it took its name) and being well ground round about the root upon the ground, or order one by another, thereby refembling the form of a ftar, from among which rife up divers hairy ftalks, about a hand's-breadth high, bearing every one a fmall, long fpikey head, like to thofe of the common plantain, having fuch like bloomings and feed after them. The root is fingle, long and fmall, with divers ftrings at it.

Place.

Place.] They grow in ſandy grounds, as in Tothil fields, by Weſtminſter, and divers other places of this land.

Time.] They flower and ſeed in May, June and July, and their green leaves do in a manner abide freſh all the Winter.

Government and Virtues.] It is under the dominion of Saturn, and is of a gallant drying and binding quality. This boiled in wine and drank, and ſome of the leaves put to the hurt place, is an excellent remedy for the biting of the viper or adder, which I take to be one and the ſame: The ſame being alſo drank, helpeth thoſe that are troubled with the ſtone in the reins or kidneys, by cooling the heat of the part afflicted, and ſtrengthening them; alſo weak ſtomachs that cannot retain, but caſt up their meat. It ſtayeth all bleeding both at mouth and noſe; bloody urine or the bloody-flux, and ſtopeth the laſk of the belly and bowels. The leaves hereof bruiſed and laid to their ſides that have an ague, ſuddenly eaſeth the fit; and the leaves and roots being beaten with ſome bay-ſalt and applied to the wriſts, worketh the ſame effects. The herb boiled in ale or wine, and given for ſome mornings and evenings together, ſtayeth the diſtillation of hot and ſharp rheums falling into the eye from the head, and helpeth all ſorts of ſore eyes.

Bucks Horn.

It is called Harts-horn, Herba-ſtella, and Herba-ſtellaria, Sanguinaria, Herb-Eve, Herb-Ivy, Wort-Treſſes, and Swine-Creſſes.

Deſcrip.] They have many ſmall and weak ſtraggling branches trailing here and there upon the ground: The leaves are many, ſmall and jagged, not much unlike to thoſe of Bucks-horn Plantain, but much ſmaller, and not ſo hairy. The flowers grow among the leaves in ſmall, rough, whitiſh cluſters: The ſeeds are ſmaller and browniſh, of a bitter taſte.

Place.] They grow in dry, barren, ſandy grounds.

Time.] they flower and ſeed when the reſt of the plantains do.

Government and Virtues.] This is alſo under the dominion of Saturn; the virtues are held to be the ſame as Bucks-

Bucks-horn plantain, and therefore by all authors it is joined with it: The leaves bruised and applied to the place, stops bleeding; the herb bruised and applied to warts, will make them consume and waste away in a short time.

BUGLE.

BESIDES the name Bugle, it is called Middle Confound and Middle Comfrey, Brown Bugle, and of some Sicklewort, and Herb-Carpenter; though in Essex we call another herb by that name.

Descript.] This hath larger leaves than those of the Self-heal, but else of the same fashion, or rather longer, in some green on the upper side, and in others more brownish, dented about the edges, somewhat hairy, as the square stalk is also, which riseth up to be half a yard high sometimes, with the leaves set by couples, from the middle almost, whereof upwards stand the flowers, together with many smaller and browner leaves than the rest, on the stalk below set at distance, and the stalk bare between them; among which flowers are also small ones of a blueish and sometimes of an ash colour, fashioned like the flowers of ground-ivy, after which come small, round blackish seeds. The root is composed of many strings, and spreadeth upon the ground.

The white flowered Bugle differeth not in form or greatness from the former, saving that the leaves and stalks are always green, and never brown, like the other, and the flowers thereof are white.

Place.] They grow in woods, copses, and fields, generally throughout England, but the white flowered Bugle is not so plentiful as the former.

Time.] They flower from May until July, and in the mean time perfect their seed. The roots and leaves next thereunto upon the ground abiding all the Winter.

Government and Virtues.] This herb belongeth to Dame Venus: If the virtues of it make you fall in love with it (as they will if you be wise) keep a syrup of it to take inwardly, and an ointment and plaister of it to use outwardly, always by you.

The decoction of the leaves and flowers made in wine, and taken, dissolveth the congealed blood in those that are bruised

bruiſed inwardly by a fall, or otherwiſe, and is very effectual for any inward wounds, thruſts or ſtabs in the body or bowels; and is an eſpecial help in all wound-drinks, and for thoſe that are liver-grown (as they call it.) It is wonderful in curing all manner of ulcers and ſores, whether new and freſh, or old and inveterate; yea, gangrenes and fiſtulas alſo, if the leaves bruiſed and applied, or their juice be uſed to waſh and bathe the place, and the ſame made into a lotion, and ſome honey and alum, cureth all ſores in the mouth and gums, be they never ſo foul, or of long continuance; and worketh no leſs powerfully and effectually for ſuch ulcers and ſores as happen in the ſecret parts of men and women. Being alſo taken inwardly, or outwardly applied, it helpeth thoſe that have broken any bone, or have any member out of joint. An ointment made with the leaves of Bugle, Scabions and Sanicle bruiſed and boiled in hog's greaſe, until the herbs be dry, and then ſtrained forth into a pot for ſuch occaſions as ſhall require; it is ſo ſingular good for all ſorts of hurts in the body, that none that know its uſefulneſs will be without it.

The truth is, I have known this herb cure ſome diſeaſes of Saturn, of which I thought good to quote one. Many times ſuch as give themſelves much to drinking are troubled with ſtrange fancies, ſtrange ſights in the night time, and ſome with voices, as alſo with the diſeaſe ephialtes, or the mare. I take the reaſon of this to be (according to Fernelius) a melancholy vapour made thin by exceſſive drinking ſtrong liquor, and ſo flies up and diſturbs the fancy, and breeds imaginations like itſelf, viz. fearful and troubleſome. Theſe I have known cured by taking only two ſpoonfuls of the ſyrup of this herb, after ſupper two hours, when you go to bed. But whether this does it by ſympathy or antipathy, is ſome doubt in aſtrology. I know there is a great antipathy between Saturn and Venus in matter of procreation; yea, ſuch a one, that the barrenneſs of Saturn can be removed by none but Venus; nor the luſt of Venus be repelled by none but Saturn; but I am not of opinion this is done this way, and my reaſon is, becauſe theſe vapours, though in quality melancholy, yet by their flying upward, ſeem to be be something aerial; therefore I rather think it is done by sympathy; Saturn being exalted in libra, in the house of Venus.

BURNET.

IT is called Sanguisorbia, Pimpinella, Bipula Solbegrella, &c. The common garden Burnet is so well known, that it needeth no description.—There is another sort which is wild, the description whereof take as followeth.

Descript.] The great wild Burnet hath winged leaves rising from the roots like the garden Burnet, but not so many; yet each of these leaves are at the least twice as large as the other, and nicked in the same manner about the edges, of a greyish colour on the under side; the stalks are greater, and rise higher, with many such like leaves set thereon, and greater heads at the top, of a brownish colour, and out of them come small dark purple flowers like the former, but greater. The root is black and long like the other, but great also: It hath almost neither scent nor taste therein, like the garden kind.

Place.] The first grows frequently in gardens. The wild kind groweth in divers counties of this island, especially in Huntingdon and Northamptonshires, in the meadows there: as also near London, by Pancras church, and by a causey-side in the middle of a field by Paddington.

Time.] They flower about the end of June, and beginning of July, and their seed is ripe in August.

Government and Virtues.] This is an herb the sun challengeth dominion over, and is a most precious herb, little inferior to Betony; the continual use of it preserves the body in health, and the spirit in vigour; for if the sun be the preserver of life under God, his herbs are the best in the world to do it by. They are accounted to be both of one property, but the lesser is more effectual because quicker and more aromatical: It is a friend to the heart, liver and other principal parts of a man's body. Two or three of the stalks, with leaves put into a cup of wine, especially claret, are known to quicken the spirits, refresh and clear the heart, and drive away melancholy: It is a special help to defend the heart from noisom vapours, and from infection of the pestilence, the juice thereof of being taken in some drink, and the party laid to sweat thereupon. They have also a drying and an astringent quality, whereby they are unvailable in all manner of fluxes of blood or humours, to stanch bleedings inward or outward, lasks, scourings, the bloody-flux, womens too abundant flux of courses, the whites, and the cholerick belchings and castings of the stomach, and is a singular wound herb for all sorts of wounds, both of the head and body, either inward or outward; for all old ulcers, running cankers, and most sores, to be used either by the juice or decoction of the herb, or by the powder of the herb or root, or the water of the distilled herb or ointment by itself, or with other things to be kept. The seed is also no less effectual both to stop fluxes, and dry up moist sores, being taken in powder inwardly in wine, or steeled water, that is, wherein hot gads of steel have been quenched; or the powder, or the seed mixed with the ointments.

The BUTTER-BUR, or PETASITIS.

Descript.] THIS riseth up in February, with a thick stalk about a foot high, whereon are set a few small leaves, or rather pieces, and at the tops a long spiked head; flowers of a blush or deep red colour, according to the soil where it groweth, and before the stalk with the flowers have abidden a month above ground, it will be withered and gone, and blown away with the wind, and the leaves will begin to spring, which being full grown, are very large and broad, being somewhat thin and almost round, whose thick red foot stalks above a foot long stand towards the middle of the leaves. The lower part being divided into two round parts, close almost one to another, and are of a pale green colour; and hairy underneath. The root is long and spreadeth under ground, being in some places no bigger than ones finger, in others much bigger, blackish on the outside, and whitish within, of a bitter and unpleasant taste.

Place and Time.] They grow in low and wet grounds by rivers and water sides. Their flower (as is said) rising and decaying in February and March, before their leaves, which appear in April.

Government and Virtues.] It is under the dominion of the Sun, and therefore is a great strengthener of the heart, and chearer of the vital spirits. The roots thereof are by long experience found to be very available against the plague and pestilential fevers, by provoking sweat; if the powder thereof be taken in wine, it also resisteth the force of any other poison. The root hereof taken with zedoary and angelica, or without them, helps the rising of the mother. The decoction of the root in wine, is singular good for those that wheese much, or are short winded. It provoketh urine also, and womens courses, and killeth the flat and broad worms in the belly. The powder of the root doth wonderfully help to dry up the moisture of the sores that are hard to be cured, and taketh away all spots and blemishes of the skin. It were well if gentlewomen would keep this root preserved, to help their poor neighbours. *It is fit the rich should help the poor, for the poor cannot help themselves.*

The BURDOCK.

THEY are also called Personata, and Loppy-major, great Burdock and Clod-bur; it is so well known, even by the little boys, who pull off the Burs to throw and stick upon one another, that I shall spare to write any description of it.

Place.] They grow plentifully by ditches and water-sides, and by the highways almost every where through this land.

Government and Virtues.] Venus challengeth this herb for her own, and by its leaf or seed you may draw the womb which way you please, either upwards by applying it to the crown of the head, in case it falls out; or downwards in fits of the mother, by applying it to the soles of the feet; or if you would stay it in its place, apply it to the navel, and that is one good way to stay the child in it. See more of it in my GUIDE FOR WOMEN. The Burdock leaves are cooling, moderately drying, and discussing withal, whereby it is good for all old ulcers and sores. A dram of the roots taken with pine-kernels, helpeth them that spit foul, mattery, and bloody phlegm. The leaves applied to the places troubled with the shrinkg of of the ſinews or arteries, give much eaſe. The juice of the leaves, or rather the roots themſelves, given to drink with old wine, doth wonderfully help the biting of any ſerpents: And the root beaten with a little ſalt, and laid on the place, ſuddenly eaſeth the pain thereof, and helpeth thoſe that are bit by a mad dog. The juice of the leaves being drank with honey, provoketh urine, and remedieth the pain of the bladder. The ſeed being drank in wine forty days together, doth wonderfully help the ſciatica. The leaves bruiſed with the white of an egg, and applied to any place burnt with fire, taketh out the fire, gives ſudden eaſe, and heals it up afterwards. The decoction of them fomented on any fretting ſore or canker, ſtayeth the corroding quality, which muſt be afterwards anointed with an ointment made of the ſame liquor, hog's greaſe, nitre and vinegar boiled together. The roots may be preſerved with ſugar, and taken faſting, or at other times, for the ſame purpoſes, and for conſumptions, the ſtone, and the laſk. The ſeed is much commended to break the ſtone, and cauſe it to be expelled by urine, and is often uſed with other ſeeds and things to that purpoſe.

CABBAGES and COLEWORTS.

I Shall ſpare a labour in writing a deſcription of theſe, ſince almoſt every one that can but write at all, may deſcribe them from his own knowledge, they being generally ſo well known, that deſcriptions are altogether needleſs.

Place.] They are generally planted in gardens.

Time.] Their flower time is towards the middle or end of July, and the ſeed is ripe in Auguſt.

Government and Virtues.] The Cabbages or Coleworts boiled gently in broth, and eaten, do open the body, but the ſecond decoction doth bind the body. The juice thereof drank in wine, helpeth thoſe that are bitten by an adder, and the decoction of the flowers bringeth down womens courſes: being taken with honey, it recovereth hoarſeneſs, or loſs of the voice. The often eating of them well boiled, helpeth thoſe that are entering into a conſumption. The pulp of the middle ribs of Coleworts boiled in almond milk, and made up into an electuary with honey, being taken often, is very profitable for those that are pursy and short-winded. Being boiled twice, an old cock boiled in the broth and drank, it helpeth the pains and the obstructions of the liver and spleen, and the stone in the kidneys. The juice boiled with honey, and dropped into the corner of the eyes, cleareth the sight, by consuming any film or cloud beginning to dim it; it also consumeth the canker growing therein. They are much commended, being eaten before meat to keep one from surfeiting, as also from being drunk with too much wine, or quickly make a man sober again that is drunk before. For (as they say) there is such an antipathy or enmity between the Vine and the Coleworts, that the one will die where the other groweth. The decoction of Coleworts taketh away the pain and ach, and allayeth the swellings of sores and gouty legs and knees, wherein many gross and watry humours are fallen, the place being bathed therewith warm. It helpeth also old and filthy sores, being bathed therewith, and healeth all small scabs, pushes, and wheals, that break out in the skin. The ashes of Colewort stalks mixed with old hog's grease, are very effectual to anoint the sides of those that have had long pains therein, or any other place pained with melancholy and windy humours. This was surely Chrysippus's God, and therefore he wrote a whole volume of them and their virtues, and that none of the least neither, for he would be no small fool: He appropriates them to every part of the body, and to every disease in every part; and honest old Cato (they say) used no other physic. I know not what metal their bodies were made of; this I am sure, Cabbages are extreme windy, whether you take them as meat or as medicine; yea, as windy meat as can be eaten, unless you eat bag-pipes or bellows, and they are but seldom eaten in our days; and Colewort-flowers are something more tolerable, and the wholesomer food of the two. The moon challengeth the dominion of the herb.

The SEA COLEWORTS.

Descript.] THIS hath divers somewhat long and broad, large, and thick wrinkled leaves, somewhat

what crumpled about the edges, and growing each upon a thick foot-ſtalk, very brittle, of a greyiſh green colour, from among which riſeth up a ſtrong thick ſtalk, two feet high, and better, with ſome leaves thereon to the top, where it branches forth much; and on every branch ſtandeth a large buſh of pale whitiſh flowers, conſiſting of four leaves a-piece; The root is ſomewhat great, ſhooteth forth many branches under ground, keeping the leaves green all the winter.

Place.] They grow in many places upon the ſea-coaſts, as well on the Kentiſh as Eſſex ſhores; as at Lid in Kent, Colcheſter in Eſſex, and divers other places, and in other counties of this land.

Time.] They flower and ſeed about the time that other kinds do.

Government and Virtues.] The moon claims the dominion of theſe alſo. The broth, or firſt decoction of the Sea Colewort, doth by the ſharp, nitrous, and bitter qualities therein, open the belly and purge the body: it cleanſeth and digeſts more powerfully than the other kind: The ſeed hereof bruiſed and drank killeth worms. The leaves or the juice of them applied to ſores or ulcers, cleanſeth and healeth them, and diſſolveth ſwellings, and taketh away inflammations.

CALAMINT, OR MOUNTAIN-MINT.

Deſcript.] THIS is a ſmall herb, ſeldom riſing above a foot high, with ſquare hairy, and woody ſtalks, and two ſmall hoary leaves ſet at a joint, about the bigneſs of majoram, or not much bigger, a little dented about the edges, and of a very fierce or quick ſcent, as the whole herb is: The flowers ſtand at ſeveral ſpaces of the ſtalks, from the middle almoſt upwards, which are ſmall and gaping like to thoſe of Mints, and of a pale bluiſh colour: After which follow ſmall, round blackiſh ſeed. The root is ſmall and woody, with divers ſmall ſtrings ſpreading within the ground, and dieth not, but abideth many years.

Place.] It groweth on heaths, and uplands, and dry grounds, in many places of this land.

Time.] They flower in July, and their seed is ripe quickly after.

Government and Virtues.] It is an herb of Mercury, and a strong one too, therefore excellent good in all afflictions of the brain; the decoction of the herb being drank, bringeth down women's courses, and provoketh urine. It is profitable for those that are bursten, or troubled with convulsions or cramps, with shortness of breath, or cholerick torments and pains in their bellies or stomach; it also helpeth the yellow jaundice, and stayeth vomiting, being taken in wine: Taken with salt and honey, it killeth all manner of worms in the body. It helpeth such as have the leprosy, either taken inwardly, drinking whey after it, or the green herb outwardly applied. It hindereth conception in women, but either burned or strewed in the chamber, it driveth away venomous serpents. It takes away black and blue marks in the face, and maketh black scars become well coloured, if the green herb (not the dry) be boiled in wine, and laid to the place, or the place washed therewith. Being applied to the huckle-bone, by continuance of time, it spends the humours, which cause the pain of the sciatica. The juice being dropped into the ears, killeth the worms in them. The leaves boiled in wine, and drank, provoke sweat, and open obstructions of the liver and spleen. It helpeth them that have a tertian ague (the body being first purged) by taking away the cold fits. The decoction hereof, with some sugar put thereto afterwards, is very profitable for those that be troubled with the overflowing of the gall, and that have an old cough, and that are scarce able to breathe by shortness of their wind; that have any cold distemper in their bowels, and are troubled with the hardness of the spleen, for all which purposes, both the powder, called Diacaluminthes, and the compound syrup of Calamint (which are to be had at the apothecaries) are the most effectual. Let not women be too busy with it, for it works very violent upon the feminine part.

CAMOMILE.

IT is so well known every where, that it is but lost time and labour to describe it. The virtues thereof are as followeth.

A de-

A decoction made of Camomile, and drank, taketh away all pains and stitches in the side. The flowers of Camomile beaten, and made up into balls with Gil, drive away all sorts of agues, if the party grieved be anointed with that oil, taken from the flowers, from the crown of the head to the sole of the foot, and afterwards laid to sweat in his bed, and that he sweats well. This is Nechessor an Egyptian's medicine. It is profitable for all sorts of agues that come either from phlegm, or melancholy, or from an inflammation of the bowels, being applied when the humours causing them shall be concocted; and there is nothing more profitable to the sides and region of the liver and spleen than it. The bathing with a decoction of Camomile taketh away weariness, easeth pains, to what part of the body soever they be applied. It comforteth the sinews that are over-strained, mollifieth all swellings: It moderately comforteth all parts that have need of warmth, digesteth and dissolveth whatsoever hath need thereof, by a wonderful speedy property. It easeth all the pains of the colic and stone, and all pains and torments of the belly, and gently provoketh urine. The flowers boiled in posset-drink provoke sweat, and help to expel all colds, aches and pains whatsoever, and is an excellent help to bring down womens courses. Syrup made of the juice of Camomile, with the flowers in white wine, is a remedy against the jaundice and dropsy. The flowers boiled in lee, are good to wash the head, and comfort both it and the brain. The oil made of the flowers of Camomile, is much used against all hard swellings, pains or aches, shrinking of the sinews, or cramps, or pains in the joints, or any other part of the body. Being used in glysters, it helps to dissolve the wind and pains in the belly; anointed also, it helpeth stitches and pains in the sides.

Nichessor saith, the Egyptians dedicated it to the sun, because it cured agues, and they were like enough to do it, for they were the arrantest apes in their religion I ever read of. Bachinus, Bena, and Lobel, commend the syrup made of the juice of it and sugar, taken inwardly, to be excellent for the spleen. Also this is certain, that it most wonderfully breaks the stone: Some take it in syrup or decoc-

decoction, others inject the juice of it into the bladder with a syringe. My opinion is, that the salt of it taken half a dram in the morning in a little white or rhenish wine, is better than either; that it is excellent for the stone, appears in this which I have seen tried, viz. That a stone that hath been taken out of the body of a man, being wrapped in Camomile, will in time dissolve, and in a little time too.

WATER-CALTROPS.

THEY are called also Tribulus Aquaticus, Tribulus Lacusoris, Tribulus Marinus, Caltrops, Saligos, Water Nuts, and Water Chesnuts.

Descript.] As for the greater sort of Water-Caltrop it is not found here, or very rarely. Two other sorts there are which I shall here describe. The first hath a long creeping and jointed root, sending forth tufts at each joint, from which joints arise long, flat, slender knotted stalks, even to the top of the water, divided towards the top into many branches, each carrying two leaves on both sides, being about two inches long, and half an inch broad, thin and almost transparent, they look as though they were torn; the flowers are long, thick and whitish, set together almost like a bunch of grapes, which being gone, there succeeds for the most part sharp pointed grains altogether, containing a small white kernel in them.

The second differs not much from this, save that it delights in more clear water; its stalks are not flat, but round; its leaves are not so long, but more pointed: As for the place we need not determine, for their name sheweth they grow in the water.

Government and Virtues.] They are under the dominion of the Moon, and being made into a poultice, are excellent for hot inflammations, swellings, cankers, sore mouths and throats, being washed with the decoction; it cleanseth and strengtheneth the neck and throat, and helps those swellings which when people have, they say the almonds of their ears are fallen down; it is excellent good for the rankness of the gums, a safe and present remedy for the king's evil; they are excellent good for the stone and gravel.

gravel, especially the nuts being dried; they also resist poison, and bitings of venomous beasts.

CAMPION WILD.

Descript. THE wild White Campion hath many long and somewhat broad dark green leaves lying upon the ground, and divers ribs therein, somewhat like plantain, but somewhat hairy, broader, and not so long: The hairy stalks rise up in the middle of them three or four feet high, and sometimes more, with divers great white joints at several places thereon, and two such like leaves thereat up to the top, sending forth branches at several joints also: All which bear on several foot-stalks white flowers at the tops of them, consisting of five broad pointed leaves, every one cut in on the end unto the middle, making them seem to be two a piece, smelling somewhat sweet, and each of them standing in a large green striped hairy husk, large and round below next to the stalk: The seed is small and greyish in the hard heads that come up afterwards. The root is white and long, spreading divers fangs in the ground.

The red wild Campion groweth in the same manner as the white, but his leaves are not so plainly ribbed, somewhat shorter, rounder, and more wooly in handling. The flowers are of the same form and bigness; but in some of a pale, in others of a bright red colour, cut in at the ends more finely, which makes the leaves look more in number than the other. The seeds and the roots are alike, the roots of both sorts abiding many years.

There are forty-five kinds of Campion more, those of them which are of a physical use, having the like virtues with those above described, which I take to be the two chiefest kinds.

Place.] They grow commonly through this land by fields and hedge-sides and ditches.

Time.] They flower in Summer, some earlier than others, and some abiding longer than others.

Government and Virtues.] They belong unto Saturn, and it is found by experience, that the decoction of the herb, either in white or red wine being drank, doth stay inward bleedings, and applied outwardly, it doth the like;

and being drank, helpeth to expel urine being ſtopped, and gravel and ſtone in the reins or kidneys. Two drams of the ſeed drank in wine, purgeth the body of cholerick humours, and helpeth thoſe that are ſtung by ſcorpions, or other venomous beaſts, and may be as effectual for the plague. It is of very good uſe in old ſores, ulcers, cankers, fiſtulas, and the like, to cleanſe and heat them, by conſuming the moiſt humours falling into them, and correcting the putrefaction of humours offending them.

CARDUUS BENEDICTUS.

IT is called Carduus Benedictus, or Bleſſed Thiſtle, or Holy Thiſtle; I ſuppoſe the name was put upon it by ſome that had little holineſs in themſelves.

I ſhall ſpare a labour in writing a deſcription of this, as almoſt every one that can but write at all, may deſcribe them from his own knowledge.

Time.] They flower in Auguſt, and ſeed not long after.

Government and Virtues.] It is an herb of Mars, and under the ſign Aries. Now, in handling this herb, I ſhall give you a rational pattern of all the reſt; and if you pleaſe to view them throughout the book, you ſhall, to your content, find it true. It helps ſwimmings and giddineſs of the head, or the diſeaſe called vertigo, becauſe Aries is in the houſe of Mars. It is an excellent remedy againſt the yellow jaundice, and other infirmities of the gall, becauſe Mars governs choler. It ſtrengthens the attractive faculty in man, and clarifies the blood, becauſe the one is ruled by Mars. The continual drinking the decoction of it, helps red faces, tetters, and ring-worms, becauſe Mars cauſeth them. It helps the plague, ſores, boils, and itch, the bitings of mad dogs and venomous beaſts, all which infirmities are under Mars; thus you ſee what it doth by ſympathy.

By antipathy to other planets it cures the French pox. By antipathy to Venus, who governs it, it ſtrengthens the memory; and cures deafneſs, by antipathy to Saturn, who hath his fall in Aries, which rules the head. It cures quartan agues, and other diſeaſes of melancholy, and aduſt choler, by ſympathy to Saturn, Mars being exalted in Capricorn.

Capricorn. Alſo it provokes urine, the ſtopping of which is uſually cauſed by Mars or the Moon.

CARROTS.

GARDEN Carrots are ſo well known, that they need no deſcription; but becauſe they are of leſs phyſical uſe than the wild kind (as indeed almoſt in all herbs the wild are moſt effectual in phyſick, as being more powerful in operation than the garden kinds) I ſhall therefore briefly deſcribe the Wild Carrot.

Deſcript.] It groweth in a manner altogether like the tame, but that the leaves and ſtalks are ſomewhat whiter and rougher. The ſtalks bear large tufts of white flowers, with a deep purple ſpot in the middle, which are contracted together when the ſeed begins to ripen, that the middle part being hollow and low, and the outward ſtalk riſing high, maketh the whole umbel to ſhew like a bird's neſt. The roots ſmall, long and hard, and unfit for meat, being ſomewhat ſharp and ſtrong.

Place.] The wild kind groweth in divers parts of this land plentifully by the field-ſides, and untilled places.

Time.] They flower and ſeed in the end of Summer.

Government and Virtues.] Wild Carrots belong to Mercury, and therefore break wind, and remove ſtitches in the ſides, provoke urine and womens courſes, and helpeth to break and expel the ſtone; the ſeed alſo of the ſame worketh the like effect, and is good for the dropſy, and thoſe whoſe bellies are ſwollen with wind; helpeth the colick, the ſtone in the kidneys, and riſing of the mother; being taken in wine, or boiled in wine, and taken, it helpeth conception. The leaves being applied with honey to running ſores or ulcers, do cleanſe them.

I ſuppoſe the ſeeds of them perform this better than the roots; and though Galen commended garden Carrots highly to break wind, yet experience teacheth they breed it firſt, and we may thank nature for expelling it, not they; the ſeeds of them expel wind indeed, and ſo mend what the root marreth.

CARRAWAY.

Deſcript.] IT beareth divers ſtalks of fine cut leaves, lying upon the ground, ſomewhat like to the leaves

leaves of carrots, but not buſhing ſo thick, of a little quick taſte in them, from among which riſeth up a ſquare ſtalk, not ſo high as the carrot, at whoſe joints are ſet the like leaves, but ſmaller and fitter, and at the top ſmall open tufts, or umbels of white flowers, which turn into ſmall blackiſh ſeed, ſmaller than the Anniſeed, and of a quicker and better taſte. The root is whitiſh, ſmall, and long, ſomewhat like unto a parſnip, but with more wrinkled bark, and much leſs, of a little hot and quick taſte, and ſtronger than the parſnip, and abideth after ſeed-time.

Place.] It is uſually ſown with us in gardens.

Time.] They flower in June and July, and ſeed quickly after.

Government and Virtues.] This is alſo a Mercurial plant. Carraway ſeed hath a moderate ſharp quality, whereby it breaketh wind, and provoketh urine, which alſo the herb doth. The root is better food than the parſnips; it is pleaſant and comfortable to the ſtomach, and helpeth digeſtion. The ſeed is conducing to all cold griefs of the head and ſtomach, bowels, or mother, as alſo the wind in them, and helpeth to ſharpen the eye-ſight. The powder of the ſeed put into a poultice, taketh away black and blue ſpots of blows and bruiſes. The herb itſelf, or with ſome of the ſeed bruiſed and fried, laid hot in a bag or double cloth, to the lower parts of the belly, eaſeth the pains of the wind colick.

The roots of Carraways eaten as men eat parſnips, ſtrengthen the ſtomachs of ancient people exceedingly, and they need not to make a whole meal of them neither, and are fit to be planted in every garden.

Carraway confects once only dipped in ſugar, and half a ſpoonful of them eaten in the morning faſting, and as many after each meal, is a moſt admirable remedy for thoſe that are troubled with wind.

CELANDINE.

Deſcript. THIS hath divers tender, round, whitiſh green ſtalks, with greater joints than ordinary in other herbs as it were knees, very brittle and eaſy to break, from whence grow branches with large tender broad leaves, divided into many parts, each of them cut

cut in on the edges, ſet at the joint on both ſides of the branches, of a dark bluiſh green colour, on the upper ſide like columbines, and of a more pale bluiſh green underneath, full of yellow ſap, when any part is broken of a bitter taſte, and ſtrong ſcent. At the flowers of four leaves a-piece, after which come ſmall long pods, with blackiſh ſeed therein. The root is ſomewhat great at the head, ſhooting forth divers long roots and ſmall ſtrings, reddiſh on the out-ſide, and yellow within, full of yellow ſap therein.

Place.] They grow in many places by old walls, hedge, and way-ſides in untilled places; and being once planted in a garden, eſpecially ſome ſhady places, it will remain there.

Time.] They flower all the Summer long, and the ſeed ripeneth in the mean time.

Government and Virtues.] This is an herb of the Sun, and under the celeſtial Lion, and is one of the beſt cures for the eyes; for, all that know any thing in aſtrology, know that the eyes are ſubject to the luminaries; let it then be gathered when the Sun is in Leo, and the Moon in Aries, applying to this time; let Leo ariſe, then may you make it into an oil or ointment, which you pleaſe, to anoint your ſore eyes with: I can prove it doth both by my own experience, and the experience of thoſe to whom I have taught it, that moſt deſperate ſore eyes have been cured by this only medicine; and then I pray, is not this far better than endangering the eyes by the art of the needle? For if this doth not abſolutely take away the film, it will facilitate the work, that it may be done without danger. The herb or root boiled in white wine and drank, a few anniſeeds being boiled therewith, openeth obſtructions of the liver and gall, helpeth the yellow jaundice; and often uſing it, helps the dropſy and the itch, and thoſe that have old ſores in their legs, or other parts of the body. The juice thereof taken faſting, is held to be of ſingular good uſe againſt the peſtilence. The diſtilled water, with a little ſugar and a little good treacle mixed therewith (the party upon the taking being laid down to ſweat a little) hath the ſame effect. The juice dropped in the eyes, cleanſeth them from films and cloudineſs which darken the ſight, but it is beſt to allay the ſharpneſs of the juice with a little breaſt-milk. It is good in old filthy corroding creeping ulcers whereſoever, to ſtay their malignity of fretting and running, and to cauſe them to heal more ſpeedily: The juice often applied to tetters, ring-worms, or other ſuch like ſpreading cankers, will quickly heal them, and rubbed often upon warts, will take them away. The herb with the roots bruiſed and bathed with oil of camomile, and applied to the navel, taketh away the griping pains in the belly and bowels, and all the pains of the mother; and applied to womens breaſts, ſtayeth the overmuch flowing of the courſes. The juice or decoction of the herb gargled between the teeth that ach, eaſeth the pain, and the powder of the dried root laid upon any aching, hollow or looſe tooth, will cauſe it to fall out. The juice mixed with ſome powder of brimſtone is not only good againſt the itch, but taketh away all diſcolourings of the ſkin whatſoever; and if it chance that in a tender body it cauſeth any itchings or inflammations, by bathing the place with a little vinegar, it is helped.

Another ill-favoured trick have phyſicians got to uſe to the eye, and that is worſe than the needle; which is to take away films by corroding or gnawing medicines. This I abſolutely proteſt againſt.

1. Becauſe the tunicles of the eyes are very thin, and therefore ſoon eaten aſunder.

2. The callus or film that they would eat away, is ſeldom of an equal thickneſs in every place, and then the tunicle may be eaten aſunder in one place, before the film be conſumed in another, and ſo be a readier way to extinguiſh the ſight than to reſtore it.

It is called Chelidonium, from the Greek word CHELIDON, which ſignifies a ſwallow, becauſe they ſay, that if you put out the eyes of young ſwallows when they are in the neſt, the old ones will recover their eyes again with this herb. This I am confident, for I have tried it, that if we mar the very apple of their eyes with a needle, ſhe will recover them again; but whether with this herb or not, I know not.

Alſo I have read (and it ſeems to be ſomewhat probable) that

that the herb being gathered as I shewed before, and the elements drawn apart from it by art of the alchymist, and after they are drawn apart rectified, the earthy quality, still in rectifying them, added to the *Terra damnata* (as Alchymists call it) or *Terra sacratissima* (as some philosophers call it) the elements so rectified are sufficient for the cure of all diseases, the humours offending being known, and the contrary element given: It is an experiment worth the trying, and can do no harm.

The Lesser CELANDINE, usually known by the name of PILEWORT and FOGWORT.

I Wonder what ailed the ancients to give this the name of Celandine, which resembles it neither in nature nor form; it acquired the name of Pilewort from its virtues, and it being no great matter where I set it down, so I set it down at all, I humoured Dr Tradition so much as to set him down here.

Descript.] This Celandine or Pilewort (which you please) doth spread many round pale green leaves, set on weak and trailing branches, which lie upon the ground, and are flat, smooth, and somewhat shining, and in some places (though seldom) marked with black spots, each standing on a long foot-stalk, among which rise small yellow flowers, consisting of nine or ten small narrow leaves, upon slender foot-stalks, very like unto Crowsfoot, whereunto the seed also is not unlike, being many small kernels like a grain of corn, sometimes twice as long as others, of a whitish colour, with some fibres at the end of them.

Place.] It groweth for the most part in moist corners of fields and places that are near water-sides, yet will abide in drier ground if they be but a little shady.

Time.] It flowereth betimes about March or April, is quite gone by May; so it cannot be found till it spring again.

Government and Virtues.] It is under the dominion of Mars, and behold here another verification of the learning of the ancients, *viz.* that the virtue of an herb may be known by its signature, as plainly appears in this; for if you dig up the root of it, you shall perceive the perfect image of the disease which they commonly call the piles.

It is certain by good experience, that the decoction of the leaves and roots doth wonderfully help piles and hæmorrhoids, alſo kernels by the ears and throat, called the king's evil, or any other hard wens or tumours.

Here's another ſecret for my countrymen and women, a couple of them together; Pilewort made into an oil, ointment, or plaiſter, readily cures both the piles, or hæmorrhoids, and the king's evil: The very herb borne about one's body next the ſkin, helps in ſuch diſeaſes, though it never touch the place grieved; let poor people make much of it for thoſe uſes; with this I cured my own daughter of the king's evil, broke the ſore, drew out a quarter of a pint of corruption, cured without any ſcar at all in one week's time.

The ordinary ſmall CENTAURY.

Deſcript.] THIS groweth up moſt uſually but with one round and ſomewhat cruſted ſtalk, about a foot high or better, branching forth at the top into many ſprigs, and ſome alſo from the joints of the ſtalks below; the flowers thus ſtand at the tops as it were in one umble or tuft, are of a pale red, tending to carnation colour, conſiſting of five, ſometimes ſix ſmall leaves, very like thoſe of St John's Wort, opening themſelves in the day time and cloſing at night, after which come ſeeds in little ſhort huſks, in form like unto wheat corn. The leaves are ſmall and ſomewhat round; the root ſmall and hard, periſhing every year. The whole plant is of an exceeding bitter taſte.

There is another ſort in all things like the former, ſave only it beareth white flowers.

Place.] They grow ordinarily in fields, paſtures, and woods, but that with the white flowers not ſo frequently as the other.

Time.] They flower in July or thereabouts, and ſeed within a month after.

Government and Virtues.] They are under the dominion of the ſun, as appears in that their flowers open and ſhut as the ſun either ſheweth or hideth his face. This herb, boiled and drank, purgeth cholerick and groſs humours, and helpeth the ſciatica; it openeth obſtructions of the liver,

liver, gall, and ſpleen, helpeth the jaundice, and eaſeth the pains in the ſides, and hardneſs of the ſpleen, uſed outwardly, and is given with very good effect in agues. It helpeth thoſe that have the dropſy, or the green-ſickneſs, being much uſed by the Italians in powder for that purpoſe. It killeth the worms in the belly, as is found by experience. The decoction thereof, *viz.* the tops of the ſtalks, with the leaves and flowers, is good againſt the colic, and to bring down womens courſes, helpeth to void the dead birth, and eaſeth pains of the mother, and is very effectual in all old pains of the joints, as the gout, cramps, or convulſions. A dram of the powder thereof taken in wine, is a wonderful good help againſt the biting and poiſon of an adder. The juice of the herb with a little honey put to it, is good to clear the eyes from dimneſs, miſts and clouds that offend or hinder ſight. It is ſingular good both for green and freſh wounds, as alſo for old ulcers and ſores, to cloſe up the one and cleanſe the other, and perfectly to cure them both, although they are hollow or fiſtulous; the green herb eſpecially being bruiſed and laid thereto. The decoction therefore dropped into the ears, cleanſeth them from worms, cleanſeth the foul ulcers and ſpreading ſcabs of the head, and taketh away all freckles, ſpots, and marks in the ſkin, being waſhed with it, the herb is ſo ſafe you cannot fail in the uſing of it, only giving it inwardly for inward diſeaſes. 'Tis very wholeſome, but not very toothſome.

There is, beſides theſe, another ſmall Centaury, which beareth a yellow flower; in all other reſpects it is like the former, ſave that the leaves are bigger, and of a darker green, and the ſtalk paſſeth through the midſt of them, as it doth the herb Thorowan. They are all of them, as I told you, under the government of the ſun; yet this, if you obſerve it, you ſhall find an excellent truth; in diſeaſes of the blood, uſe the red Centaury; if of choler, uſe the yellow; but if phlegm or water, you will find the white beſt.

The Cherry-Tree.

I Suppoſe there are few but know this tree, for its fruit's ſake; and therefore, I ſhall ſpare writing a deſcription thereof.

Place.] For the place of its growth, it is afforded room in every orchard.

Government and Virtues.] It is a tree of Venus. Cherries, as they are of different taſtes, ſo they are of different qualities. The ſweet paſs through the ſtomach and the belly more ſpeedily, but are of little nouriſhment; the tart or ſour are more pleaſing to an hot ſtomach, procure appetite to meat, and help to cut tough phlegm, and groſs humours; but when theſe are dried, they are more binding to the belly than when they are freſh, being cooling in hot diſeaſes, and welcome to the ſtomach, and provoke urine. The gum of the Cherry-tree, diſſolved in wine, is good for a cold, cough, and hoarſeneſs of the throat; mendeth the colour in the face, ſharpeneth the eye-ſight, provoketh appetite, and helpeth to break and expel the ſtone; the Black Cherries bruiſed with the ſtones, and diſſolved, the water thereof is much uſed to break the ſtone, and to expel gravel and wind.

WINTER-CHERRIES.

Deſcript.] THE Winter Cherry hath a running or creeping root in the ground, of the bigneſs many times of one's little finger, ſhooting forth at ſeveral joints in ſeveral places, whereby it quickly ſpreads a great compaſs of ground. The ſtalk riſeth not above a yard high, whereon are ſet many broad and long green leaves, ſomewhat like nightſhade, but larger; at the joints whereof come forth whitiſh flowers made of five leaves a piece, which afterwards turn into green berries incloſed with thin ſkins, which change to be reddiſh when they grow ripe, the berry likewiſe being reddiſh, and as large as a cherry; wherein are contained many flat and yellowiſh ſeeds lying within the pulp, which being gathered and ſtrung up, are kept all the year to be uſed upon occaſion.

Place.] They grow not naturally in this land, but are cheriſhed in gardens for their virtues.

Time.] They flower not until the middle or latter end of July; and the fruit is ripe about Auguſt, or the beginning of September.

Government and Virtues.] This alſo is a plant of Venus. They

They are of great uſe in phyſic: The leaves being cooling, may be uſed in inflammations, but not opening as the berries and fruit are; which by drawing down the urine provoke it to be avoided plentifully when it is ſtopped or grown hot, ſharp, and painful in the paſſage; it is good alſo to expel the ſtone and gravel out of the reins, kidneys, and bladder, helping to diſſolve the ſtone, and voiding it by grit or gravel ſent forth in the urine; it alſo helpeth much to cleanſe inward impoſthumes or ulcers in the reins or bladder, or in thoſe that void a bloody or foul urine. The diſtilled water of the fruit, or the leaves together with them, or the berries, green or dry, diſtilled with a little milk and drank morning and evening with a little ſugar, is effectual to all the purpoſes before ſpecified and eſpecially againſt the heat and ſharpneſs of the urine. I ſhall only mention one way, amongſt many others, which might be uſed for ordering the berries, to be helpful for the urine and the ſtone; which is this: Take three or four good handfuls of the berries, either green or freſh, or dried, and having bruiſed them, put them into ſo many gallons of beer or ale when it is new tunned up: This drink, taken daily, hath been found to do much good to many, both to eaſe the pains and expel urine and the ſtone, and to cauſe the ſtone not to engender. The decoction of the berries in wine and water is the moſt uſual way; but the powder of them taken in drink is more effectual.

CHERVIL.

IT is called Cerefolium, Mirrhis, and Mirrha, Chervel, Sweet Chervil, and Sweet Cicely.

Deſcript.] The garden Chervil doth at firſt ſomewhat reſemble Parſley, but after it is better grown, the leaves are much cut in and jagged, reſembling hemlock, being a little hairy and of a whitiſh green colour, ſometimes turning reddiſh in the Summer, with the ſtalks alſo; it riſeth a little above half a foot high, bearing white flowers in ſpiked tufts, which turn into long and round ſeeds pointed at the ends, and blackiſh when they are ripe; of a ſweet taſte, but no ſmell, though the herb itſelf ſmelleth reaſonably well. The root is ſmall and long, and periſheth every year, and muſt be ſown a-new in ſpring, for ſeed after July or Autumn fails.

The

The wild Chervil groweth two or three feet high, with yellow ſtalks and joints, ſet with broader and more hairy leaves, divided into ſundry parts, nicked about the edges, and of a dark green colour, which likewiſe grow reddiſh with the ſtalks; at the tops whereof ſtand ſmall white tufts of flowers, afterwards ſmaller and longer ſeed. The root is white, hard, and enduring long. This hath little or no ſcent.

Place.] The firſt is ſown in gardens for a ſallet herb; the ſecond groweth wild in many of the meadows of this land, and by the hedge ſides, and on heaths.

Time.] They flower and ſeed early, and thereupon are ſown again in the end of Summer.

Government and Virtues.] The garden Chervil being eaten, doth moderately warm the ſtomach, and is a certain remedy (ſaith Tragus) to diſſolve congealed or clotted blood in the body, or that which is clotted by bruiſes, falls, &c. The juice or diſtilled water thereof being drank, and the bruiſed leaves laid to the place, being taken either in meat or drink, it is good help to provoke urine, or expel the ſtone in the kidneys, to ſend down womens courſes, and to help the pleuriſy and pricking of the ſides.

The wild Chervil bruiſed and applied, diſſolveth ſwellings in any part, or the marks of congealed blood by bruiſes or blows, in a little ſpace.

SWEET CHERVIL, OR SWEET CICELY.

Deſcrip.] THIS groweth very like the great hemlock, having large ſpread leaves cut into divers parts, but of a freſher green colour than the hemlock, taſting as ſweet as the anniſeed. The ſtalks riſe up a yard high, or better, being creſſed or hollow, having leaves at the joints, but leſſer; and at the tops of the branched ſtalks, umbels or tufts of white flowers; after which comes large and long creſted black ſhining ſeed, pointed at both ends, taſting quick, yet ſweet and pleaſant. The root is great and white, growing deep in the ground, and ſpreading ſundry long branches therein, in taſte and ſmell ſtronger than the leaves or ſeeds, and continuing many years.

Place.] This groweth in gardens.

Government and Virtues.] Theſe are all three of them

of

of the nature of Jupiter, and under his dominion. This whole plant, besides its pleasantness in sallets, hath its physical virtue. The root boiled, and eaten with oil and vinegar, (or without oil) do much please and warm old and cold stomachs oppressed with wind or phlegm, or those that have the phthisick or consumption of the lungs. The same drank with wine is a preservation from the plague. It provoketh womens courses, and expelleth the after-birth, procureth an appetite to meat, and expelleth wind. The juice is good to heal the ulcers of the head and face; the candied roots hereof are held as effectual as Angelica, to preserve from infection in the time of a plague, and to warm and comfort a cold weak stomach. It is so harmless you cannot use it amiss.

CHESNUT TREE.

IT were as needless to describe a tree so commonly known, as to tell a man he had gotten a mouth; therefore take the government and virtues of them thus:

The tree is abundantly under the dominion of Jupiter, and therefore the fruit must needs breed good blood, and yield commendable nourishment to the body; yet, if eaten over-much, they make the blood thick, procure head-ach, and bind the body; the inner skin, that covereth the nut, is of so binding a quality, that a scruple of it being taken by a man, or ten grains by a child, soon stops any flux whatsoever: The whole nut being dried and beaten into powder, and a dram taken at a time, is a good remedy to stop the terms in women. If you dry Chesnuts, (only the kernels I mean) both the barks being taken away, beat them into powder, and make the powder up into an electuary with honey, so have you an admirable remedy for the cough and spitting of blood.

EARTH CHESNUTS.

THEY are called Earth Nuts, Earth Chesnuts, Ground Nuts, Ciper-nuts, and in Sussex Pig-nuts. A description of them were needless, for every child knows them.

Government and Virtues.] They are something hot and dry in quality, under the dominion of Venus, they provoke lust exceedingly, and stir up to those sports she is mistress

mistress of; the seed is excellent good to provoke urine; and so also is the root, but it doth not perform it so forcibly as the seed doth. The root being dried and beaten into powder, and the powder made into an electuary, is as singular a remedy for spitting and pissing of blood, as the former Chesnut was for coughs.

CHICKWEED.

IT is so generally known to most people, that I shall not trouble you with the description thereof, nor myself with setting forth the several kinds, since but only two or three are considerable for their usefulness.

Place.] They are usually found in moist and watery places, by woodsides, and elsewhere.

Time.] They flower about June, and their seed is ripe in July.

Government and Virtues.] It is a fine soft pleasing herb, under the dominion of the Moon. It is found to be effectual as Purslain to all the purposes whereunto it serveth, except for meat only. The herb bruised, or the juice applied (with cloths or sponges dipped therein) to the region of the liver, and as they dry, to have it fresh applied, doth wonderfully temperate the heat of the liver, and is effectual for all imposthumes and swellings whatsoever, for all redness in the face, wheals, pushes, itch, scabs; the juice either simply used, or boiled with hog's grease and applied, helpeth cramps, convulsions, and palsy. The juice, or distilled water, is of much good use for all heats and redness in the eyes, to drop some thereof into them; as also into the ears, to ease pains in them; and is of good effect to ease pains from the heat and sharpness of the blood in the piles, and generally all pains in the body that arise of heat. It is used also in hot and virulent ulcers and sores in the privy parts of men or women, or on the legs, or elsewhere. The leaves boiled with marshmallows, and made into a poultice with fenugreek and linseed, applied to swellings or imposthumes, ripen and break them, or assuage the swellings and ease the pains. It helpeth the sinews when they are shrunk by cramps, or otherwise, and to extend and make them pliable again by this medicine, boil a handful of Chickweed, and a handful

ful of red rose leaves dried, in a quart of mascadine, until a fourth part be consumed; then put to them a pint of oil of trotters or sheep's feet; let them boil a good while, still stirring them well; which being strained, anoint the grieved place therewith, warm against the fire, rubbing it well with one hand; and bind also some of the herb (if you will) to the place, and, with God's blessing, it will help it in three times dressing.

CHICK-PEASE, or CICERS.

Descript.] THE garden sorts, whether red, black, or white, bring forth stalks a yard long, whereon do grow many small and almost round leaves, dented about the edges, set on both sides of a middle rib: At the joints come forth one or two flowers, upon sharp foot stalks, pease-fashion, either white or whitish, or purplish red, lighter or deeper, according as the pease that follow will be, that are contained in small, thick, and short pods, wherein lie one or two pease, more usually pointed at the lower end, and almost round at the head, yet a little cornered or sharp; the root is small and perisheth yearly.

Place and Time.] They are sown in gardens, or fields, as pease, being sown later than pease, and gathered at the same time with them, or presently after.

Government and Virtues.] They are both under the dominion of Venus. They are less windy than beans, but nourish more; they provoke urine, and are thought to increase sperm; they have a cleansing faculty, whereby they break the stone in the kidneys. To drink the cream of them, being boiled in water, is the best way. It moves the belly downwards, provokes womens courses and urine, increases both milk and seed. One ounce of Cicers, two ounces of French barley, and a small handful of marshmallow roots, clean washed and cut, being boiled in the broth of a chicken, and four ounces taken in the morning, and fasting two hours after, is a good medicine for a pain in the sides. The white Cicers are used more for meat than medicine, yet have the same effect, and are thought more powerful to increase milk and seed. The wild Cicers are so much more powerful than the garden

kinds,

kinds, by how much they exceed them in heat and dryneſs; whereby they do more open obſtructions, break the ſtone, and have all the properties of cutting, opening, digeſting, and diſſolving; and this more ſpeedily and certainly than the former.

CINQUEFOIL, *or* Five-leaved Graſs; *called in ſome Counties* Five-fingered Graſs.

Deſcript.] IT ſpreads and creeps far upon the ground, with long ſlender ſtrings like ſtrawberries, which take root again, and ſhoot forth many leaves made of five parts, and ſometimes of ſeven, dented about the edges, and ſomewhat hard. The ſtalks are ſlender, leaning downwards, and bear many ſmall yellow flowers thereon, with ſome yellow threads in the middle, ſtanding about a ſmooth green head, which, when it is ripe, is a little rough, and containeth ſmall browniſh ſeed. The root is of a blackiſh brown colour, as big as one's little finger, but growing long, with ſome threads thereat; and by the ſmall ſtrings it quickly ſpreadeth over the ground.

Place.] It groweth by wood ſides, hedge ſides, the pathway in fields, and in the borders and corners of them, almoſt through all this land.

Time.] It flowereth in Summer, ſome ſooner, ſome later.

Government and Virtues.] This is an herb of Jupiter, and therefore ſtrengthens the part of the body it rules; let Jupiter be angular and ſtrong when it is gathered; and if you give but a ſcruple (which is but twenty grains) of it at a time, either in white wine, or in white wine vinegar, you ſhall very ſeldom miſs the cure of an ague, be it what ague ſoever, in three fits, as I have often proved, to the admiration both of myſelf and others; let no man deſpiſe it becauſe it is plain and eaſy, the ways of God are all ſuch. It is an eſpecial herb uſed in all inflammations and fevers, whether infectious or peſtilential; or among other herbs to cool and temper the blood and humours in the body. As alſo for all lotions, gargles, infections, and the like, for ſore mouths, ulcers, cancers, fiſtulas, and other corrupt, foul, or running ſores. The juice hereof drank, about four ounces at a time, for certain days together, cureth the quinſey and yellow jaundice;

and

and taken for thirty days together, cureth the fallen ſickneſs. The roots boiled in milk and drank, is a moſt effectual remedy for all fluxes in man or woman, whether the white or red, as alſo the bloody-flux. The roots boiled in vinegar, and the decoction thereof held in the mouth, eaſeth the pains of the tooth-ach. The juice or decoction taken with a little honey, helpeth the hoarſeneſs of the throat, and is very good for the cough of the lungs. The diſtilled water of both roots and leaves is alſo effectual to all the purpoſes aforeſaid; and if the hands be often waſhed therein, and ſuffered at every time to dry in of itſelf without wiping, it will in a ſhort time help the palſy, or ſhaking in them. The root boiled in vinegar, helpeth all knots, kernels, hard ſwellings, and lumps growing in any part of the fleſh, being thereto applied; as alſo inflammations, and St. Anthony's fire, all impoſthumes, and painful ſores with heat and putrefaction, the ſhingles alſo, and all other ſorts of running and foul ſcabs, ſores, and itch. The ſame alſo boiled in wine, and applied to any joint full of pain, ach, or the gout in the hands or feet, or the hip gout, called the Sciatica, and the decoction thereof drank the while, doth cure them, and eaſeth much pain in the bowels. The roots are likewiſe effectual to help ruptures or burſtings, being uſed with other things available to that purpoſe, taken either inwardly or outwardly, or both; as alſo bruiſes or hurts by blows, falls, or the like, and to ſtay the bleeding of wounds in any parts inward or outward.

Some hold that one leaf cures a quotidian, three a tertian, and four a quartan ague, and a hundred to one if it be not Dioſcorides; for he is full of whimſies. The truth is, I never ſtood ſo much upon the number of the leaves, nor whether I gives it in powder or decoction: If Jupiter were ſtrong, and the Moon applying to him, or his good aſpect at the gathering, I never knew it miſs the deſired effects.

CIVES.

CALLED alſo Ruſh Leeks, Chives, Civet, and Sweth. *Temperature and Virtues.*] I confeſs I had not added theſe, had it not been for a country gentleman, who by a letter certified me, that amongſt other herbs, I had left theſe out; they are indeed a kind of leeks, hot and dry in the fourth degree as they are, and ſo under the dominion of Mars; if they be eaten raw, (I do not mean raw, oppoſite to roaſted or boiled, but raw, oppoſite to chymical preparation) they ſend up very hurtful vapours to the brain, cauſing troubleſome ſleep, and ſpoiling the eye-ſight, yet of them, prepared by the art of the alchymiſt, may be made an excellent remedy for the ſtoppage of urine.

CLARY, or more properly CLEAR-EYE.

Deſcript.] OUR ordinary garden Clary hath four ſquare ſtalks, with broad, rough, wrinkled, whitiſh or hoary green leaves, ſomewhat evenly cut in on the edges, and of a ſtrong ſweet ſcent, growing ſome near the ground, and ſome by couples upon ſtalks. The flowers grow at certain diſtances, with two ſmall leaves at the joints under them, ſomewhat like unto the flowers of Sage, but ſmaller, and of a whitiſh blue colour. The ſeed is browniſh, and ſomewhat flat, or not ſo round as the wild. The roots are blackiſh, and ſpread not far, and periſh after the ſeed time. It is uſually ſown, for it ſeldom riſes of its own ſowing.

Place.] This groweth in gardens.

Time.] It flowereth in June and July, ſome a little later than others, and their ſeed is ripe in Auguſt, or thereabouts.

Government and Virtues.] It is under the dominion of the Moon. The ſeed put into the eyes clears them from motes and ſuch like things gotten within the lids to offend them, as alſo clears them from white and red ſpots on them. The mucilage of the ſeed made with water, and applied to tumours, or ſwellings, diſperſeth and taketh them away; as alſo draweth forth ſplinters, thorns, or other things gotten into the fleſh. The leaves uſed with vinegar, either by itſelf, or with a little honey, doth help boils, felons, and the hot inflammations that are gathered by their pains, if applied before it be grown too great. The powder of the dried root put into the noſe, provoketh ſneezing, and thereby purgeth the head and brain of much rheum and corruption. The ſeed or leaves taken

in

in wine, provoketh to venery. It is of much uſe both for men and women that have weak back, and helpeth to ſtrengthen the reins, uſed either by itſelf, or with other herbs conducing to the ſame effect, and in tanſies often. The freſh leaves dipped in a batter of flour, eggs, and a little milk, and fried in butter, and ſerved to the table, is not unpleaſant to any, but exceeding profitable for thoſe that are troubled with weak backs, and the effects thereof. The juice of the herb put into ale or beer, and drank, bringeth down womens courſes, and expelleth the after-birth.

It is an uſual courſe with many men, when they have gotten the running of the reins, or women the whites, they run to the buſh of Clary; Maid, bring hither the frying-pan, fetch me ſome butter quickly, then for eating fried Clary, juſt as hogs eat acorns; and this they think will cure their diſeaſe (forſooth) whereas when they have devoured as much Clary as will grow upon an acre of ground, their backs are as much the better, as though they had piſſed in their ſhoes; nay, perhaps much worſe.

We will grant that Clary ſtrengthens the back; but this we deny, that the cauſe of the running of the reins in men, or the whites in women, lies in the back (though the back may ſometimes be weakened by them) and therefore the medicine is as proper, as for me when my toe is ſore, to lay a plaiſter on my noſe.

WILD CLARY.

WILD Clary is moſt blaſphemouſly called Chriſt's eye, becauſe it cures diſeaſes of the eyes. I could wiſh from my ſoul, blaſphemy, ignorance and tyranny were ceaſed among phyſicians, that they may be happy, and I joyful.

Deſcript.] It is like the other Clary, but leſſer, with many ſtalks about a foot and an half high. The ſtalks are ſquare and ſomewhat hairy; the flowers of a bluſh colour: He that knows the common Clary cannot be ignorant of this.

Place.] It grows commonly in this nation in barren places; you may find it plentifully if you look in the fields near Gray's-Inn, and the fields near Chelſea.

Time.] They flower from the beginning of June till the latter end of Auguſt.

Government and Virtues.] It is ſomething hotter and drier than the garden Clary is, yet nevertheleſs under the dominion of the Moon, as well as that; the ſeeds of it being beaten to powder, and drank with wine, is an admirable help to provoke luſt. A decoction of the leaves being drank, warms the ſtomach, and it is a wonder if it ſhould not, the ſtomach being under Cancer, the houſe of the Moon. Alſo it helps digeſtion, ſcatters congealed blood in any part of the body. The diſtilled water hereof cleanſeth the eyes of redneſs, wateriſhneſs and heat: It is a gallant remedy for dimneſs of ſight, to take one of the ſeeds of it, and put into the eyes, and there let it remain till it drops out of itſelf, the pain will be nothing to ſpeak on; it will cleanſe the eyes of all filthy and putrefied matter, and in often repeating it, will take off a film which covereth the ſight; a handſomer, ſafer, and eaſier remedy by a great deal, than to tear it off with a needle.

CLEAVERS.

IT is alſo called Aparine, Gooſe-ſhare, Gooſe-graſs, and Cleavers.

Deſcript.] The common Cleavers have divers very rough ſquare ſtalks, not ſo big as the top of a point, but riſing up to be two or three yards high ſometimes, if it meet with any tall buſhes or trees whereon it may climb, yet without any claſpers, or elſe much lower, and lying on the ground full of joints, and at every one of them ſhooteth forth a branch, beſides the leaves thereat which are uſually ſix, ſet in a round compaſs like a ſtar, or a rowel of a ſpur; From between the leaves or the joints towards the tops of the branches, come forth very ſmall white flowers, at every end upon ſmall thready foot-ſtalks, which after they have fallen, there do ſhew two ſmall round and rough ſeeds joined together like two teſticles, which, when they are ripe, grow hard and whitiſh, having a little hole on the ſide, ſomething like unto a navel. Both ſtalks, leaves, and ſeeds are ſo rough, that they will cleave to any thing that ſhall touch them. The root is ſmall and thready.

thready, ſpreading much to the ground, but dieth every year.

Place.] It groweth by the hedge and ditch ſides in many places of this land, and is ſo troubleſome an inhabitant in gardens, that it rampeth upon, and is ready to choak whatever grows near it.

Time.] It flowereth in June or July, and the ſeed is ripe and falleth again in the end of July or Auguſt, from whence it ſpringeth up again, and not from the old roots.

Government and Virtues.] It is under the dominion of the Moon. The juice of the herb and the ſeed together taken in wine, helpeth thoſe bitten with an adder, by preſerving the heart from the venom. It is familiarly taken in broth to keep them lean and lank, that are apt to grow fat. The diſtilled water drank twice a-day helpeth the yellow jaundice, and the decoction of the herb, in experience, is found to do the ſame, and ſtayeth laſks and bloody-fluxes. The juice of the leaves, or they a little bruiſed and applied to any bleeding wounds, ſtayeth the bleeding. The juice alſo is very good to cloſe up the lips of green wounds, and the powder of the dried herb ſtrewed thereupon doth the ſame, and likewiſe helpeth old ulcers. Being boiled in hog's greaſe, it helpeth all ſorts of hard ſwellings or kernels in the throat, being anointed therewith. The juice dropped into the ears taketh away the pain of them.

It is a good remedy in the Spring, eaten (being firſt chopped ſmall, and boiled well) in water-gruel, to cleanſe the blood, and ſtrengthen the liver, thereby to keep the body in health, and fitting it for that change of ſeaſon that is coming.

CLOWNS WOODWORT.

Deſcript.] IT groweth up ſometimes to two or three feet high, but uſually about two feet, with ſquare, green, rough ſtalks, but ſlender, joined ſomewhat far aſunder, and two very long, ſomewhat narrow dark green leaves bluntly dented about the edges thereof ending in a long point. The flowers ſtand towards the tops, compaſſing the ſtalks at the joints with the leaves, and end likewiſe in a ſpiked top, having long and much gaping

H 3 hoods,

hoods of a purplish red colour, with whitish spots in them, standing in somewhat round husks, wherein afterwards stand blackish round seeds. The root is composed of many long strings, with some tuberous long knobs growing among them, of a pale yellowish or whitish colour, yet some times of the year these knobby roots in many places are not seen in this plant: The plant smelleth somewhat strong.

Place.] It groweth in sundry counties of this land, both north and west, and frequently by path-sides in the fields near about London, and within three or four miles distant about it, yet it usually grows in or near ditches.

Time.] It flowereth in June or July, and the seed is ripe soon after.

Government and Virtues.] It is under the dominion of the planet Saturn. It is singularly effectual in all fresh and green wounds; and therefore beareth not this name for nought. And it is very available in stenching of blood, and to dry up the fluxes of humours in old fretting ulcers, cankers, &c. that hinder the healing of them.

A syrup made of the juice of it, is inferior to none for inward wounds, ruptures of veins, bloody flux, vessels broken, spitting, pissing, or vomiting blood: Ruptures are excellently and speedily, even to admiration, cured by taking now and then a little of the syrup, and applying an ointment or plaister of this herb to the place. Also, if any vein or muscle be swelled, apply a plaister of this herb to it, and if you add a little Comfrey to it, it will not do amiss, I assure thee the herb deserves commendations, though it has gotten such a clownish name; and whosoever reads this, (if he try it as I have done) will commend it; only take notice that it is of a dry earthy quality.

COCK's HEAD, Red Fitching, or Medick Fetch.

Descript.] THIS hath divers weak but rough stalks, half a yard long, leaning downwards, but set with winged leaves, longer and more pointed than those of lintels and whitish underneath; from the tops of these stalks arise up other slender stalks, naked without leaves unto the tops, where there grow many small flowers

flowers in manner of a spike, of a pale reddish colour, with some blueness among them; after which rise up in their places, round, rough, and somewhat flat heads. The root is tough, and somewhat woody, yet liveth and shooteth a-new every year.

Place.] It groweth under hedges, and sometimes in the open fields, in divers places of this land.

Time.] They flower all the months of July and August, and the seed ripeneth in the mean while.

Government and Virtues.] It is under the dominion of Venus. It hath power to rarify and digest; and therefore the green leaves bruised and laid as a plaister, disperse knots, nodes, or kernels in the flesh; and if when dry it be taken in wine, it helpeth the strangura; and being anointed with oil, it provoketh sweat. It is a singular food for cattle, to cause them to give store of milk; and why then may it not do the like, being boiled in ordinary drink for nurses?

COLUMBINES.

THESE are so well known, growing almost in every garden, that I think I may save the expence of time in writing a description of them.

Time.] They flower in May, and abide not for the most part when June is past, perfecting their seed in the mean time.

Government and Virtues.] It is also an herb of Venus. The leaves of Columbines are commonly used in lotions with good success for sore mouths and throats. Tragus saith, that a dram of the seed taken in wine with a little saffron, openeth obstructions of the liver, and is good for the yellow jaundice, if the party after the taking thereof be laid to sweat well in bed. The seed also taken in wine causeth a speedy delivery of women in childbirth; if one draught suffice not, let her drink the second, and it is effectual: The Spaniards used to eat a piece of the root thereof in a morning fasting, many days together, to help them when troubled with the stone in the reins or kidneys.

COLTSFOOT.

CALLED also Coughwort, Foals-foot, Horse-hoof, and Bull's-foot.

Descript.

Descript.] This shooteth up a slender stalk, with small yellowish flowers somewhat earlier, which fall away quickly, and after they are past, come up somewhat round leaves, sometimes dented about the edges, much lesser, thicker, and greener than those of butter-bur, with a little down or frieze over the green leaf on the upper side, which may be rubbed away, and whitish or meally underneath. The root is small and white, spreading much under gound, so that where it taketh it will hardly be driven away again, if any little piece be abiding therein; and from thence spring fresh leaves.

Place.] It groweth as well in wet grounds as in drier places.

Time.] And flowereth in the end of February, the leaves begin to appear in March.

Government and Virtues.] The plant is under Venus, the fresh leaves or juice, or a syrup thereof is good for a hot dry cough, or wheesing, and shortness of breath. The dry leaves are best for those that have thin rheums and distillations upon their lungs, causing a cough, for which also the dried leaves taken as tobacco, or the root is very good. The distilled water hereof simply, or with elder flowers and nightshade, is a singular good remedy against all hot agues, to drink two ounces at a time, and apply cloths wet therein to the head and stomach, which also does much good, being applied to any hot swellings and inflammations: It helpeth St Anthony's fire and burnings, and is singular good to take away wheals and small pushes that arise thro' heat; as also the burning heat of the piles, or privy parts, cloths wet therein being thereunto applied.

COMFREY.

Descript.] THE common Great Comfrey hath divers very large hairy green leaves lying on the ground, so hairy or prickly, that if they touch any tender parts of the hands, face, or body, it will cause it to itch; the stalk that riseth from among them, being two or three feet high, hollow and cornered, is very hairy also, having many such like leaves as grow below, but lesser and lesser up to the top: At the joints of the stalks it is divided into many branches, with some leaves thereon, and at the

ends

ends ſtand many flowers in order one above another, which are ſomewhat long and hollow like the finger of a glove, of a pale whitiſh colour, after which come ſmall black ſeeds. The roots are great and long, ſpreading great thick branches under ground, black on the outſide, and whitiſh within, ſhort and eaſy to break, and full of glutinous or clammy juice, of little or no taſte at all.

There is another ſort in all things like this, only ſomewhat leſs, and beareth flowers of a pale purple colour.

Place.] They grow by ditches and water-ſides, and in divers fields that are moiſt, for therein they chiefly delight to grow. The firſt generally through all the land, and the other but in ſome places. By the leave of my authors, I know the firſt grows often in dry places.

Time.] They flower in June or July, and give their ſeed in Auguſt.

Government and Virtues.] This is an herb of Saturn, and I ſuppoſe under the ſign Capricorn, cold, dry, and earthy in quality. What was ſpoken of clowns woundwort may be ſaid of this. The Great Comfrey helpeth thoſe that ſpit blood, or make a bloody urine. The root boiled in water or wine, and the decoction drank, helps all inward hurts, bruiſes, wounds, and ulcers of the lungs, and cauſeth the phlegm that oppreſſeth them to be eaſily ſpit forth: It helpeth the defluction of rheum from the head upon the lungs, the fluxes of blood or humours by the belly, womens immodeerate courſes, as well the reds as the whites, and the running of the reins, happening by what cauſe ſoever. A ſyrup made thereof is very effectual for all thoſe inward griefs and hurts, and the diſtilled water for the ſame purpoſe alſo, and for outward wounds and ſores in the fleſhy or ſinewy part of the body whatſoever, as alſo to take away the fits of agues, and allay the ſharpneſs of humours. A decoction of the leaves hereof is available to all the purpoſes, though not ſo effectual as the roots. The roots being outwardly applied, help freſh wounds or cuts immediately, being bruiſed and laid thereto; and is ſpecial good for ruptures and broken bones; yea, it is ſaid to be ſo powerful to conſolidate and knit together, that if they be boiled with diſſevered pieces of fleſh in a pot, it will join them together again. It is good to

be

be applied to womens breasts that grow sore by the abundance of milk coming into them; also to repress the overmuch bleeding of the hæmorrhoids, to cool the inflammation of the parts thereabouts, and to give ease of the pains. The roots of Comfrey taken fresh, beaten small, and spread upon leather, and laid upon any place troubled with the gout, doth presently give ease of the pains; and applied in the same manner, giveth ease to pained joints, and profiteth very much for running and moist ulcers, gangrenes, mortifications, and the like, for which it hath by often experience been found helpful.

CORALWORT.

IT is also called by some Toothwort, Tooth Violet, Dog Teeth Violet, and Dentaria.

Descript.] Of the many sorts of this herb two of them may be found growing in this nation; the first of which shooteth forth one or two winged leaves, upon long brownish foot-stalks, which are doubled down at their first coming out of the ground; when they are fully opened they consist of seven leaves, most commonly of a sad green colour, dented about the edges, set on both sides the middle rib one against another, as the leaves of the ash tree; the stalk beareth no leaves on the lower half of it; the upper half beareth sometimes three or four, each consisting of five leaves, sometmes of three; on the top stand four or five flowers upon short foot-stalks, with long husks, the flowers are very like the flowers of stock Gilliflowers, of a pale purplish colour, consisting of four leaves a-piece, after which come small cods, which contain the seed; the root is very smooth, white and shining; it doth not grow downwards, but creeping along under the upper crust of the ground, and consisteth of divers small round knobs set together; towards the top of the stalk there grows some single leaves, by each of which cometh a small cloven bulb, which when it is ripe, if it be set in the ground, it will grow to be a root.

As for the other Coralwort which groweth in this nation, 'tis more scarce than this, being a very small plant, much like crowfoot, therefore some think it to be one of the

the ſorts of crowfoot; I know not where to direct you to it, therefore I ſhall forbear the deſcription.

Plac.] The firſt groweth in Mayfield in Suſſex, in a wood called Highread, and in another wood there alſo, called Fox-holes.

Time.] They flower from the latter end of April to the middle of May, and before the middle of July they are gone, and not to be found.

Government and Virtues.] It is under the dominion of the Moon. It cleanſeth the bladder, and provoketh urine, expels gravel, and the ſtone; it eaſeth pains in the ſides and bowels, is excellent good for inward wounds, eſpecially ſuch as are made in the breaſt or lungs, by taking a dram of the powder of the root every morning in wine; the ſame is excellent good for ruptures, as alſo to ſtop fluxes; an ointment of it is excellent good for wounds and ulcers, for it ſoon dries up the watry humours which hinder the cure.

COSTMARY, or Alcoſt, or Balſam Herb.

THIS is ſo frequently known to be an inhabitant in almoſt every garden, that I ſuppoſe it needleſs to write a deſcription thereof.

Time.] It flowereth in June and July.

Government and Virtues.] It is under the dominion of Jupiter. The ordinary Coſtmary, as well as Maudlin, provoketh urine abundantly, and moiſteneth the hardneſs of the mother; it gently purgeth choler and phlegm, extenuating that which is groſs, and cutting that which is tough and glutinous, cleanſeth that which is foul, and hindereth putrefaction and corruption; it diſſolveth without attraction, openeth obſtructions, and helpeth their evil effects, and it is a wonderful help to all ſorts of dry agues. It is aſtringent to the ſtomach, and ſtrengtheneth the liver, and all the other inward parts; and taken in whey worketh more effectually. Taken faſting in the morning, it is very profitable for pains in the head that are continual, and to ſtay, dry up, and conſume all thin rheums or diſtillations from the head into the ſtomach, and helpeth much to digeſt raw humours that are gathered therein. It is very prpfitable for thoſe that are fallen in-

to

to a continual evil disposition of the whole body, called Cachexia, but especially in the beginning of the disease. It is an especial friend and help to evil, weak and cold livers. The seed is familiarly given to children for the worms, and so is the infusion of the flowers in white wine given them to the quantity of two ounces at a time; it maketh an excellent salve to cleanse and heal old ulcers, being boiled with oil of olive, and adders tongue with it, and after it is strained, put a little wax, rosin, and turpentine, to bring it to a convenient body.

CUDWEED, or COTTONWEED.

BESIDES Cudweed and Cottonweed, it is also called Chaffweed, Dwarff Cotton, and Petty Cotton..

Descript.] The common Cudweed riseth up with one stalk sometimes, and sometimes with two or three, thick set on all sides with small, long and narrow whitish or woody leaves, from the middle of the stalk almost up to the top, with every leaf standeth a small flower of a dun or brownish yellow colour, or not so yellow as others; in which herbs, after the flowers are fallen, come small seed wrapped up, with the down therein, and is carried away with the wind; the root is small and thready.

There are other sorts hereof, which are somewhat lesser than the former, not much different, save only that the stalks and leaves are shorter, so the flowers are paler and more open.

Place.] They grow in dry, barren, sandy, and gravelly grounds, in most places of this land.

Time.] They flower about July, some earlier, some latter, and their seed is ripe in August.

Government and Virtues.] Venus is Lady of it. The plants are all astringent, binding, or drying, and therefore profitable for defluctions of rheum from the head, and to stay fluxes of blood wheresoever, the decoction being made into red wine and drank, or the powder taken therein. It also helpeth the bloody-flux, and easeth the torments that come thereby, stayeth the immoderate courses of women, and is also good for inward or outward wounds, hurts and bruises, and helpeth children both of burstings and the worms, and being either drank or injected, for the

the diseafe called Tenefmus, which is an often provocation to the ftool without doing any thing. The green leaves bruifed, and laid to any green wound, ftayeth the bleeding, and healeth it up quickly. The juice of the herb taken in wine and milk is, as Pliny faith, a fovereign remedy againft the mumps and quinfey; and further faith, That whofoever fhall fo take it, fhall never be troubled with that difeafe again.

COWSLIPS, OR PEAGLES.

BOTH the wild and garden Cowflips are fo well known that I will neither trouble myfelf nor the reader with a defcription of them.

Time.] They flower in April and May.

Government and Virtues.] Venus lays claim to this herb as her own, and it is under the fign Aries, and our city dames know well enough the ointment or diftilled water of it adds beauty, or at leaft reftores it when it is loft. The flowers are held to be more effectual than the leaves, and the roots of little ufe. An ointment being made of them, taketh away fpots and wrinkles of the fkin, fun-burning and freckles, and adds beauty exceedingly; they remedy all infirmities of the head coming of heat and wind, as vertigo, ethialtes, falfe apparitions, phrenzies, falling fickness, palfies, convulfions, cramps, pains in the nerves; the roots eafe pains in the back and bladder, and open the paffages of urine. The leaves are good in wounds, and the flowers take away trembling. If the flowers be not well dried, and kept in a warm place, they will foon putrefy and look green: Have a fpecial eye over them. If you let them fee the fun once a month, it will do neither the fun nor them harm.

Becaufe they ftrengthen the brain and nerves, and remedy palfies, the Greeks gave them the name Paralifis: The flowers preferved or conferved and the quantity of a nutmeg eaten every morning, is a fufficient dofe for inward difeafes; but for wounds, fpots, wrinkles, and fun-burnings, an ointment is made of the leaves, and hog's greafe.

CRABS CLAWS.

CALLED alfo Water Sengreen, Knights Pond Water, Water Houfeleek, Pond Weed, and Frefh-water Soldier.

Descript.] It hath sundry long narrow leaves, with sharp prickles on the edges of them also, very sharp-pointed; the stalks which bear flowers seldom grow so high as the leaves, bearing a forked head like a Crab's Claws, out of which comes a white flower, consisting of three leaves with divers yellowish hairy threeds in the middle; it taketh root in the mud in the bottom of the water.

Place.] It groweth plentifully in the fens in Lincolnshire.

Time.] It flowers in June, and usually from thence till August.

Government and Virtues.] 'Tis a plant under the dominion of Venus, and therefore a great strengthener of the reins; it is excellent good in that inflammation which is commonly called St. Anthony's fire; It assuageth all inflammations, and swellings in wounds and an ointment made of it, is excellent good to heal them; there is scarce a better remedy growing than this is, for such as have bruised their kidneys, and upon that account pissing blood; a dram of the powder of the herb taken every morning, is a very good remedy to stop the terms.

Black Cresses.

Descript.] IT hath long leaves deeply cut and jagged on both sides, not much unlike wild mustard; the stalks small, very limber, though very tough; you may twist them round as you may a willow, before they break. The stones be very small and yellow, after which come small cods, which contain the seed.

Place.] It is a common herb, grows usually by the way-sides, and sometimes upon mud walls about London, but it delights most to grow among stones and rubbish.

Time.] It flowers in June and July, and the seed is ripe in August and September.

Government and Virtues.] It is a plant of a hot and biting nature under the dominion of Mars. The seed of Black Cresses strengthens the brain exceedingly, being in performing that office, little inferior to mustard seed, if at all; they are excellent good to stay those rheums which may fall down from the head upon the lungs; you may beat the seed into powder, if you please, and make it up into an electuary with honey; so you have an excellent remedy by you, not only for the premises, but also for the cough, yellow jaundice, and sciatica. The herb boiled into a poultice, is an excellent remedy for inflammations both in womens breasts and mens testicles.

SCIATICA CRESSES.

Descript.] THESE are of two kinds: The first riseth up with a round stalk, about two feet high, spread into divers branches, whose lower leaves are somewhat larger than the upper, yet all of them cut or torn on the edges, somewhat like garden cresses, but smaller; the flowers are small and white, growing at the tops of branches, where afterwards grow husks, with small brownish seed therein, very strong and sharp in taste, more than the cresses of the garden; the root is long, white, and woody.

The other hath the lower leaves whole, somewhat long and broad, not torn at all, but only somewhat deeply dented about the edges towards the ends; but those that grow up higher are lesser. The flowers and seeds are like the former, and so is the root likewise, and both root and seeds as sharp as it.

Place.] They grow by the way-sides in untilled places, and by the sides of old walls.

Time.] They flower in the end of June, and their seed is ripe in July.

Government and Virtues.] It is a Saturnine plant. The leaves, but especially the root, taken fresh in Summer-time, beaten or made into a poultice or salve with old hog's grease, and applied to the places pained with the sciatica, to continue thereon four hours, if it be on a man, and two hours on a woman; the place afterwards bathed with wine and oil mixed together, and then wrapped with wool or skins after they have sweat a little, will assuredly not only cure the same disease in hips, huckle-bone or other of the joints, as gout in the hands or feet, but all other old griefs of the head, (as inveterate rheums) and other parts of the body that are hard to be cured. And if of the former griefs any parts remain, the same medicine after twenty days is to be applied again. The same is alſo effectual in the diſeaſes of the ſpleen; and applied to the ſkin, it taketh away the blemiſhes thereof, whether they be ſcars, leproſy, ſcabs, or ſcurf, which although it ulcerate the part, yet that is to be helped afterwards with a ſalve made of oil and wax. Eſteem this as another ſecret.

WATER CRESSES.

Deſcript.] OUR ordinary Water Creſſes ſpread forth with many weak, hollow, ſappy ſtalks, ſhooting out fibres at the joints, and upwards long winged leaves, made of ſundry broad ſappy almoſt round leaves, of a browniſh colour. The flowers are many and white, ſtanding on long foot-ſtalks, after which come ſmall yellow ſeed contained in ſmall long pods like horns. The whole plant abideth green in the winter, and taſteth ſomewhat hot and ſharp.

Place.] They grow (for the moſt part) in ſmall ſtanding waters, yet ſometimes in ſmall rivulets of running water.

Tim.] They flower and ſeed in the beginning of Summer.

Government and Virtues.] It is an herb under the dominion of the Moon. They are more powerful againſt the ſcurvey, and to cleanſe the blood and humours, than Brooklime is, and ſerve in all the other uſes in which Brooklime is available, as to break the ſtone, and provoke urine and womens courſes. The decoction thereof cleanſeth ulcers, by waſhing them therewith. The leaves bruiſed, or the juice is good, to be applied to the face or other parts troubled with freckles, pimples, ſpots, or the like, at night, and waſhed away in the morning. The juice mixed with vinegar, and the forepart of the head bathed therewith, is very good for thoſe that are dull and drouſy, or have the lethargy.

Watercreſs pottage is a good remedy to cleanſe the blood in the ſpring, and help head-achs, and conſume the groſs humours winter hath left behind; thoſe that would live in health, may uſe it if they pleaſe, if they will not, I cannot help it. If any fancy not pottage, they may eat the herb as a ſallet.

CROSSWORT.

CROSSWORT.

Descript.] COMMON Crosswort groweth up with square hairy brown stalks a little above a foot high, having four small broad and pointed, hairy, yet smooth green leaves, growing at every joint, each against other cross-way, which has caused the name. Towards the tops of the stalks at the joints, with the leaves in three or four rows downwards, stand small, pale, yellow flowers, after which come small blackish round seeds, four for the most part, set in every husk. The root is very small and full of fibres, or threads, taking good hold of the ground, and spreading with the branches a great deal of ground, which perish not in winter, although the leaves die every year, and spring again anew.

Place.] It groweth in many moist grounds, as well meadows as untilled places about London, in Hampstead church-yard, at Wye in Kent, and sundry other places.

Time.] It flowers from May all the Summer long, in one place or other, as they are more open to the sun; the seed ripeneth soon after.

Government and Virtues.] It is under the dominion of Saturn. This is a singular good wound herb, and is used inwardly, not only to stay bleeding of wounds, but to consolidate them, as it doth outwardly any green wound, which it quickly soldereth up, and healeth. The decoction of the herb in wine helpeth to expectorate phlegm out of the chest, and is good for obstructions in the breast, stomach or bowels, and helpeth a decayed appetite. It is also good to wash any wound or sore with, to cleanse and heal it. The herb bruised, and then boiled, applied outwardly for certain days together, renewing it often; and in the mean time the decoction of the herb in wine, taken inwardly every day, doth certainly cure the rupture in any, so as it be not too inveterate; but very speedily, if it be fresh and lately taken.

CROWFOOT.

MANY are the names this furious biting herb hath obtained, almost enough to make up a Welshman's pedigree, if he fetch no farther than John of Gaunt, or

William the Conqueror; for it is called Frogsfoot from the Greek name Barrakion: Crowfoot, Gold Knobs, Gold Cups, King's Knob, Baffiners, Troilflowers, Polts, Locket Goulions, and Butterflowers.

So abundant are the ſorts of this herb, that to deſcribe them all would try the patience of Socrates himſelf; but becauſe I have not yet attained to the ſpirits of Socrates, I ſhall but deſcribe the moſt uſual.

Deſcript.] The moſt common Crowfoot hath many dark green leaves, cut into divers parts, in taſte biting and ſharp, biting and bliſtering the tongue: it bears many flowers, and thoſe of a bright, reſplendent, yellow colour. I do not remember that I ever ſaw any thing yellower. Virgins in ancient time uſed to make powder of them to furrow bride beds; after which flowers come ſmall heads, ſome ſpiked and rugged like a Pine-Apple.

Place.] They grow very common every where; unleſs you turn your head into a hedge, you cannot but ſee them as you walk.

Time.] They flower in May and June, even till September.

Government and Virtues] This fiery and hot ſpirited herb of Mars is no way fit to be given inwardly, but an ointment of the leaves or flowers will draw a bliſter, and may be ſo fitly applied to the nape of the neck to draw back rheum from the eyes. The herb being bruiſed and mixed with a little muſtard, draws a bliſter as well, and as perfectly as Cantharides, and with far leſs danger to the veſſels of urine, which Cantharides naturally delights to wrong: I knew the herb once applied to a peſtilential riſing that was fallen down, and it ſaved life even beyond hope; it were good to keep an ointment and plaiſter of it, if it were but for that.

CUCKOW-POINT.

IT is called Alron, Janus, Barba-aron, Calves-foot, Ramp, Starchwort, Cuckow-pintle, Prieſts-pintle, and Wake Robin.

Deſcrip.] This ſhooteth forth three, four, or five leaves at the moſt, from one root, every one whereof is ſomewhat large and long, broad at the bottom next the ſtalk, and forked, but ending in a point, without a cut on the edge,

edge, of a full green colour, each ſtanding upon a thick round ſtalk, of a hand-breadth long, or more, among which, after two or three months that they begin to wither, riſeth up a bare, round, whitiſh green ſtalk, ſpotted and ſtreaked with purple, ſomewhat higher than the leaves: At the top whereof ſtandeth a long hollow huſk, cloſe at the bottom, but open from the middle upwards, ending in a point; in the middle whereof ſtand the ſmall long peſtle or clapper, ſmaller at the bottom than at the top, of a dark purple colour, as the huſk is on the inſide, though green without; which, after it hath ſo abided for ſome time, the huſk with the clapper decayeth, and the foot or bottom thereof groweth to be a ſmall long bunch of berries, green at the firſt, and of a yellowiſh red colour when they are ripe, of the bigneſs of a hazel nut kernel, which abideth thereon almoſt until Winter; the root is round, and ſomewhat long, for the moſt part lying along, the leaves ſhooting forth at the largeſt end, which, when it beareth his berries, are ſomewhat wrinkled and looſe, another growing under it, which is ſolid and firm, with many ſmall threads hanging thereat. The whole plant is of a very ſharp biting taſte, pricking the tongue as nettles do the hands, and ſo abideth for a great while without alteration. The root thereof was anciently uſed inſtead of ſtarch to ſtarch linen with.

There is another ſort of Cuckow-point, with leſſer leaves than the former, and ſometimes harder, having blackiſh ſpots upon them, which for the moſt part abide longer green in Summer than the former, and both leaves and roots are more ſharp and fierce than it: In all things elſe it is like the former.

Place.] Theſe two ſorts grow frequently almoſt under every hedge-ſide in many places of this land.

Time.] They ſhoot forth leaves in the Spring, and continue but until the middle of Summer, or ſomewhat later; their huſks appearing before they fall away, and their fruit ſhewing in April.

Government and Virtues.] It is under the dominion of Mars. Tragus reporteth, that a dram weight, or more, if need be, of the ſpotted Wake Robin, either freſh and green, or dried, being eaten and taken, is a preſent and

ſure

ſure remedy for poiſon and the plague. The juice of the herb taken to the quantity of a ſpoonful hath the ſame effect. But if there be a little vinegar added thereto, as well as to the root aforeſaid, it ſomewhat allayeth the ſharp biting taſte thereof upon the tongue. The green leaves bruiſed, and laid upon any boil or plague ſore, doth wonderfully help to draw forth the poiſon: A dram of the powder of the dried root taken with twice ſo much ſugar in the form of a licking electuary, or the green root, doth wonderfully help thoſe that are purſy and ſhort-winded, as alſo thoſe that have a cough; it breaketh, digeſteth, and riddeth away phlegm from the ſtomach, cheſt and lungs. The milk wherein the root hath been boiled is effectual alſo for the ſame purpoſe. The ſaid powder taken in wine or other drink, or the juice of the berries, or the powder of them, or the wine wherein they have been boiled, provoketh urine, and bringeth down womens courſes, and purgeth them effectually after child-bearing, to bring away the after-birth. Taken with ſheeps milk, it healeth the inward ulcers of the bowels. The diſtilled water thereof is effectual to all the purpoſes aforeſaid. A ſpoonful taken at a time healeth the itch; and an ounce or more taken at a time for ſome days together, doth help the rupture: The leaves, either green or dry, or the juice of them, doth cleanſe all manner of rotten and filthy ulcers, in what part of the body ſoever; and healeth the ſtinking ſores in the noſe, called Polypus. The water wherein the root hath been boiled, dropped into the eyes, cleanſeth them from any film or ſkin, cloud or miſts, which begin to hinder the ſight, and helpeth the watering and redneſs of them, or when, by ſome chance, they become black and blue. The root mixed with bean-flour, and applied to the throat or jaws that are inflamed, helpeth them. The juice of the berries boiled in oil of roſes, or beaten into powder mixed with the oil, and dropped into the ears, eaſeth pains in them. The berries, or the roots beaten with hot ox-dung, and applied, eaſeth the pains of the gout. The leaves and roots boiled in wine with a little oil, and applied to the piles, or the falling down of the fundament, eaſeth them, and ſo doth ſitting over the hot fumes thereof. The freſh roots bruiſed and

diſtilled

diſtilled with a little milk, yieldeth a moſt ſovereign water to cleanſe the ſkin from ſcurf, freckles, ſpots, or blemiſhes whatſoever therein.

Authors have left large commendations of this herb you ſee, but for my part, I have neither ſpoken with Dr Reaſon nor Dr Experience about it.

CUCUMBERS.

Government and Virtues.] THERE is no diſpute to be made, but that they are under the dominion of the Moon, though they are ſo much cried out againſt for their coldneſs, and if they were but one degree colder they would be poiſon. The beſt of Galeniſts hold them to be cold and moiſt in the ſecond degree, and then not ſo hot as either lettuces or purſlain: They are excellent good for a hot ſtomach, and hot liver; the unmeaſurable uſe of them fills the body full of raw humours, and ſo indeed the unmeaſurable uſe of any thing elſe doth harm. The face being waſhed with their juice, cleanſeth the ſkin, and is excellent good for hot rheums in the eyes; the ſeed is excellent good to provoke urine, and cleanſeth the paſſages thereof when they are ſtopped; there is not a better remedy for ulcers in the bladder growing, than Cucumbers are. The uſual courſe is, to uſe the ſeeds in emulſions, as they make almond milk; but a far better way (in my opinion) is this: When the ſeaſon of the year is, Take the Cucumbers and bruiſe them well, and diſtil the water from them, and let ſuch as are troubled with ulcers in the bladder drink no other drink. The face being waſhed with the ſame water, cureth the reddiſt face that is; it is alſo excellent good for ſun-burning, freckles, and morphew.

DAISIES.

THESE are ſo well known almoſt to every child, that I ſuppoſe it needleſs to write any deſcription of them. Take therefore the virtues of them as follow.

Government and Virtues.] The herb is under the ſign Cancer, and under the dominion of Venus, and therefore excellent good for wounds in the breaſt, and very fitting to be kept both in oils, ointments, and plaiſters, as alſo

in

in syrup. The greater wild Daisey is a wound herb of good respect, often used in those drinks or salves that are for wounds, either inward or outward. The juice or distilled water of these, or the small Daisey, doth much temper the heat of choler, and refresh the liver, and the other inward parts. A decoction made of them, and drank, helpeth to cure the wounds made in the hollowness of the breast. The same also cureth all ulcers and pustules in the mouth or tongue, or in the secret parts. The leaves bruised and applied to the cods, or to any other parts that are swoln and hot, doth dissolve it, and temper the heat. A decoction made thereof, of walwort and agrimony, and the places fomented or bathed therewith warm, giveth great ease to them that are troubled with the palsy, sciatica, or the gout. The same also disperseth and dissolveth the knots or kernels that grow in the flesh of any part of the body, and bruises and hurts that come of falls and blows; they are also used for ruptures, and other inward burnings, with very good success. An ointment made thereof doth wonderfully help all wounds that have inflammations about them, or by reason of moist humours having access unto them, are kept long from healing, and such are those, for the most part, that happen to joints of the arms or legs. The juice of them dropped into the running eyes of any, doth much help them.

DANDELION, vulgarly called PISS-A-BEDS.

Descript.] IT is well known to have many long and deep gashed leaves, lying on the ground round about the head of the roots; the ends of each gash or jag, on both sides looking downwards towards the roots; the middle rib being white, which being broken, yieldeth abundance of bitter milk, but the root much more; from among the leaves, which always abide green, arise many slender, weak, naked foot-stalks, every one of them bearing at the top one large yellow flower, consisting of many rows of yellow leaves, broad at the points, and nicked in with deep spots of yellow in the middle, which growing ripe, the green husk wherein the flowers stood turns itself down to the stalk, and the head of down becomes as round as a ball; with long reddish seed underneath, bearing

ing a part of the down on the head of every one, which together is blown away with the wind, or may be at once blown away with one's mouth. The root growing downwards, exceeding deep, which being broken off within the ground, will yet ſhoot forth again, and will hardly be deſtroyed where it hath once taken deep root in the ground.

Place.] It groweth frequently in all meadows and paſture-grounds.

Time.] It flowereth in one place or other almoſt all the year long.

Government and Virtue.] It is under the dominion of Jupiter. It is of an opening and cleanſing quality, and therefore very effectual for the obſtructions of the liver, gall and ſpleen, and the diſeaſes that ariſe from them, as the jaundice and hypochondriac; it openeth the paſſages of the urine both in young and old; powerfully cleanſeth impoſthumes and inward ulcers in the urinary paſſage, and by its drying and temperate quality doth afterwards heal them; for which purpoſe the decoction of the roots or leaves in white wine, or the leaves chopped as potherbs, with a few aliſanders, and boiled in their broth, are very effectual. And whoever is drawing towards a conſumption or an evil diſpoſition of the whole body, called Cachexia, by the uſe hereof for ſome time together, ſhall find a wonderful help: It helpeth alſo to procure reſt and ſleep to bodies diſtempered by the heat of ague fits, or otherwiſe: The diſtilled water is effectual to drink in peſtilential fevers, and to waſh the ſores.

You ſee here what virtues this common herb hath, and that is the reaſon the French and Dutch ſo often eat them in the ſpring: and now, if you look a little farther, you may ſee plainly, without a pair of ſpectacles, that foreign phyſicians are not ſo ſelfiſh as ours are, but more communicative of the virtues of plants to people.

DARNEL.

IT is called Jum and Wray; in Suſſex they call it Crop; it being a peſtilent enemy among corn.

Deſcript.] This hath all the winter long, ſundry long, flat, and rough leaves, which, when the ſtalk riſeth, which is ſlender and jointed, are narrower, but rough ſtill; on the

the top groweth a long spike, composed of many heads set one above another, containing two or three husks, with sharp but short beards of awns at the end; the seed is easily shaked out of the ear, the husk itself being somewhat rough.

Place.] The country husbandmen do know this too well to grow among their corn, or in the borders and path-ways of the other fields that are fallow.

Government and Virtues.] It is a malicious part of sullen Saturn. As it is not without some vices, so hath it also many virtues. The meal of Darnel is very good to stay gangrenes, and other such like fretting and eating cankers, and putrid sores: It also cleanseth the skin of all leprosies, morphews, ringworms, and the like, if it be used with salt and reddish roots. And being used with quick brimstone and vinegar, it dissolveth knots and kernels, and breaketh those that are hard to be dissolved, being boiled in wine with pigeons-dung and linseed: A decoction thereof made with water and honey, and the places bathed therewith, is profitable for the sciatica. Darnel meal applied in a poultice draweth forth splinters and broken bones in the flesh: The red Darnel, boiled in red wine and taken, stayeth the lask and all other fluxes, and women's bloody issues; and restraineth urine that passeth away too suddenly.

DILL.

Descript.] THE common Dill groweth up with seldom more than one stalk, neither so high, nor so great usually as Fennel, being round and fewer joints thereon, whose leaves are sadder, and somewhat long, and so like Fennel that it deceiveth many, but harder in handling, and somewhat thicker, and of a stronger unpleasant scent: The tops of the stalks have four branches, and smaller umbels of yellow flowers, which turn into small seed, somewhat flatter and thinner than Fennel seed. The root is somewhat small and woody, perisheth every year after it hath borne seed; and is also unprofitable, being never put to any use.

Place.] It is most usually sown in gardens and grounds for the purpose, and is also found wild in many places.

Govern.

Government and Virtues.] Mercury hath the dominion of this plant, and therefore to be sure it strengthens the brain. The Dill being boiled and drank, is good to ease swellings and pains; it also stayeth the belly and stomach from casting. The decoction thereof helpeth women that are troubled with the pains and windiness of the mother, if they sit therein. It stayeth the hiccough, being boiled in wine, and but smelled unto, being tied in a cloth. The seed is of more use than the leaves, and more effectual to digest raw and viscous humours, and is used in medicines that serve to expel wind and the pains proceeding therefrom. The seed, being roasted or fried, and used in oils or plaisters, dissolve the imposthumes, in the fundament; and drieth up all moist ulcers, especially in the fundament; an oil made of Dill is effectual to warm, or dissolve humours and impostumes, to ease pains and procure rest. The decoction of Dill, be it herb or seed (only if you boil the seed you must bruise it) in white wine, being drank, it is a gallant expeller of wind, and provoker of the terms.

DEVIL'S-BIT.

Descript.] THIS rises up with a round, green, smooth stalk, about two feet high, set with divers long and somewhat narrow, smooth, dark green leaves, somewhat nip'd about the edges, for the most part, being else all whole, and not divided at all, or but very seldom, even to the tops of the branches, which yet are smaller than those below, with one rib only in the middle. At the end of each branch standeth a round head of many flowers set together in the same manner, or more neatly than Scabions, and of a more bluish purple colour, which being past, there followeth seed that falleth away. The root is somewhat thick, but short and blackish, with many strings, abiding after seed time many years. This root was longer, until the devil (as the friars say) bit away the rest of it from spite, envying its usefulness to mankind; for sure he was not troubled with any disease for which it is proper.

There are two other sorts hereof, in nothing unlike

the former, save that the one beareth white, and the other blush-coloured flowers.

Place.] The first groweth as well in dry meadows and fields as moist, in many places of this land: But the other two are more rare, and hard to be met with, yet they are both found growing wild about Appledore, near Rye in Kent.

Time.] They flower not usually until August.

Government and Virtues.] The plant is venereal, pleasing and harmless. The herb or the root (all that the devil hath left of it) being boiled in wine, and drank, is very powerful against the plague, and all pestilential diseases or fevers, poisons also, and the bitings of venomous beasts: It helpeth also those that are inwardly bruised by any casuality or outwardly by falls or blows, dissolving the clotted blood; and the herb or root beaten and outwardly applied, taketh away the black and blue marks that remain in the skin. The decoction of the herb, with honey of roses put therein, is very effectual to help the inveterate tumours and swellings of the almonds and throat, by often gargling the mouth therewith. It helpeth also to procure women's courses, and easeth all pains of the mother, and to break and discuss wind therein, and in the bowels. The powder of the root taken in drink, driveth forth worms in the body. The juice or distilled water of the herb, is effectual for green wounds, or old sores, and cleanseth the body inwardly, and the seed outwardly from sores, scurf, itch, pimples, freckles, morphew, or other deformities thereof, especially if a little vitriol be dissolved therein.

DOCK.

MANY kinds of these are so well known, that I shall not trouble you with a description of them: My book grows big too fast.

Government and Virtues.] All docks are under Jupiter, of which the Red Dock, which is commonly called Bloodwort, cleanseth the blood, and strengthens the liver; but the yellow Dock-root is best to be taken when either the blood or liver is affected by choler. All of them have a kind of cooling (but not all alike) drying quality, the sorrel

rel being moſt cold, and the blood-worts moſt drying. Of the Burdock I have ſpoke already by itſelf. The ſeed of moſt of the other kinds, whether the gardens or fields, do ſtay laſks and fluxes of all ſorts, the loathing of the ſtomach through choler, and is helpful for thoſe that ſpit blood. The roots boiled in vinegar help the itch, ſcabs, and breaking out of the ſkin, if it be bathed therewith. The diſtilled water of the herb and roots have the ſame virtue, and cleanſeth the ſkin from freckles, morphews, and all other ſpots, and diſcolourings therein.

All Docks being boiled with meat, make it boil the ſooner: Beſides, Blood-wort is exceeding ſtrengthening to the liver, and procures good blood, being as wholeſome a pot-herb as any grows in a garden; yet ſuch is the nicety of our times (forſooth) that women will not put it into a pot, becauſe it makes the pottage black; pride and ignorance (a couple of monſters in the creation) prefering nicety before health.

DODDER of THYME, EPITHYMUM, and other DODDERS.

Deſcript.] THIS firſt from ſeed giveth roots in the ground, which ſhooteth forth threads or ſtrings, groſſer or finer, as the property of the plant wherein it groweth, and the climate doth ſuffer, creeping and ſpreading on that plant whereon it faſteneth, be it high or low. The ſtrings have no leaves at all upon them, but wind and interlace themſelves ſo thick upon a ſmall plant, that it taketh away all comfort of the ſun from it; and is ready to choak or ſtrangle it. After theſe ſtrings are riſen up to that height, that they may draw nouriſhment from that plant, they ſeem to be broken off from the ground, either by the ſtrength of their riſing, or withered by the heat of the ſun. Upon theſe ſtrings are found cluſters of ſmall heads or huſks, out of which ſhoot forth whitiſh flowers, which afterwards give ſmall pale coloured ſeed, ſomewhat flat, and twice as big as a Poppy-ſeed. It generally participates of the nature of the plant which it climbeth upon; but the Dodder of Thyme is accounted the beſt, and is the only true Epithymum.

Government and Virtues.] All Dodders are under Saturn,

turn. Tell not me of physicians crying up Epithymum, or that Dodder which grows upon Thyme, (most of which comes from Hemetius in Greece, or Hybla in Sicily, because those mountains abound with Thyme) he is a physician indeed, that hath wit enough to choose his Dodder, according to the nature of the disease and humour peccant. We confess, Thyme is the hottest herb it usually grows upon; and therefore that which grows upon Thyme, is hotter than that which grows upon colder herbs; for it draws nourishment from what it grows upon, as well as from the earth where its root is, and thus you see old Saturn is wise enough to have two strings to his bow. This is accounted the most effectual for melancholy diseases, and to purge black or burnt choler, which is the cause of many diseases of the head and brain, as also for the trembling of the heart, faintings and swoonings. It is helpful in all diseases and griefs of the spleen, and melancholy that arises from the windiness of the hypochondria. It purgeth also the reins or kidneys by urine; it openeth obstructions of the gall, whereby it profiteth them that have the jaundice; as also the leaves the spleen: Purging the veins of the cholerick and phlegmatick humours, and helpeth children in agues, a little worm seed being put thereto.

The other Dodders do (as I said before) participate of the nature of those plants whereon they grow: As that which hath been found growing upon nettles in the west-country, hath by experience been found very effectual to procure plenty of urine, where it hath been stopped or hindered. And so of the rest.

Sympathy and antipathy are two hinges upon which the whole model of physick turns; and that physician which minds them not, is like a door off from the hooks, more like to do a man mischief, than to secure him. Then all the diseases Saturn causeth, this helps by sympathy, and strengthens all the parts of the body he rules; such as be caused by Sol, it helps by antipathy. What those diseases are, see my judgment of diseases by astrology; and if you be pleased to look the herb wormwood, you shall find a rational way for it.

Dog's

Dog's-Grass, or Couch-Grass.

Descrip.] IT is well known, that the Grass creepeth far about under ground, with long white jointed roots, and small fibres almost at every joint, very sweet in taste, as the rest of the herb is, and interlacing one another, from whence shoot forth many fair grassy leaves, small at the ends, and cutting or sharp on the edges. The stalks are jointed like corn, with the like leaves on them, and a large spiked head, with a long husk in them, and hard rough seed in them. If you know it not by this description, watch the dogs when they are sick, and they will quickly lead you to it.

Place.] It groweth commonly through this land in divers ploughed grounds, to the no small trouble of the husbandman, as also of the gardeners, in gardens, to weed it out, if they can; for it is a constant customer to the place it gets footing in.

Government and Virtues.] 'Tis under the dominion of Jupiter, and is most medicinable of all the Quick-grasses. Being boiled and drank, it openeth obstructions of the liver and gall, and the stopping of urine, and easeth the gripping pains of the belly, and inflammations; wasteth the matter of the stone in the bladder, and the ulcers thereof also. The roots bruised and applied do consolidate wounds. The seed doth more powerfully expel urine, and stayeth the lask and vomiting. The distilled water alone, or with a little worm-seed, killeth the worms in children.

The way of use is to bruise the roots, and having well boiled them in white wine, drink the decoction; 'tis opening not purging, very safe: 'Tis a remedy against all diseases coming of stopping, and such are half those that are incident to the body of man; and altho' a gardener be of another opinion, yet a physician holds half an acre of them to be worth five acres of Carrots twice told over.

Doves-Foot, or Cranes-Bill.

Descript.] THIS hath divers small, round, pale-green leaves, cut in about the edges, much like mallows, standing upon long, reddish, hairy stalks, lying in a round compass upon the ground; among which rise up two, or three, or more reddish jointed, slender, weak, hairy stalks, with such like leaves thereon, but smaller, and more cut in up to the tops, where grow many very small bright red flowers of five leaves a piece; after which follow small heads, with small short beaks pointed forth, as all other sorts of those herbs do.

Place.] It groweth in pasture grounds, and by the path-sides in many places, and will also be in gardens.

Time.] It flowereth in June, July, and August, some earlier and some later; and the seed is ripe quickly after.

Government and Virtues.] It is a very gentle, though martial plant. It is found by experience to be singular good for the wind cholic, as also to expel the stone and gravel in the kidneys. The decoction thereof in wine, is an excellent good cure for those that have inward wounds, hurts, or bruises, both to stay the bleeding, to dissolve and expel the congealed blood, and to heal the parts, as also to cleanse and heal outward sores, ulcers, and fistulas, and for green wounds, many do only bruise the herb, and apply it to the place, and it healeth them quickly. The same decoction in wine fomented to any place pained with the gout, or to joint-achs, or pain of the sinews, giveth much ease. The powder or decoction of the herb taken for some time together, is found by experience to be singular good for ruptures and burstings in people, either young or old.

Ducks Meat.

THIS is so well known to swim on the top of standing waters, as ponds, pools, and ditches, that it is needless further to describe it.

Government and Virtues.] Cancer claims the herb, and the Moon will be Lady of it; a word is enough to a wise man. It is effectual to help inflammations, and St Anthony's fire, as also the gout, either applied by itself, or in a poultice with barley meal. The distilled water by some is highly esteemed against all inward inflammations and pestilent fever; as also to help the redness of the eyes, and swellings of the cods, and of the beasts before they be grown too much. The fresh herb applied to the forehead, easeth the pains of the head-ach coming of heat.

DOWN, or COTTON-THISTLE.

Descript.] THIS hath large leaves lying on the ground, somewhat cut in, and as it were crumpled on the edges, of a green colour on the upper side, but covered with long hairy wool, or Cotton Down, set with most sharp and cruel pricks, from the middle of whose heads of flowers, thrust forth many purplish crimson threads, and sometimes (altho' very seldom) white ones. The seed that followeth in the heads, lying in a great deal of white down, is somewhat large, long, and round, like the seed of Ladies Thistle, but somewhat paler. The root is great and thick, spreading much, yet it usually dieth after seed-time.

Place.] It groweth in divers ditches, banks, and in corn fields and high-ways, generally every where throughout the land.

Time.] It flowereth and beareth seed about the end of Summer, when other thistles do flower and seed.

Government and Virtues.] Mars owns the plant, and manifests to the world, that though it may hurt your finger, it will help your body; for I fancy it much for the ensuing virtues. Pliny and Dioscorides write, That the leaves and roots thereof taken in drink, help those that have a crick in their neck; whereby they cannot turn their neck, but their whole body must turn also (sure they do not mean those that have got a crick in their neck by being under the hangman's hand.) Galen saith, that the root and leaves hereof are of a heating quality, and good for such persons as have their bodies drawn together by some spasm or convulsions, as it is with children that have the rickets, or rather (as the college of physicians will have it) the Rachites, for which name of the disease they have (in a particular treatise lately set forth by them) learnedly disputed and put forth to public view, that the world may see they have took much pains to little purpose.

DRAGONS.

THEY are so well known to every one that plants them in their gardens, they need no description;

if not, let them look down to the lower end of the ſtalks, and ſee how like a ſnake they look.

Government and Virtue.] The plant is under the dominion of Mars, and therefore it would be a wonder if it ſhould want ſome obnoxious quality or other; in all herbs of that quality, the ſafeſt way is either to diſtil the herb in an alembick, in what vehicle you pleaſe, or elſe to preſs out the juice, and diſtil that in a glaſs ſtill in ſand. It ſcoureth and cleanſeth the internal parts of the body mightily, and it cleareth the external parts alſo, being externally applied, from freckles, morphew, and ſun-burning: Your beſt way to uſe it externally, is to mix it with vinegar; an ointment of it is held to be good in wounds and ulcers; it conſumes cankers, and that fleſh growing in the noſtrils, which they call Polipus: Alſo the diſtilled water being dropped into the eyes, taketh away ſpots there, or the pin and web, and mends the dimneſs of ſight; it is excellent good againſt peſtilence and poiſon. Pliny and Dioſcorides affirm, that no ſerpent will meddle with him that carries this herb about him.

The ELDER-TREE.

I Hold it needleſs to write any deſcription of this, ſince every boy that plays with a pot-gun will not miſtake another tree inſtead of Elder. I ſhall therefore in this place only deſcribe the Dwarf-Elder, called alſo Deadwort, and Wall-wort.

The DWARF-ELDER.

Deſcript.] THIS is but an herb every year, dying with his ſtalks to the ground, and riſing freſh every Spring, and is like unto the Elder both in form and quality, riſing up with a ſquare rough hairy ſtalk, four feet high, or more ſometimes. The winged leaves are ſomewhat narrower than the Elder, but elſe like them. The flowers are white with a daſh of purple ſtanding in umbels, very like the elder alſo, but more ſweet in ſcent; after which come ſmall blackiſh berries full of juice while they are freſh, wherein is ſmall hard kernels, or ſeed. The root doth creep under the upper cruſt of the ground,

ſpringing

divers places, being of the bigness of one's
ımb sometimes.
he Elder-tree groweth in hedges, being plant-
:rengthen the fences and partitions of ground,
the banks by ditches and water-courses.
rf Elder grows wild in many places of Eng-
being once gotten into a ground, it is not
forth again.
oft of the Elder Trees flower in June, and
ripe for the most part in August. But the
, or Wallwort, flowereth somewhat later, and
ıot ripe until September.
nt and Virtues.] Both Elder and Dwarf Tree
: dominion of Venus. The first shoots of the
er boiled like Asparagus, and the young leaves
iled in fat broth, doth mightily carry forth
choler. The middle or inward bark boiled in
iven in drink, worketh much more violently;
es, either green or dry, expel the same humour,
n given with good success to help the dropsy;
:he root boiled in wine, or the juice thereof
:th the same effects but more powerfully than
aves or fruit. The juice of the root taken,
y procure vomitings, and purgeth the watry
:he dropsy. The decoction of the root taken,
iting of an adder, and biting of mad dogs. It
e hardness of the mother, if women sit there-
neth their veins, and bringeth down their
e berries boiled in wine, performeth the same
the hair of the head washed therewith, is
The juice of the green leaves applied to the
ations of the eyes assuageth them; the juice
snuffed up into the nostrils, purgeth the tuni-
rain; the juice of the berries boiled with ho-
pped into the ears, helpeth the pains of them;
n of the berries in wine being drank provok-
he distilled water of the flowers, is of much
the skin from sun-burning, freckles, mor-
e like; and taketh away the head-ach, com-
cause, the head being bathed therewith. The
wers distilled in the month of May, and the
legs

legs often washed with the said distilled water, it taketh away the ulcers and sores of them. The eyes washed therewith, it taketh away the redness and blood shot; and the hands washed morning and evening therewith, helpeth the palsy, and shaking of them.

The Dwarf Elder is more powerful than the common Elder in opening and purging choler, phlegm, and water; in helping the gout, piles, and womens diseases, coloureth the hair black, helpeth the inflammations of the eyes, and pains in the ears, the biting of serpents, or mad dogs, burnings and scaldings, the wind colick, colick and stone, the difficulty of urine, the cure of old sores, and fistulous ulcers. Either leaves or bark of Elder stripped upwards as you gather it, causeth vomiting. Also Dr Butler in a manuscript of his commends Dwarf Elder to the sky for dropsies, viz. to drink it, being boiled in white wine; to drink the decoction I mean, not the Elder.

The Elm Tree.

THIS tree is so well known, growing generally in all counties of this land, that it is needless to describe it.

Government and Virtues.] It is a cold and Saturnine plant. The leaves thereof bruised and applied heal green wounds, being bound thereon with its own bark. The leaves or the bark used with vinegar, cure scurf and leprosy very effectually: The decoction of the leaves, bark, or root, being bathed, heals broken bones. The water that is found in the bladders on the leaves, while it is fresh, is very effectual to cleanse the skin, and make it fair; and if cloths be often wet therein, and applied to the ruptures of children, it healeth them, if they be well bound up with a truss. The said water put into a glass, and set into the ground, or else in dung for twenty-five days, the mouth thereof being close stopped, and the bottom set upon a lay of ordinary salt, that the fœces may settle and water become clear, is a singular and sovereign balm for green wounds, being used with soft tents: The decoction of the bark of the root fomented, mollifieth hard tumours, and the shrinking of the sinews. The roots of the Elm boiled for a long time in water, and the fat arising on the top thereof, being clean scummed off, and the place

place anointed therewith that is grown bald, and the hair fallen away, will quickly restore them again. The said bark ground with brine and pickle, until it come to the form of a poultice, and laid on the place pained with the gout, giveth great ease. The decoction of the bark in water, is excellent to bathe such places as have been burnt with fire.

ENDIVE.

Descript.] COMMON garden Endive beareth a longer and larger leaf than succory, and abideth but one year, quickly running up to stalk and seed, and then perisheth; it hath blue flowers, and the seed of the ordinary Endive is so like succory seed, that it is hard to distinguish them.

Government and Virtues.] It is a fine cooling, cleansing, jovial plant. The decoction of the leaves, or the juice, or the distilled water of Endive, serveth well to cool the excessive heat of the liver and stomach, and in the hot fits of agues, and all other inflammations in any part of the body; it cooleth the heat and sharpness of the urine, and excoriations in the urinary parts. The seeds are of the same property, or rather more powerful, and besides are available for fainting, swoonings, and passions of the heart. Outwardly applied, they serve to temper the sharp humours of fretting ulcers, hot tumours, swellings, and pestilential sores; and wonderfully help not only the redness and inflammations of the eyes, but the dimness of the sight also; they are also used to allay the pains of the gout. You cannot use it amiss; a syrup of it is a fine cooling medicine for fevers. See the end of this book, and the English Dispensatory.

ELECAMPANE.

Descript.] IT shooteth forth many large leaves, long and broad, lying near the ground, small at both ends, somewhat soft in handling, of a whitish green on the upper side, and grey underneath, each set upon a short foot-stalk, from among which rise up divers great and strong hairy stalks, three or four feet high, with some leaves thereupon compassing them about at the lower end, and are branched towards the tops, bearing divers great and large flowers, like those of the corn marigold, both the border of leaves, and the middle thrum being yellow, which turn into down, with long, small, brownish seeds among it, and is carried away with the wind. The root is great and thick, branched forth divers ways, blackish on the outside, and whitish within. of a very bitter taste, and strong, but good scent, especially when they are dried, no part else of the plant having any smell.

Place.] It groweth in moist grounds and shadowy places oftener than in the dry and open borders of fields and lanes, and in other waste places, almost in every county of this land.

Time.] It flowereth in the end of June and July, and the seed is ripe in August. The roots are gathered for use, as well in the Spring before the leaves come forth, as in Autumn or Winter.

Government and Virtues.] It is a plant under the dominion of Mercury. The fresh roots of Elecampane preserved with sugar, or made into a syrup or conserve, are very effectual to warm a cold windy stomach, or the pricking therein, and stitches in the sides caused by the spleen; and to help the cough, shortness of breath, and wheezing in the lungs. The dried root made into powder, and mixed with sugar and taken, serveth to the same purpose, and is also profitable for those who have their urine stopped, or the stopping of womens courses, the pains of the mother and of the stone in the reins, kidneys, or bladder; it resisteth poison, and stayeth the spreading of the venom of serpents, as also putrid and pestilential fevers, and the plague itself. The roots and herbs beaten and put into new ale or beer, and daily drank, cleareth, strengtheneth, and quickeneth the sight of the eyes wonderfully. The decoction of the roots in wine, or the juice taken therein, killeth and driveth forth all manner of worms in the belly, stomach, and maw; and gargled in the mouth, or the root chewed, fasteneth loose teeth, and helps to keep them from putrefaction; and being drank is good for those that spit blood, helpeth to remove cramps or convulsions, gout, sciatica, pains in the joints applied outwardly or inwardly, and is also good for those that are bursten,

burſten, or have any inward bruiſe. The root boiled well in vinegar, beaten afterwards, and made into an ointment with hog's ſuet, or oil of trotters, is an excellent remedy for ſcabs or itch in young or old; the places alſo bathed or waſhed with the decoction doth the ſame; it alſo helpeth all ſorts of filthy old putrid ſores or cankers whatſoever. In the roots of this herb lieth the chief effect for the remedies aforeſaid. The diſtilled water of the leaves and roots together, is very profitable to cleanſe the ſkin of the face, or other parts, from any morphew, ſpots, or blemiſhes therein, and make it clear.

ERINGO, or SEA HOLLY.

Deſcript.] THE firſt leaves of our ordinary Sea Holly are nothing ſo hard and prickly as when they grow old, being almoſt round, and deeply dented about the edges, hard and ſharp pointed, and a little crumpled, of a bluiſh green colour, every one upon a long footſtalk; but thoſe that grow up higher with the ſtalk, do as it were compaſs it about. The ſtalk itſelf is round and ſtrong, yet ſomewhat creſted with joints, and leaves ſet thereat, but more divided, ſharp and prickly; and branches riſing from thence, which have likewiſe other ſmall branches, each of them having ſeveral bluiſh round prickly heads, with many ſmall, jagged, prickly leaves under them, ſtanding like a ſtar, and ſometimes found greeniſh or whitiſh: The root groweth wonderful long, even to eight or ten feet in length, ſet with rings and circles toward the upper part, cut ſmooth and without joints down lower, browniſh on the outſide, and very white within, with a pith in the middle, of a pleaſant taſte, but much more, being artificially preſerved, and candied with ſugar.

Place.] It is found about the ſea coaſt in almoſt every county of this land which bordereth upon the ſea.

Time.] It flowereth in the end of Summer, and giveth ripe ſeed within a month after.

Government and Virtues.] The plant is venereal, and breedeth ſeed exceedingly, and ſtrengthens the ſpirit procreative; it is hot and moiſt, and under the celeſtial Balance. The decoction of the root hereof in wine, is very effectual to open obſtructions of the ſpleen and liver, and helpeth yellow jaundice, dropsy, pains of the loins, and wind colick, provoketh urine, and expelleth the stone, procureth womens courses. The continued use of the decoction for fifteen days, taken fasting, and next to bedward, doth help the strangury, the pissing by drops, the stopping of urine, and stone, and all defects of the reins and kidneys; and if the said drink be continued longer, it is said that it cureth the stone; it is found good against the French-pox. The roots bruised and applied outwardly, helpeth the kernels of the throat, commonly called the king's evil; or taken inwardly, and applied to the place stung or bitten by any serpent, healeth it speedily. If the roots be bruised, and boiled in old hog's grease, or salted lard, and applied to broken bones, thorns, &c. remaining in the flesh, they do not only draw them forth, but heal up the place again, gathering new flesh where it was consumed. The juice of the leaves dropped into the ear, helpeth imposthumes therein. The distilled water of the whole herb, when the leaves and stalks are young, is profitably drank for all the purposes aforesaid; and helpeth the melancholy of the heart, and is available in quartan and quotidian agues; as also for them that have their necks drawn awry, and cannot turn them without turning their whole body.

EYEBRIGHT.

Descript.] COMMON Eyebright is a small low herb, rising up usually but with one blackish green stalk a span high, or not much more, spread from the bottom into sundry branches, whereon are small and almost round, yet pointed, dark green leaves, finely snipped about the edges, two always set together, and very thick: At the joints with the leaves, from the middle upward, come forth small white flowers, steeped with purple and yellow spots, or stripes; after which follow small round heads, with very small seed therein. The root is long, small, and thready at the end.

Place.] It groweth in meadows, and grassy places in this land.

Government and Virtues.] It is under the sign of the Lion, and Sol claims dominion over it. If the herb was but

but as much used as it is neglected, it would half spoil the spectacle-makers trade; and a man would think, that reason should teach people to prefer the preservation of their natural before artificial spectacles; which that they may be instructed how to do, take the virtues of Eyebright as followeth:

The juice, or distilled water of Eyebright, taken inwardly in white wine or broth, or dropped into the eyes, for divers days together, helpeth all infirmities of the eyes that cause dimness of sight. Some make conserve of the flowers to the same effect. Being used any of the ways, it also helpeth a weak brain, or memory. This tunned up with strong beer that it may work together, and drank; or the powder of the dried herb mixed with sugar, a little mace, and Fennel seed, and drank, or eaten in broth; or the said powder made into an electuary with sugar, and taken, hath the same powerful effect to help and restore the sight decayed through age: and Arnoldus de Villa Nova saith, it hath restored sight to them that have been blind a long time before.

FERN.

Descript.] OF this there are two kinds principally to be treated of, viz. the Male and Female. The Female groweth higher than the Male, but the leaves thereof are lesser, and more divided or dented, and of as strong a smell as the Male; the virtue of them are both alike, and therefore I shall not trouble you with any description or distinction of them.

Place.] They grow both in heaths and in shady places near the hedge-sides in all counties of this land.

Time.] They flower and give their seed at Mid-summer.

The Female Fern is that plant which is in Sussex called Brakes, the seed of which some authors hold to be so rare: Such a thing there is I know, and may be easily had upon Midsummer Eve, and for ought I know, two or three days after it, if not more.

Government and Virtues.] It is under the dominion of Mercury, both Male and Female. The roots of both those sorts of Fern being bruised and boiled in mead, or honeyed water, and drank, killeth both the broad and long worms in the body, and abateth the ſwelling and hardneſs of the ſpleen. The green leaves eaten, purge the belly and cholerick and wateriſh humours that trouble the ſtomach. They are dangerous for women with child to meddle with, by reaſon they cauſe abortions. The roots bruiſed and boiled in oil, or hog's greaſe, make a very profitable ointment to heal wounds, or pricks gotten in the fleſh. The powder of them uſed in foul ulcers, drieth np their malignant moiſture, and cauſeth their ſpeedier healing. Fern being burned, the ſmoak thereof driveth away ſerpents, gnats, and other noiſome creatures, which in fenny countries do, in the night time, trouble and moleſt people lying in their beds with their faces uncovered; it cauſeth barrenneſs.

OSMOND ROYAL, or WATER FERN.

Deſcript.] THIS ſhooteth forth in ſpring time (for in the Winter the leaves periſh) divers rough hard ſtalks, half round, and yellowiſh, or flat on the other ſide, two feet high, having divers branches of winged yellowiſh green leaves on all ſides, ſet one againſt another, longer, narrower, and not nicked on the edges as the former. From the top of ſome of theſe ſtalks grow forth a long buſh of ſmall, and more yellow, green, ſcaly aglets, ſet in the ſame manner on the ſtalks as the leaves are, which are accounted the flowers and ſeeds. The root is rough, thick and ſcabby, with a white pith in the middle, which is called the heart thereof.

Place.] It groweth on moors, bogs, and watery places, in many parts of this land.

Time.] It is green all the ſummer, and the root only abideth in winter.

Government and Virtues.] Saturn owns the plant. This hath all the virtues mentioned in the former Ferns, and is much more effectual than they, both for inward and outward griefs, and is accounted ſingular good in wounds, bruiſes, or the like. The decoction to be drank, or boiled into an ointment of oil, as a balſam or balm, and ſo it is ſingular good againſt bruiſes, and bones broken, or out of joint, and giveth much eaſe to the colick and ſplenetick diſeaſes; as alſo for ruptures or burſtings. The decoction

tion of the root in white wine, provokes urine exceedingly, and cleanseth the bladder and passages of urine.

FEVERFEW, or FEATHERFEW.

Descript.] COMMON Featherfew hath large, fresh, green leaves, much torn or cut on the edges. The stalks are hard and round, set with many such like leaves, but smaller, and at the tops stand many single flowers, upon small foot stalks, consisting of many small white leaves standing round about a yellow thrum in the middle. The root is somewhat hard and short, with many strong fibres about it. The scent of the whole plant is very strong and stuffing, and the taste is very bitter.

Place.] This grows wild in many places of the land, but is for the most part nourished in gardens.

Time.] It flowereth in the months of June and July.

Government and Virtues.] Venus commands this herb, and hath commended it to succour her sisters (women) and to be a general strengthener of their wombs, and remedy such infirmities as a careless midwife hath there caused; if they will but be pleased to make use of her herb boiled in white wine, and drink the decoction; it cleanseth the womb, expels the after-birth, and doth a woman all the good she can desire of an herb. And if any grumble because they cannot get the herb in winter, tell them, if they please, they may make a syrup of it in summer; it is chiefly used for the disease of the mother, whether it be the strangling or rising of the mother, or hardness or inflammations of the same, applied outwardly thereunto. Or a decoction of the flowers in wine, with a little nutmeg or mace put therein, and drank often in a day, is an approved remedy to bring down womens courses speedily, and helpeth to expel the dead birth and after-birth. For a woman to sit over the hot fumes of the decoction of the herb made in water or wine, is effectual for the same; and in some cases, to apply the boiled herb warm to the privy parts. The decoction thereof made, with some sugar or honey put thereto, is used by many with good success to help the cough and stuffing of the chest, by colds, as also to cleanse the reins and bladder, and helps to expel the stone in them. The powder of the herb taken in wine, with some Oxymel, purgeth both choler and phlegm, and is available for those that are short winded, and are troubled with melancholy and heaviness, or sadness of spirits. It is very effectual for all pains in the head coming of a cold cause, the herb being bruised and applied to the crown of the head: As also for the vertigo, that is a running or swimming of the head. The decoction thereof drank warm, and the herb bruised with a few corns of Bay-salt, and applied to the wrists before the coming of the ague fits, doth take them away. The distilled water taketh away freckles, and other spots and deformities in the face. The herb bruised and heated on a tile, with some wine to moisten it, or fried with a little wine and oil in a frying-pan, and applied warm outwardly to the places, helpeth the wind and colic in the lower part of the belly. It is an especial remedy against opium taken too liberally.

FENNEL.

EVERY garden affordeth this so plentifully, that it needs no description.

Government and Virtues.] One good old fashion is not yet left off, viz. to boil Fennel with fish; for it consumes that phlegmatick humour, which fish most plentifully afford and annoy the body with, though few that use it know wherefore they do it; I suppose the reason of its benefit this way is, because it is an herb of Mercury, and under Virgo, and therefore bears antipathy to Pisces. Fennel is good to break wind, to provoke urine, and ease the pains of the stone, and helps to break it. The leaves or seed, boiled in barley water and drank, are good for nures, to increase their milk, and make it more wholesome for the child. The leaves, or rather the seeds, boiled in water, stayeth the hiccough, and taketh away the loathings which oftentimes happen to the stomachs of sick and feverish persons, and allayeth the heat thereof. The seed boiled in wine and drank, is good for those that are bitten with serpents, or have eaten poisonous herbs, or mushrooms. The seed and the roots much more help to open obstructions of the liver, spleen, and gall, and thereby help the painful and windy swellings of the spleen, and

and the yellow jaundice; as alſo the gout and cramps. The ſeed is of good uſe in medicines to help ſhortneſs of breath and wheezing by ſtopping of the lungs. It helpeth alſo to bring down the courſes, and to cleanſe the parts after delivery. The roots are of moſt uſe in phyſic drinks and broths that are taken to cleanſe the blood, to open obſtructions of the liver, to provoke urine, and amend the ill colour in the face after ſickneſs, and to cauſe a good habit through the body. Both leaves, ſeeds, and roots thereof are much uſed in drink or broth, to make people more lean that are too fat. The diſtilled water of the whole herb, or the condenſate juice diſſolved, but eſpecially the natural juice, that in ſome counties iſſueth out hereof of its own accord, dropped into the eyes, cleanſeth them from miſts and films that hinder the ſight. The ſweet Fennel is much weaker in phyſical uſes than the common Fennel. The wild Fennel is ſtronger and hotter than the tame, and therefore moſt powerful againſt the ſtone, but not ſo effectual to increaſe milk, becauſe of its dryneſs.

SOW-FENNEL, or HOG'S FENNEL.

BESIDES the common name in Engliſh, Hog's Fennel, and the Latin name Peucidanum, it is called Hoarſtrange, and Hoar-ſtrong, Sulphur-wort, and Brimſtonewort.

Deſcript.] The common Sow-Fennel hath divers branched ſtalks of thick and ſomewhat long leaves, three for the moſt part joined together at a place, among which ariſeth a creſted ſtreight ſtalk, leſs than Fennel, with ſome joints thereon, and leaves growing thereat, and towards the tops ſome branches iſſuing from thence; likewiſe on the tops of the ſtalks and branches ſtand divers turfs of yellow flowers, whereafter grows ſomewhat flat, thin, and yellowiſh ſeed, bigger than Fennel ſeed. The roots grow great and deep, with many other parts and fibres about them of a ſtrong ſcent like hot brimſtone, and yield forth a yellowiſh milk, or clammy juice, almoſt like a gum.

Place.] It groweth plentifully in the ſalt low marſhes near Feverſham in Kent.

Time.] It flowereth plentifully in July and Auguſt.

Govern-

Government and Virtues.] This is also an herb of Mercury. The juice of Sow-Fennel (saith Dioscorides, and Galen,) used with vinegar and rose water, or the juice with a little euphorbium put to the nose, helpeth those that are troubled with the lethargy, frenzy, giddiness of the head, the falling-sickness, long and inveterate head-ach, the palsy, sciatica, and the cramp, and generally all the diseases of the sinews, used with oil and vinegar. The juice dissolved in wine, or put into an egg, is good for a cough, or shortness of breath, and for those that are troubled with wind in the body. It purgeth the belly gently, expelleth the hardness of the spleen, giveth ease to women that have sore travail in child-birth, and easeth the pains of the reins and bladder, and also the womb. A little of the juice dissolved in wine, and dropped into the ears, easeth much of the pains in them, and put into a hollow tooth, easeth the pains thereof. The root is less effectual to all the aforesaid disorders; yet the powder of the root cleanseth foul ulcers, being put into them, and taketh out splinters of broken bones, or other things in the flesh, and healeth them up perfectly; as also, drieth up old and inveterate running sores, and is of admirable virtue in all green wounds.

FIG-WORT, OR THROAT-WORT.

Descript.] COMMON great Fig-wort sendeth divers great strong, hard, square brown stalks, three or four feet high, whereon grow large, hard and dark green leaves, two at a joint, harder and larger than nettle leaves, but not stinging; at the tops of the stalks stand many purple-flowers set in husks, which are sometimes gaping and open, somewhat like those of Water Betony; after which come hard round heads, with a small point in the middle, wherein lie small brownish seed. The root is great, white, and thick, with many branches at it, growing aslope under the upper crust of the ground, which abideth many years, but keepeth not his green leaves in Winter.

Place.] It groweth frequently in moist and shadowy woods, and in the lower parts of the fields and meadows.

Time.] It flowereth about July, and the seed will be ripe about a month after the flowers are fallen.

Government

Government and Virtues.] Some Latin authors call it Cervicaria, becaufe it is appropriated to the neck; and we Throat-wort, becaufe it is appropriated to the throat. Venus owns the herb, and the Celeftial Bull will not deny it; therefore a better remedy cannot be for the king's evil, becaufe the Moon that rules the difeafe is exalted there. The decoction of the herb taken inwardly, and the bruifed herb applied outwardly, diffolveth, clotted and congealed blood within the body, coming by any wounds, bruife, or fall; and is no lefs effectual for the king's evil, or any other knobs, kernels, bunches, or wens growing in the flefh wherefoever; and for the hæmorrhoids, or piles. An ointment made hereof may be ufed at all times when the frefh herb is not to be had. The diftilled water of the whole plant, roots and all, is ufed for the fame purpofes, and drieth up the fuperfluous, virulent moifture of hollow and corroding ulcers; it taketh away all rednefs, fpots, and freckles in the face, as alfo the fcurf, and any foul deformity therein, and the leprofy likewife.

FILIPENDULA, or DROP-WORT.

Defcript.] THIS fendeth forth many leaves, fome bigger, fome leffer, fet on each fide of a middle rib, and each of them dented about the edges, fomewhat refembling wild Tanfy, or rather Agrimony, but harder in handling; among which rife up one or more ftalks, two or three feet high, with the leaves growing thereon, and fometimes alfo divided into other branches fpreading at the top into many white, fweet fmelling flowers, confifting of five leaves a-piece with fome threads in the middle of them ftanding together, in a pith or umbel, each upon a fmall foot-ftalk, which, after they have deen blown upon a good while, do fall away, and in their places appear fmall, round, chaffy heads like buttons, wherein are the chaffy feeds fet and placed. The root confifts of many fmall, black, tuberous pieces faftened together by many fmall, long, blackifh ftrings, which run from one to another.

Place.] It groweth in many places of this land, in the corners of dry fields and meadows, and the hedge-fides.

Time.

Time.] They flower in June and July, and their ſeed is ripe in Auguſt.

Government and Virtues.] It is under the dominion of Venus. It effectually opens the paſſages of the urine, helpeth the ſtrangury; the ſtone in the kidneys or bladder, the gravel, and all other pains of the bladder and reins, by taking the roots in powder, or a decoction of them in white wine, with a little honey. The roots made into powder, and mixed with honey in the form of an electuary, doth much help thoſe whoſe ſtomachs are ſwollen, diſſolving and breaking the wind which was the cauſe thereof; and is alſo very effectual for all the diſeaſes of the lungs, as ſhortneſs of breath, wheezing, hoarſeneſs of the throat, and the cough; and to expectorate tough phlegm, or any other parts thereabout. It is called dropwort, becauſe it helps ſuch as piſs by drops.

The FIG-TREE.

FOR to give a deſcription of a tree ſo well known to every body that keeps it in his garden, were needleſs. They proſper very well in our Engliſh gardens, yet are fitter for medicine, than for any other profit that is gotten by the fruit of them.

Government and Virtues.] The tree is under the dominion of Jupiter. The milk that iſſueth out from the leaves or branches where they are broken off, being dropped upon warts, taketh them away. The decoction of the leaves is excellent good to waſh ſore heads with: and there is ſcarcely a better remedy for the leproſy than it is. It clears the face alſo of morphew, and the body of white ſcurf, ſcabs and running ſores. If it be dropped into old fretting ulcers, it cleanſeth out the moiſture, and bringeth up the fleſh; becauſe you cannot have the leaves green all the year, you may make an ointment of them whilſt you may. A decoction of the leaves being drank inwardly, or rather a ſyrup made of them, diſſolves congealed blood cauſed by bruiſes or falls, and helps the bloody flux. The aſhes of the wood made into an ointment with hog's greaſe, help kibes and chilblains. The juice being put into an hollow tooth, eaſeth pain; as alſo pain and noiſe in the ears, being dropped into them; and deafneſs. An ointment

of the juice and hog's greafe, is as excellent a
the biting of mad dogs, or other venomous
oft are. A fyrup made of the leaves, or green
llent good for coughs, hoarfnefs, or fhortnefs
nd all difeafes of the breaft and lungs; it is
it good for the dropfy and falling ficknefs.
it the Fig-Tree, as well as the Bay-Tree, is
y lightening; as alfo if you tie a bull be he
to a Fig-Tree, he will quickly become tame
As for fuch figs as come from beyond fea,
to fay, becaufe I write not of exoticks; yet
fay, the eating of them makes people loufy.

v WATER-FLAG, or FLOWER-DE-LUCE.

THIS groweth like the Flower-de-luce, but
it hath much longer and narrower fad
jointed together in that fafhion; the ftalk
oftentimes as high, bearing fmall yellow
ed like the Flower-de-luce, with three falling
other three arched that cover their bottoms;
f the three upright leaves, as the Flower-de-
his hath only three fhort pieces ftanding in
after which fucceed thick and long three
, containing in each part fomewhat big and
e thofe of the Flower-de-luce. The root is
ider, of a pale brownifh colour on the out-
horfe flefh colour on the infide, with many
hereat, and very harfh in tafte.
ufually grows in watery ditches, ponds, lakes,
es, which are always overflowed with water.
flowereth in July, and the feed is ripe in

it and Virtues.] It is under the dominion of
The root of this Water-flag is very aftringent,
drying; and thereby helps all lafks and fluxes,
lood or humours, as bleeding at the mouth,
r parts, bloody-flux, and the immoderate flux
courfes. The diftilled water of the whole
and roots, is a fovereign good remedy for
s, both to be dropped into them, and to have
nges wetted therein, and applied to the forehead

head: It alſo helpeth the ſpots and blemiſhes that happen in and about the eyes, or in any other parts: The ſaid water fomented on ſwellings and hot inflammations of womens breaſts, upon cankers alſo, and thoſe ſpreading ulcers called *Noli me tangere,* do much good: It helpeth alſo foul ulcers in the privities of man or woman; but an ointment made of the flowers is better for thoſe external applications.

FLAX-WEED, or TOAD-FLAX.

Deſcript.] OUR common Flax-weed hath divers ſtalks full fraught with long and narrow aſh coloured leaves, and from the middle of them almoſt upward, ſtored with a number of pale yellow flowers, of a ſtrong unpleaſant ſcent, with deeper yellow mouths, and blackiſh flat ſeed in round heads. The root is ſomewhat woody and white, eſpecially the main downright one, with many fibres, abiding many years, ſhooting forth roots every way round about, and new branches every year.

Place.] This groweth throughout this land, both by the way-ſides and in meadows, as alſo by hedge-ſides, and upon the ſides of banks, and borders of fields.

Time.] It flowereth in Summer, and the ſeed is ripe uſually before the end of Auguſt.

Government and Virtues.] Mars owns the herb: In Suſſex we call it Gallwort, and lay it in our chickens water to cure them of the gall; it relieves them when they are drooping. This is frequently uſed to ſpend the abundance of thoſe watery humours by urine, which cauſe the dropſy. The decoction of the herb, both leaves and flowers, in wine taken and drank, doth ſomewhat move the belly downwards, openeth obſtructions of the liver, and helpeth the yellow jaundice; expelleth poiſon, provoketh womens courſes, driveth forth the dead child, and after birth. The diſtilled water of the herb and flowers is effectual for all the ſame purpoſes; being drank with a dram of the powder of the ſeeds of bark or the roots of Wall-wort, and a little cinnamon, for certain days together, it is held a ſingular remedy for the dropſy. The juice of the herb, or the diſtilled water, dropped into the eyes, is a certain remedy for all heat, inflammation, and redneſs

redness in them. The juice or water put into foul ulcers, whether they be cancerous or fistulous, with tents rolled therein, or parts washed and injected therewith, cleanseth them thoroughly from the bottom, and healeth them up safely. The same juice or water also cleanseth the skin wonderfully of all sorts of deformity, as leprosy, morphew, scurf, wheals, pimpels, or spots, applied of itself, or used with some powder of Lupines.

FLEA-WORT.

Descript.] ORDINARY Flea-wort riseth up with a stalk two feet high or more, full of joints and branches on every side up to the top, and at every joint two small, long, and narrow whitish green leaves somewhat hairy: At the top of every branch stand divers small, short, scaly, or chaffy heads, out of which come forth small whitish yellow threads, like to those of the plantain herbs, which are the bloomings of flowers. The seed inclosed in these heads is small and shining while it is fresh, very like unto fleas both for colour and bigness, but turning black when it groweth old. The root is not long, but white, hard, and woody, perishing every year, and rising again of its own seed for divers years, if it be suffered to shed: The whole plant is somewhat whitish and hairy, smelling somewhat like rosin.

There is another sort hereof, differing not from the former in the manner of growing, but only that this stalk and branches being somewhat greater, do a little more bow down to the ground: The leaves are somewhat greater, the heads somewhat lesser, the seed alike; and the root and leaves abide all winter and perish not as the former.

Place.] The first groweth only in gardens, the second plentifully in fields that are near the sea.

Time.] They flower in July, or thereabouts.

Government and Virtues.] The herb is cold, dry, and Saturnine. I suppose it obtained the name of Flea-wort, because the seeds are so like fleas. The seed fried, and taken, stayeth the flux or lask of the belly, and the corrosions that come by reason of hot cholerick, or sharp and malignant humours, or by too much purging of any violent medicine, as Scammony, or the like. The mucilage of the feed made with Rosewater, and a little sugar-candy put thereto, is very good in all hot agues and burning fevers, and other inflammations, to cool the thirst, and lenify the dryness and roughness of the tongue and throat. It helpeth also hoarseness of the voice, and diseases of the breast and lungs caused, by heat, or sharp salt humours, and the plurisy also. The mucilage of the seed made with plantain water, whereunto the yolk of an egg or two, and a little populeon are put, is a most safe and sure remedy to ease the sharpness, pricking, and pains of the hæmorrhoids or piles, if it be laid on a cloth and bound thereto It helpeth all inflammations in any part of the body, and the pains that come thereby, as the head-ach and megrims, and all hot imposthumes, swellings, and breaking out of the skin, as blains, wheals, pushes, purples and the like; as also the joints of those that are out of joint, the pains of the gout and sciatica, the bursting of young children, and the swelling of the navel, applied with oil of roses and vinegar. It is also good to heal the nipples and sore breasts of women, being often applied thereunto. The juice of the herb with a little honey put into the ears, helpeth the running of them, and the worms breeding in them: The same also mixed with hog's grease, and applied to corrupt and filthy ulcers, cleanseth and healeth them.

FLUXWEED.

Descript.] IT riseth up with a round uprigt hard stalk, four or five feet high, spread into sundry branches, whereon grow many greyish green leaves, very finely cut and severed into a number of short and almost round parts. The flowers are very small and yellow, growing spike fashion, after which come small long pods, with small yellowish seed in them. The root is long and woody perishing every year.

There is another sort, differing in nothing, save only it hath somewhat broader leaves; they have a strong evil savour, being smelled unto, and are of a drying taste.

Place.] They flower wild in the fields by hedge-sides and high-ways, and among rubbish and other places.

Time.] They flower and seed quickly after, namely in June and July.

Govern-

Government and Virtues.] This herb is Saturnine alſo. Both the herb and ſeed of Fluxweed is of excellent uſe to ſtay the flux and laſk of the belly, being drank in water wherein are gads of ſteel heated have been often quenched; and is no leſs effectual for the ſame porpoſe than plantain or comfrey, and to reſtrain any other flux of blood in man or woman, as alſo to conſolidate bones broken or out of joint. The juice thereof drank in wine, or the decoction of the herb drank, doth kill the worms in the ſtomach or belly, or the worms that grow in putrid and filthy ulcers; and made into a ſalve doth quickly heal all old ſores, how foul and malignant ſoever they be. The diſtilled water of the herb worketh the ſame effects, although ſomewhat weaker, yet it is a fair medicine, and more acceptable to be taken. It is called fluxweed becauſe it cures the flux, and for its uniting broken bones, &c. Paracelſus extols it to the ſkies. It is fitting that ſyrup, ointment, and plaiſters of it were kept in your houſes.

FLOWER-DE-LUCE.

IT is ſo well known, being nouriſhed up in moſt gardens, that I ſhall not need to ſpend time in writing a deſcription thereof.

Time.] The flaggy kinds thereof have the moſt phyſical uſes; the dwarf kinds thereof flower in April the greater ſorts in May.

Government and Virtues.] The herb is Lunar. The juice or decoction of the green root of the flaggy kind of Flower-de-luce, with a little honey drank, doth purge and cleanſe the ſtomach of groſs and tough phlegm and choler therein; it helpeth the jaundice and the dropſy, evacuating thoſe humours both upwards and downwards; and becauſe it ſomewhat hurts the ſtomach, is not to be taken without honey and ſpikenard. The ſame being drank, doth eaſe the pains and torments of the belly and ſides, the ſhaking of agues, the diſeaſes of the liver and ſpleen, the worms of the belly, the ſtone in the reins, convulſions and cramps that come of old humours; it alſo helps thoſe whoſe ſeed paſs from them unawares: It is a remedy againſt the bitings and ſtingings of venomous creatures, being boiled in water and vinegar and drank: Boiled in water and drank,

 it

it provoketh urine, helpeth the colick, bringeth down womens courſes; and made up into a peſſary with honey, and put up into the body, draweth forth the dead child. It is much commended againſt the cough, to expectorate tough phlegm; it much eaſeth pains in the head, and procureth ſleep; being put into the noſtrils it procureth ſneezing, and thereby purgeth the head of phlegm: The juice of the root applied to the piles or hæmorrhoids, giveth much eaſe. The decoction of the roots gargled in the mouth, eaſeth the tooth-ach, and helpeth a ſtinking breath. Oil called Oleum Irinum, if it be rightly made of the great broad flag Flower-de-luce (and not of the great bulbus blue Flower-de-luce, as is uſed by ſome apothecaries) and roots of the ſame of the flaggy kinds, is very effectual to warm and comfort all cold joints and ſinews, as alſo the gout and ſciatica, and mollifieth, diſſolveth and conſumeth tumours and ſwellings in any part of the body, as alſo of the matrix; it helpeth the cramp, or convulſions of the ſinews: The head and temples anointed therewith, helpeth the catarrh of thin rheum diſtilled from thence; and uſed upon the breaſt or ſtomach, helpeth to extenuate the cold tough phlegm; it helpeth alſo the pains and noiſe in the ears, and the ſtench of the noſtrils. The root itſelf, either green or in powder, helpeth to cleanſe, heal, and incarnate wounds, and to cover the naked bones with fleſh again, that ulcers have made bare; and is alſo very good to cleanſe and heal up fiſtulas and cankers that are hard to be cured.

FLUELLIN, or LLUELLIN.

Deſcript.] IT ſhooteth forth many long branches partly lying upon the ground, and partly ſtanding upright, ſet with almoſt red leaves, yet a little pointed, and ſometimes more long than round, without order thereon, ſomewhat hairy, and of an evil greeniſh white colour; at the joints all along the ſtalks, and with the leaves come forth ſmall flowers, one at a place, upon a very ſmall ſhort foot-ſtalk, gaping ſomewhat like ſnapdragons, or rather like toad-flax, with the upper jaw of a yellow colour, and the lower of a purpliſh, with a ſmall heel or ſpur behind; after which come forth ſmall round heads,

heads, containing ſmall black ſeed. The root is ſmall and thready, dying every year, and raiſeth itſelf again of its own ſowing.

There is another ſort of Lluellin which hath longer branches wholly trailing upon the ground, two or three feet long, and ſomewhat more thin, ſet with leaves thereon, upon ſmall foot-ſtalks. The leaves are a little larger, and ſomewhat round, and cornered ſometimes in ſome places on the edges; but the lower part of them being the broadeſt, hath on each ſide a ſmall point, making it ſeem as if they were ears, ſometimes hairy, but not hoary, and of a better green colour than the former. The flowers come forth like the former, but the colours therein are more white than yellow, and the purple not ſo far: It is a large flower, and ſo are the ſeed and ſeed-veſſels. The root is like the other, and periſheth every year.

Place.] They grow in divers corn-fields, and in borders about them, and in other fertile grounds about Southfleet in Kent abundant; at Buchrite, Hamerton, and Richmanworth in Huntingdonſhire, and in divers other places.

Time.] They are in flower about June and July, and the whole plant is dry and withered before Auguſt be done.

Government and Virtues.] It is a Lunar herb. The leaves bruiſed and applied with barley-meal to watering eyes, that are hot and inflamed by defluctions from the head, do very much help them, as alſo the fluxes of blood or humours, as the laſk, bloody-flux, womens courſes, and ſtayeth all manner of bleeding at noſe, mouth, or any other place, or that cometh by any bruiſe or hurt, or burſting a vein; it wonderfully helpeth all thoſe inward parts that need conſolidating or ſtrengthening, and is no leſs effectual both to heal and cloſe green wounds, than to cleanſe and heal all foul or old ulcers, fretting or ſpreading cankers or the like. Bees are induſtrious, and go abroad to gather honey from each plant and flower, but drones lie at home, and eat up what the bees have taken pains for: Juſt ſo do the college of phyſicians lie at home and domineer, and ſuck out the ſweetneſs of other mens labours and ſtudies, themſelves being as ignorant in the knowledge of herbs as a child of four years old, as I can make appear to any rational man by their last dispensatory. Now then to hide their ignorance, there is no readier way in the world than to hide knowledge from their countrymen, that so no body might be able so much as to smell out their ignorance. When simples were in use, mens bodies were better in health by far than now they are, or shall be, if the college can help it. The truth is, this herb is of a fine cooling, drying quality, and an ointment or plaister of it might do a man a courtesey that hath any hot virulent sores: 'Tis admirable for the ulcers of the French-pox; if taken inwardly, may cure the disease. It was first called Female Speedwell, but a shentleman of Wales, whose nose was almost eaten off with the pox, and so near the matter, that the doctors commanded it to be cut off, being cured only by the use of this herb; and to honour the herb, for saving hur nose whole, gave it one of hur country names, Fluellin.

FOX-GLOVES.

Descript.] IT hath many long and broad leaves lying upon the ground dented upon the edges, a little soft or wooly, and of a hoary green colour, among which riseth up sometimes sundry stalks, but one very often, bearing such leaves thereon from the bottom to the middle, from whence to the top it is stored with large and long hollow reddish purple flowers, a little more long and imminent at the lower edge, with some white spots within them, one above another, with small green leaves at every one, but all of them turning their heads one way, and hanging downwards, having some threads also in the middle, from whence rise round heads, pointed sharp at the ends, wherein small brown seed lieth. The roots are so many small fibers, and some greater strings among them; the flowers have no scent, but the leaves have a bitter hot taste

Place.] It groweth on dry sandy ground for the most part, and as well on the higher as the lower places under hedge-sides in almost every county of this land.

Time.] It seldom flowereth before July, and the seed is ripe in August.

Government and Virtues.] The plant is under the domi-

nion

nion of Venus, being of a gentle cleanſing nature, and withal very friendly to nature. The herb is familiarly and frequently uſed by the Italians to heal any freſh or green wound, the leaves being but bruiſed and bound thereon; and the juice thereof is alſo uſed in old ſores, to cleanſe, dry, and heal them. The decoction hereof made up with ſome ſugar or honey, is available to cleanſe and purge the body both upwards and downwards, ſometimes of tough phlegm and clammy humours, and to open obſtructions of the liver and ſpleen. It hath been found by experience to be available for the king's evil, the herb bruiſed and applied, or an ointment made with the juice thereof, and ſo uſed; and a decoction of two handfuls thereof, with four ounces of Polypody in ale, hath been found by late experience to cure divers of the falling ſickneſs, that have been troubled with it above twenty years. I am confident that an ointment of it is one of the beſt remedies for a ſcabby head that is.

FUMITORY.

Deſcript.] OUR common Fumitory is a tender ſappy herb, ſendeth forth from one ſquare, a ſlender weak ſtalk, and leaning downwards on all ſides, many branches two or three feet long, with finely cut and jagged leaves of whitiſh, or rather bluiſh ſea-green colour: At the tops of the branches ſtand many ſmall flowers, as it were in a long ſpike one above another, made like little birds, of a reddiſh purple colour, with whitiſh bellies, after which come ſmall round huſks, containing ſmall black ſeeds. The root is yellow, ſmall, and not very long, full of juice while it is green, but quickly periſhes with the ripe ſeed. In the corn-fields in Cornwall, it beareth white flowers.

Place.] It groweth in corn fields almoſt every where, as well as in gardens.

Time.] It flowereth in May, for the moſt part, and the ſeed ripeneth ſhortly after.

Government and Virtues.] Saturn owns the herb, and preſents it to the world as a cure for his own diſeaſe, and ſtrengthener of the parts of the body he rules. If by my aſtrological judgment of diſeaſes, from the decumbiture, you

you find Saturn author of the disease, or if by direction from a nativity you fear a Saturnine disease approaching, you may by this herb prevent it in the one, and cure it in the other, and therefore it is fit you keep a syrup of it always by you. The juice or syrup made thereof, or the decoction made in whey by itself, with some other purging or opening herbs and roots to cause it to work the better (itself being but weak) is very effectual for the liver and spleen, opening the obstuctions thereof, and clarifying the blood from saltish, cholerick, and adust humours, which cause leprosy, scabs, tetters, and itches, and such like breakings-out of the skin, and after the purgings doth strengthen all the inward parts. It is also good against the yellow jaundice, and spendeth it by urine, which it procureth in abundance. The powder of the dried herb given for some time together, cureth melancholy, but the seed is strongest in operation for all the former diseases. The distilled water of the herb is also of good effect in the former diseases, and conduceth much against the plague and pestilence, being taken with good treacle. The distilled water also, with a little water and honey of roses, helpeth all the sores of the mouth or throat, being gargled often therewith. The juice dropped into the eyes, cleareth the sight, and taketh away redness and other defects in them, although it procureth some pain for the present, and cause tears. Dioscorides saith it hindereth any fresh springing of hairs on the eye-lids (after they are pulled away) if the eye-lids be anointed with the juice hereof with Gum Arabic dissolved therein. The juice of the Fumitory and Docks mingled with vinegar, and the places gently washed or wet therewith, cureth all sorts of scabs, pimples, blotches, wheals, and pushes which arise on the face or hands, or any other parts of the body.

The Furz Bush.

IT is as well known by this name, as it is in some counties by the name of Gorz or Whins, that I shall not need to write any discription thereof, my intent being to teach my countrymen what they know not, rather than to tell them again of that which is generally known before.

Place.

Place.] They are known to grow on dry barren heaths, and other waste, gravely or sandy grounds, in all counties of this land.

Time.] They also flower in the Summer months.

Government and Virtues.] Mars owns the herb. They are hot and dry, and open obstructions of the liver and spleen. A decoction made with the flowers thereof hath been found effectual against the jaundice, as also to provoke urine, and cleanse the kidneys from gravel or stone engendered in them. Mars doth also this by sympathy.

GARLICK.

THE offensiveness of the breath of him that hath eaten Garlick, will lead you by the nose to the knowledge hereof, and (instead of a description) direct you to the place where it groweth in gardens, which kinds are the best, and most physical.

Government and Virtues.] Mars owns this herb. This was anciently accounted the poor man's treacle, it being a remedy for all diseases and hurts (except those which itself breeds.) It provoketh urine and womens courses, helpeth the biting of mad dogs, and other venomous creatures; killeth worms in children, cutteth and voideth tough phlegm, purgeth the head, helpeth the lethargy, is a good preservative against, and a remedy for any plague, sore, or foul ulcer; taketh away spots and blemishes in the skin, easeth pains in the ears, ripeneth and breaketh impostumes, or other swellings. And for all those diseases the onions are as effectual. But the Garlick hath some more peculiar virtues besides the former, viz. it hath a special quality to discuss inconveniencies coming by corrupt agues or mineral vapours, or by drinking corrupt or stinking waters; as also by taking wolf-bane, hen-bane, hemlock, or other poisonous and dangerous herbs. It is also held good in hydropick diseases, the jaundice, falling-sickness, cramps, convulsions, the piles or hæmorrhoids, or other cold diseases. Many authors quote many diseases this is good for; but conceal its vices. Its heat is very vehement, and all vehement hot things send up but ill-favoured vapours to the brain. In cholerick men it will add fuel to the fire; in men oppressed by melancholy, it will attenuate the humour, and send up strong fancies, and as many strange visions to the head; therefore let it be taken inwardly with great moderation; outwardly you may make more bold with it.

GENTIAN, FELWORT, or BALDMONY.

IT is confessed that Gentian, which is most used amongst us, is brought over from beyond sea, yet we have two sorts of it growing frequently in our nation, which besides the reasons so frequently alledged why English herbs should be fittest for English bodies, hath been proved by the experience of divers physicians, to be not a whit inferior in virtue to that which cometh from beyond sea, therefore be pleased to take the description of them as followeth.

Descript.] The greater of the two hath many small long roots thrust down deep into the ground, and abiding all the Winter. The stalks are sometimes more, sometimes fewer, of a brownish green colour, which is sometimes two feet high, if the ground be fruitful, having many long, narrow, dark green leaves, set by couples up to the top; the flowers are long and hollow, of a purple colour, ending in fine corners. The smaller sort which is to be found in our land, groweth up with sundry stalks, not a foot high, parted into several small branches, whereon grow divers small leaves together, very like those of the lesser Centaury, of a whitish green colour; on the tops of these stalks grow divers perfect blue flowers, standing in long husks, but not so big as the other; the root is very small, and full of threads.

Place.] The first groweth in divers places of both the East and West countries, and as well in wet as in dry grounds, as near Long-field by Gravesend, near Cobham in Kent, near Lillinstone in Kent, also in a chalk pit hard by a paper-mill not far from Dartford in Kent. The second groweth also in divers places in Kent, as about Southfleet and Longfield; upon Barton's Hills in Bedfordshire; also not far from St Albans, upon a piece of waste chalky ground, as you go out of Dunstable way towards Gorhambury.

Time.] They flower in August.

Government and Virtues.] They are under the dominion of

of Mars, and one of the most principal herbs he is ruler of. They resist putrefactions, poison, and a more sure remedy cannot be found to prevent the pestilence than it is; it strengthens the stomach exceedingly, helps digestion, comforts the heart, and preserves it against faintings and swoonings: The powder of the dry roots helps the biting of mad dogs and venomous beasts, opens obstructions of the liver, and restoreth an appetite of their meat to such as have lost it. The herb steeped in wine, and the wine drank, refresheth such as be over-weary with travel, and grow lame in their joints, either by cold or evil lodgings; it helps stitches, and griping pains in the sides; is an excellent remedy for such as are bruised by falls; it provokes urine and the terms exceedingly, therefore let it not be given to women with child: The same is very profitable for such as are troubled with cramps and convulsions, to drink the decoction: Also they say it breaks the stone, and helps ruptures most certainly; it is excellent in all cold diseases, and such as are troubled with tough phlegm, scabs, itch, or any fretting sores and ulcers; it is an admirable remedy to kill the worms, by taking half a dram of the powder in a morning in any convenient liquor; the same is excellent good to be taken inwardly for the king's evil. It helps agues of all sorts, and the yellow jaundice, as also the bots in cattle; when kine are bitten on the udder by any venomous beast, do but stroke the place with the decoction of any of these, and it will instantly heal them.

GLOVE GILLIFLOWERS.

IT is vain to describe an herb so well known.

Government and Virtues.] They are gallant, fine, temperate flowers, of the nature and under the dominion of Jupiter; yea, so temperate, that no excess, neither in heat, cold, dryness, nor moisture, can be perceived in them; they are great strengtheners both of the brain and heart, and will therefore serve either for cordials or cephalicks, as your occasion will serve. There is both a syrup and a conserve made of them alone, commonly to be had at every apothecary's. To take now and then a little of either, strengthens nature much, in such as are in consumptions. They are also excellent good in hot pestilent fevers, and expel poison.

GERMANDER.

Descript.] COMMON Germander shooteth forth sundry stalks, with small and somewhat round leaves, dented about the edges. The flowers stand at the tops of a deep purple colour. The root is composed of divers sprigs, which shoot forth a great way round about, quickly overspreading a garden.

Place.] It groweth usually with us in gardens.

Time.] And flowereth in June and July.

Government and Virtues.] It is a most prevalent herb of Mercury, and strengthens the brain and apprehension exceedingly; (you may see what human virtues are under Mercury, in the latter end of my Ephemeris for 1652,) strengthens them when weak, and relieves them when drooping. This taken with honey (saith Dioscorides) is a remedy for coughs, hardness of the spleen, and difficulty of urine, and helpeth those that are fallen into a dropsy, especially at the beginning of the disease, a decoction being made thereof when it is green, and drank. It also bringeth down womens courses, and expelleth the dead child. It is most effectual against the poison of all serpents, being drank in wine, and the bruised herb outwardly applied; used with honey, it cleanseth old and foul ulcers; and made into an oil, and the eyes anointed therewith, taketh away the dimness and moistness. It is likewise good for the pains in the sides and cramps. The decoction thereof taken for four days together, driveth away and cureth both tertian and quartan agues. It is also good against all diseases of the brain, as continual headach falling sickness, melancholy, drousiness and dulness of the spirits, convulsions and palsies. A dram of the seed taken in powder purgeth by urine, and is good against the yellow jaundice. The juice of the leaves dropped into the ears killeth the worms in them. The tops thereof, when they are in flowers, steeped twenty-four hours in in a draught of white wine, and drank, killeth the worms in the belly.

STINKING

STINKING GLADWIN.

Descript.] THIS is one of the kinds of Flower-de-luce, having divers leaves arising from the roots, very like a Flower-de-luce, but that they are sharp-edged on both sides, and thicker in the middle, of a deeper green colour, narrower and sharper pointed, and a strong ill scent, if they be bruised between the fingers. In the middle riseth up a reasonable strong stalk, a yard high at the least, bearing three or four Flowers at the top, made somewhat like the flowers of the Flower-de-luce, with three upright leaves, of a dead purplish ash colour, with some veins discoloured in them; the other three do not fall down, nor are the three other small ones so arched, nor cover the lower leaves as the Flower-de-luce doth, but stand loose or asunder from them. After they are past, there come up three square hard husks, opening wide into three parts when they are ripe, wherein lie reddish seed, turning back when it hath abidden long. The root is like that of the Flower-de-luce, but reddish on the outside, and whitish within, very sharp and hot in the taste, of as evil scent as the leaves.

Place.] This groweth as well in upland grounds as in moist places, woods, and shadowy places by the sea-side in many places of this land, and is usually nursed up in gardens.

Time.] It flowereth not until July, and the seed is ripe in August or September, yet the husks after they are ripe, opening themselves, will hold their seed with them for two or three months, and not shed them.

Government and Virtues.] It is supposed to be under the dominion of Saturn. It is used by many country people to purge corrupt phlegm and choler which they do by drinking the decoction of the roots; and some, to make it more gentle, do but infuse the sliced roots in ale; and some take the leaves, which serve well for the weaker stomachs: The juice hereof put up, or snuffed up the nose, causeth sneezing, and draweth from the head much corruption; and the powder thereof doth the same. The powder thereof drank in wine, helpeth those that are troubled with cramps and convulsions, or with the gout and sciatica, and giveth ease to those that have griping pains in their body and belly, and helpeth those that have the stranguary, It is given with much profit to those that have had long fluxes by the sharp and evil quality of humours, which it stayeth, having first cleansed and purged them by the drying and binding property therein. The root boiled in wine and drank, doth effectually procure women's courses, and used as a pessary, worketh the same effect, but causeth abortion in women with child. Half a dram of the seed beaten to powder, and taken in wine, doth speedily cause one to piss, which otherwise cannot. The same taken with vinegar, dissolveth the hardness and swellings of the spleen. The root is very effectual in all wounds, especially of the head; as also to draw forth any splinters, thorns, or broken bones, or any other thing sticking in the flesh, without causing pains, being used with a little verdigrease and honey, and the great Centaury root. The same boiled in vinegar, and laid upon any tumour or swelling, doth very effectually dissolve and consume them; yea, even the swellings of the throat called king's evil; the juice of the leaves or roots healeth the itch, and all running or spreading scabs, sores, blemishes, or scars in the skin, wheresoever they be.

GOLDEN ROD.

Descript.] THIS ariseth up with brownish small round stalks, two feet high, and sometimes more, having thereon many narrow and long dark green leaves, very seldom with any dents about the edges, or any stalks or white spots therein, yet they are sometimes so found divided at the tops into many small branches, with divers small yellow flowers on every one of them, all which are turned one way, and being ripe, do turn into down, and are carried away by the wind. The root consists of many small fibres, which grows not deep in the ground, but abideth all the winter therein, shooting forth new branches every year, the old one lying down to the ground.

Place.] It groweth in the open places of woods and copses, both moist and dry grounds, in many places of this land.

Time.] It flowereth about the month of July.

Government and Virtues.] Venus claims the herb, and therefore to be sure it respects beauty lost. Arnoldus de Villa

Villa Nova commends it much against the stone in the reins and kidneys, and to provoke urine in abundance, whereby also the gravel and stone may be voided. The decoction of the herb, green or dry, or the distilled water thereof, is very effectual for inward bruises, as also to be outwardly applied, it stayeth bleeding in any part of the body, and of wounds; also the fluxes of humours, the bloody-flux, and womens courses; and is no less prevalent in all ruptures or burstings, being drank inwardly, and outwardly applied. It is a sovereign wound herb, inferior to none, both for inward and outward hurts; green wounds, old sores and ulcers, are quickly cured therewith. It also is of especial use in all lotions for sores or ulcers in the mouth, throat, or privy parts of man or woman. The decoction also helpeth to fasten the teeth that are loose in the gums.

GOUTWORT, or HERB GERRARD.

Descript.] IT is a low herb, seldom rising half a yard high, having sundry leaves standing on brownish green stalks by three, snipped about, and of a strong unpleasant savour: The umbels of the flowers are white, and the seed blackish, the root runneth in the ground, quickly taking a great deal of room.

Place.] It groweth by hedge and wall-sides, and often in the border and corners of fields, and in gardens also.

Time.] It flowereth and seedeth about the end of July.

Government and Virtues.] Saturn rules it. Neither is it to be supposed Goutwort hath its name for nothing, but upon experiment to heal the gout and sciatica; as also joint-achs, and other cold griefs. The very bearing of it about one easeth the pains of the gout, and defends him that bears it from the disease.

GROMEL.

OF this I shall briefly describe their kinds, which are principally used in physick, the virtues whereof are alike, though somewhat different in their manner and form of growing.

Descript.] The greater Gromel groweth up with slender hard and hairy stalks, trailing and taking root in the

 ground,

ground, as it lieth thereon, and parted into many other small branches with hairy dark green leaves thereon. At the joints with the leaves come forth very ſmall blue flowers, and after them hard ſtony roundiſh ſeed. The root is long and woody, abiding the Winter, and ſhooteth forth freſh ſtalks in the ſpring.

The ſmaller wild Gromel ſendeth forth divers upright hard branched ſtalks, two or three feet high, full of joints, at every one of which groweth ſmall, long, hard, and rough leaves like the former, but leſſer; among which leaves come forth ſmall white flowers, and after them greyiſh round ſeed like the former; the root is not very big, but with many ſtrings thereat.

The garden Gromel hath divers upright, ſlender, woody, hairy ſtalks, blown and creſſed, very little branched, with leaves like the former, and white flowers; after which, in rough brown huſks, is contained a white, hard, round ſeed, ſhining like pearls, and greater than either of the former; the root is like the firſt deſcribed, with divers branches and ſprigs thereat, which continueth (as the firſt doth) all the Winter.

Place.] The two firſt grow wild in barren or untilled places, and by the way ſides in many places of this land. The laſt is a nurſling in the gardens of the curious.

Time.] They all flower from Midſummer until September ſometimes and in the mean time the ſeed ripeneth.

Government and Virtues.] The herb belongs to Dame Venus; and therefore if Mars cauſe the colick or ſtone, as uſually he doth, if in Virgo, this is your cure. Theſe are accounted to be of as ſingular force as any herb or ſeed whatſoever, to break the ſtone and to void it, and the gravel either in the reins or bladder, as alſo to provoke urine being ſtopped, and to help the ſtranguary. The ſeed is of greateſt uſe, being bruiſed and boiled in white wine or in broth, or the like, or the powder of the ſeed taken therein. Two drams of the ſeed in powder taken with womens breaſt milk, is very effectual to procure a very ſpeedy delivery to ſuch women as have ſore pains in their travail, and cannot be delivered: The herb itſelf, (when the ſeed is not to be had) either boiled, or the juice thereof drank,

drank, is effectual to all the purposes aforesaid, but not so powerful or speedy in operation.

GOOSEBERRY BUSH.

CALLED also Feapberry, and in Sussex Dewberry Bush, and in some counties Wineberry.

Government and Virtues.] They are under the dominion of Venus. The berries, while they are unripe, being scalded, or baked, are good to stir up a fainting or decayed appetite, especially such whose stomachs are afflicted by cholerick humours: They are excellent good to stay longings of women with child. You may keep them preserved with sugar all the year long. The decoction of the leaves of the tree cools hot swellings and inflammations; as also St Anthony's fire. The ripe Goosberries being eaten, are an excellent remedy to allay the violent heat both of the stomach and liver. The young and tender leaves break the stone, and expel gravel both from the kidneys and bladder. All the evils they do to the body of man is, they are supposed to breed crudities, and by crudities, worms.

WINTER-GREEN.

Descript.] THIS sends forth seven, eight, or nine leaves from a small brown creeping root, every one standing upon a long foot stalk, which are almost as broad as long, round pointed, of a sad green colour, and hard in handling, and like the leaf of a Pear-tree; from whence ariseth a slender weak stalk, yet standing upright, bearing at the top many small white sweet-smelling flowers, laid open like a star, consisting of five round pointed leaves, with many yellowish threads standing in the middle about a green head, and a long stalk with them, which in time groweth to be the seed-vessel, which being ripe is found five square, with a small point at it, wherein is contained seed as small as dust.

Place.] It groweth seldom in fields, but frequent in the woods northwards, viz. in Yorkshire, Lancashire, and Scotland.

Time.] It flowereth about June and July.

Government and Virtues.] Winter-green is under the

dominion of Saturn, and is a singular good wound herb, and an especial remedy for to heal green wounds speedily, the green leaves being bruised and applied, or the juice of them. A salve made of the green herb stamped, or the juice boiled with hog's lard, or with salid oil and wax, and some turpintine added unto it, is a sovereign salve, and highly extolled by the Germans, who use it to heal all manner of wounds and sores. The herb boiled in wine and water, and given to drink to them that have any inward ulcers in their kidneys, or neck of the bladder, doth wonderfully help them. It stayeth all fluxes, as the lask, bloody fluxes, womens courses, and bleeding of wounds, and taketh away any inflammations rising upon pains of the heart; it is no less helpful for foul ulcers hard to be cured; as also for cankers or fistulas. The distilled water of the herb doth effectually perform the same things.

GROUNDSEL.

Descript.] OUR common Groundsel hath a round green and somewhat brownish stalk, spreading toward the top into branches, set with long and somewhat narrow green leaves, cut in on the edges, somewhat like the oak-leaves, but lesser, and round at the end. At the tops of the branches stand many small green heads, out of which grow many small, yellow threads or thumbs, which are the flowers, and continue many days blown in that manner, before it pass away into down, and with the seed is carried away in the wind. The root is small and thready, and soon perisheth, and as soon riseth again of its own sowing, so that may be seen many months in the year, both green and in flower, and seed; for it will spring and seed twice in a year at least, if it be suffered in a garden.

Place.] This groweth almost every where, as well on tops of walls, as at the foot, amongst rubbish and untilled grounds, but especially in gardens.

Time.] It flowereth, as is said before, almost in every month throughout the year.

Government and Virtues.] This herb is Venus's mistress-piece, and is as gallant and universal medicine for all diseases

eaſes coming of heat, in what part of the body ſoever they be, as the ſun ſhines upon; it is very ſafe and friendly to the body of man; yet cauſeth vomiting if the ſtomach be afflicted; if not, purging; and it doth it with more gentleneſs than can be expected; it is moiſt, and ſomething cold withal, thereby cauſing expulſion, and repreſſing the heat cauſed by the motion of the internal parts in purges and vomits. Lay by our learned receipts; take ſo much Sena, ſo much Scammony, ſo much Colocynthis, ſo much infuſion of Crocus Metallorum, &c. this herb alone preſerved in a ſyrup, in a diſtilled water, or in an ointment, ſhall do the deed for you in all hot diſeaſes, and, ſhall do it, 1. Safely, 2. Speedily.

The decoction of the herb (ſaith Dioſcorides) made with wine, and drank, helpeth the pains of the ſtomach, proceeding of choler, (which it may well do by a vomit) as daily experience ſheweth. The juice thereof taken in drink, or the decoction of it in ale, gently performeth the ſame. It is good againſt the jaundice and falling ſickneſs, being taken in wine; as alſo againſt difficulty of making water. It provokes urine, expelleth gravel in the reins or kidneys; a dram thereof given in oxymel, after ſome walking or ſtirring of the body. It helpeth alſo the ſciatica, griping of the belly, the colick; defects of the liver, and provoketh womens courſes. The freſh herb boiled, and made into a poultice, applied to the breaſts of women that are ſwolen with pain and heat, as alſo the privy parts of man or woman, the ſeat or fundament, or the arteries, joints, and ſinews, when they are inflamed and ſwolen, doth much eaſe them; and uſed with ſome ſalt, helpeth to diſſolve knots or kernels in any part of the body. The juice of the herb, or (as Dioſcorides ſaith) the leaves and flowers, with ſome fine frankincenſe in powder, uſed in wounds of the body, nerves or ſinews, do ſingularly help to heal them. The diſtilled water of the herb performeth well all the aforſaid cures, but eſpecially for inflammations or watering of the eyes, by reaſon of the defluction of rheum into them.

HEART'S-EASE.

THIS is that herb which such physicians as are licensed to blaspheme by authority, without danger of having their tongues burned through with an hot iron, called an herb of the Trinity. It is also called by those that are more moderate, Three Faces in a Hood, Live in Idleness, Cull me to you; and in Sussex we call them Pancies.

Place.] Besides those which are brought up in gardens, they grow commonly wild in the fields, especially in such as are very barren; sometimes you may find it on the tops of the high hills.

Time.] They flower all the Spring and Summer long.

Government and Virtues.] The herb is really Saturnine, something cold, viscous, and slimy. A strong decoction of the herbs and flowers (if you will, you may make it into syrup) is an excellent cure for the French-pox, the herb being a gallant antivenerean; and that antivenereans are the best cure for that disease, far better and safer than to torment them with the flux, divers foreign physicians have confessed. The spirit of it is excellent good for the convulsions in children, as also for the falling-sickness, and a gallant remedy for the inflammation of the lungs and breasts, plurisy, scabs, itch, &c. It is under the celestial sign Cancer.

ARTICHOKES.

THE Latins call them Cinera, only our college calls them Artichocus.

Government and Virtues.] They are under the dominion of Venus, and therefore it is no marvel if they provoke lust, as indeed they do, being something windy meat; and yet they stay the involuntary course of natural seed in man, which is commonly called nocturnal pollutions. And here I care not greatly if I quote a little of Galen's nonsense in his treatise of the faculties of nourishment. He saith, they contain plenty of cholerick juice (which notwithstanding I can scarely believe) of which he saith is engendered melancholy juice, and of that melancholy juice thin cholerick blood. But to proceed; this is certain,

tain, that the decoction of the root boiled in wine, or the root bruised and distilled in wine in an alembick, and being drank, purgeth by urine exceedingly.

HARTS-TONGUE.

Descript.] THIS hath divers leaves arising from the root, every one severally, which fold themselves in their first springing and spreading; when they are full grown, are about a foot long, smooth and green above, but hard and with little sap in them, and streaked on the back, thwart on both sides of the middle rib, with small and somewhat long and brownish marks; the bottoms of the leaves are a little bowed on each side of the middle rib, somewhat narrow with the length, and somewhat small at the end. The root is of many black threads, folded or interlaced together.

Time.] It is green all the Winter; but new leaves spring every year.

Government and Virtues.] Jupiter claims dominion over this herb, therefore it is a singular remedy for the liver, both to strengthen it when weak, and ease it when afflicted, you shall do well to keep it in a syrup all the year: For though authors say it is green all the year, I scarce believe it. Harts-Tongue is much commended against the hardness and stoppings of the spleen and liver, and against the heat of the liver and stomach, and against lasks, and the bloody-flux. The distilled water thereof is also very good against the passions of the heart, and to stay the hiccough, to help the falling of the palate, and to stay the bleeding of the gums, being gargled in the mouth. Dioscorides saith, it is good against the stinging or biting of serpents. As for the use of it, my direction at the latter end will be sufficient, and enough for those that are studious in physick, to whet their brains upon for one year or two.

HAZEL-NUT.

HAZEL Nuts are so well known to every body, that they need no description.

Government and Virtues.] They are under the dominion of Mercury. The parted kernels made into an electuary,

lectuary, or the milk drawn from the kernels with mead or honeyed water, is very good to help an old cough; and being parched, and a little pepper put to them and drank, digesteth the distillations of rheum from the head. The dried husks and shells, to the weight of two drams, taken in red wine, stayeth lasks and womens courses, and so doth the red skin that covers the kernels, which is more effectual to stay womens courses.

And if this be true, as it is, then why should the vulgar so familiarly affirm, that eating Nuts causeth shortness of breath, than which nothing is falser? For, how can that which strengthens the lungs, cause shortness of breath? I confess, the opinion is far older than I am; I knew tradition was a friend to error before, but never that he was the father of slander: Or are mens tongues so given to slandering one another, that they must slander Nuts too, to keep their tongues in use? If any thing of the Hazel Nut be stopping, it is the husks and shells, and no body is so mad to eat them, unless physically; and the red skin which covers the kernel, you may easily pull off. And so thus have I made an apology for Nuts, which cannot speak for themselves.

HAWK-WEED.

Descript.] IT hath many large leaves lying upon the ground, much rent or torn on the sides into gashes like Dandelion, but with greater parts, more like the smooth Sow Thistle, from among which riseth a hollow, rough stalk, two or three feet high, branched from the middle upward, whereon are set at every joint longer leaves, little or nothing rent or cut, bearing on their top sundry pale, yellow flowers, consisting of many small, narrow leaves, broad pointed, and nicked in at the ends, set in a double row or more, the outermost being larger than the inner, which from most of the Hawkweeds (for there are many kinds of them) do hold, which turn into down, and with the small brownish seed is blown away with the wind. The root is long, and somewhat greater, with many small fibres thereat. The whole plant is full of bitter milk.

Place.

weth in divers places about the field-sides, ays in dry grounds.
vereth and flies away in Summer Months.
nd Virtues.] Saturn owns it. Hawk-weed es) is cooling, somewhat drying and bind-re good for the heat of the stomach, and n; for inflammations, and the hot fits of aice thereof in wine, helpeth digestion, , hindereth crudities abiding in the sto-peth the difficulty of making water, the ous serpents, and stinging of the scorpion, lso outwardly applied to the place, and is ast all other poisons. A scruple of the n in wine and vinegar, is profitable for the dropsy. The decoction of the herb ey, degesteth the phlegm in the chest or hyssop helpeth the cough. The decoc-d of wild succory, made with wine, and he wind colic and hardness of the spleen; t and sleep, hindereth venery and vener-ling heats, purgeth the stomach, increas-helpeth the diseases of reins and bladder. ied, it is singularly good for all the defects the eyes, used with some womens milk; good success in fretting or creeping ulcers, beginning. The green leaves bruised, e salt applied to any place burnt with fire, lo arise, helpeth them; as also inflamma-ony's fire, and all pushes and eruptions, legm. The same applied with meal and anner of a poultice, to any place affected s and the cramp, such as are out of joint, and ease. The distilled water cleanseth keth away freckles, spots, morphew, or face.

HAWTHORN.

ntent to trouble you with a description of nich is so well known that it needeth none. but a hedge bush, although being pruned groweth to a tree of a reasonable height.

As

As for the Hawthorn Tree at Glastenbury, which is said to flower yearly on Christmas-day, it rather shews the superstition of those that observe it for the time of its flowering, than any great wonder, since the like may be found in divers other places of this land; as in Whey-street in Romney Marsh, and near unto Nantwich in Cheshire, by a place called White Green, where it flowereth about Christmas and May. If the weather be frosty, it flowereth not until January or that the hard weather be over.

Government and Virtues.] It is a Tree of Mars. The seeds in the berries beaten to powder being drank in wine, are held singular good against the stone, and are good for the dropsy. The distilled water of the flowers stayeth the lask. The seed cleared from the down, bruised and boiled in wine, and drank, is good for inward tormenting pains. If cloths and spunges be wet in the distilled water, and applied to any place wherein thorns and splinters, or the like, do abide in the flesh, it will notably draw them forth.

And thus you see the thorn gives a medicine for his own pricking, and so doth almost every thing else.

HEMLOCK.

Descript.] THE common great Hemlock groweth up with a green stalk, four or five feet high, or more, full of red spots sometimes, and at the joints very large winged leaves set at them, which are divided into many other winged leaves one set against the other, dented about the edges, of a sad green colour, branched towards the top, where it is full of umbels of white flowers, and afterwards with whitish flat seed: The root is long, white, and sometimes crooked, and hollow within. The whole plant, and every part, hath a strong, heady, and ill-favoured scent, much offending the senses.

Place.] It groweth in all counties of this land, by walls and hedge-sides, in waste grounds and untilled places.

Time.] It flowereth and seedeth in July, or thereabouts.

Government and Virtues.] Saturn claims dominion over this herb, yet I wonder why it may not be applied to the privities in a Priapism, or continual standing of the yard, it being very beneficial to that disease: I suppose, my author's thor's judgment was firſt upon the oppoſite diſpoſition of Saturn to Venus in thoſe faculties, and therefore he forbad the applying of it to thoſe parts, that it might not cauſe barrenneſs, or ſpoil the ſpirit procreative; which if it do, yet applied to the privities, it ſtops its luſtful thoughts. Hemlock is exceedingly cold, and very dangerous, eſpecially to be taken inwardly. It may ſafely be applied to inflammations, tumours, and ſwellings in any part of the body (ſave the privy parts) as alſo to St Anthony's fire, wheals, puſhes, and creeping ulcers that ariſe of hot ſharp humours, by cooling and repelling the heat; the leaves bruiſed and laid to the brow or forehead are good for their eyes that are red and ſwollen; as alſo to take away a pin and web growing in the eye; this is a tried medicine: Take a ſmall handful of this herb, and half ſo much Bay ſalt, beaten together, and applied to the contrary wriſt of the hand, for 24 hours, doth remove it in thrice dreſſing. If the root thereof be roaſted under the embers, wrapped in double wet paper, until it be ſoft and tender, and then applied to the gout in the hands or fingers, it will quickly help this evil. If any through miſtake eat the herb Hemlock inſtead of Parſley, or the roots inſtead of a Parſnip (both of which it is very like) whereby happeneth a kind of frenzy, or perturbation of the ſenſes, as if they were ſtupid and drunk, the remedy is (as Pliny ſaith) to drink of the beſt and ſtrongeſt pure wine, before it ſtrikes to the heart, or gentian put in wine, or a draught of vinegar, wherewith Tragus doth affirm, that he cured a woman that had eaten the root.

HEMP.

THIS is ſo well known to every good houſe-wife in the country, that I ſhall not need to write any deſcription of it.

Time.] It is ſown in the end of March, or beginning of April, and is ripe in Auguſt or September.

Government and Virtues.] It is a plant of Saturn, and good for ſomething elſe, you ſee, than to make halters only. The ſeed of hemp conſumeth wind, and by too much uſe thereof diſperſeth it ſo much, that it drieth up the natural ſeed for procreation; yet being boiled in milk, and taken, helpeth ſuch as have a hot dry cough. The Dutch make an emulſion out of the ſeed, and give it with good ſucceſs to thoſe that have the jaundice, eſpecially in the beginning of the diſeaſe, if there be no ague accompanying it, for it openeth obſtructions of the gall, and cauſeth digeſtion of choler. The emulſion or decoction of the ſeed ſtayeth laſks and continual fluxes, eaſeth the colic, and allayeth the troubleſome humours in the bowels, and ſtayeth bleeding at the mouth, noſe, or other places, ſome of the leaves being fried with the blood of them that bleed, and ſo given them to eat. It is held very good to kill the worms in men or beaſts; and the juice dropped into the ears killeth worms in them; and draweth forth earwigs, or other living creatures gotten into them. The decoction of the root allayeth inflammations of the head, or any other parts; the herb itſelf, or the diſtilled water thereof, doth the like. The decoction of the roots eaſeth the pains of the gout, the hard humours of knots in the joints, the pains and ſhrinking of the ſinews, and the pains of the hips. The freſh juice mixed with a little oil and butter, is good for any place that hath been burnt with fire, being thereto applied.

HENBANE.

Deſcript.] OUR common Henbane hath very large, thick, ſoft, woolly leaves, lying on the ground, much cut in, or torn on the edges, of a dark, ill greyiſh green colour; among which ariſe up divers thick and ſhort ſtalks, two or three feet high, ſpread into divers ſmall branches, with leſſer leaves on them, and many hollow flowers, ſcarce appearing above the huſk, and uſually torn on one ſide, ending in five round points, growing one above another, of a deadiſh yellowiſh colour, ſomewhat paler towards the edges, with many purpliſh veins therein, and of a dark, yellowiſh purple in the bottom of the flower, with a ſmall point of the ſame colour in the middle, each of them ſtanding in a hard cloſe huſk, which after the flowers is paſt, groweth very like the huſk of Aſarabacca, and ſomewhat ſharp at the top points, wherein is contained much ſmall ſeed, very like Poppy Seed, but of a duſky, greyiſh colour. The root is great, white, and thick, branching forth divers ways under ground, ſo like Parſnip root (but that it is not ſo white) that it hath deceived others. The whole plant, more than the root, hath a very heavy, ill, ſoporiferous ſmell, ſomewhat offenſive.

Place.] It commonly groweth by the way-ſides, and under hedge-ſides and walls.

Time.] It flowereth in July, and ſpringeth again yearly of its own ſeed. I doubt my author's miſtook July for June if not for May.

Government and Virtues.] I wonder how aſtrologers could take on them to make this an herb of Jupiter; and yet Mezaldus, a man of a penetrating brain, was of that opinion as well as the reſt; the herb is indeed under the dominion of Saturn, and I prove it by this argument: All the herbs which delight moſt to grow in Saturnine places, are Saturnine herbs. But Henbane delights moſt to grow in Saturnine places, and whole cart loads of it may be found near the places where they empty the common Jacks, and ſcarce a ditch to be found without it growing by it. Ergo, it is an herb of Saturn. The leaves of Henbane do cool all hot inflammations in the eyes, or any other part of the body; and are good to aſſuage all manner of ſwellings of the cods, or womens breaſts, or elſewhere, if they be boiled in wine, and either applied themſelves, or the fomentation warm; it alſo aſſuageth the pain of the gout, the ſciatica, and other pains in the joints which ariſe from a hot cauſe. And applied with vinegar to the forehead and temples, helpeth the head-ach and want of ſleep in hot fevers. The juice of the herb or ſeed, or the oil drawn from the ſeed, does the like. The oil of the ſeed is helpful for deafneſs, noiſe, and worms in the ears, being dropped therein; the juice of the herb or root doth the ſame. The decoction of the herb or ſeed, or both, killeth lice in man or beaſt. The fume of the dried herb, ſtalks and ſeed, burned, quickly healeth ſwellings, chilblains or kibes in the hands or feet, by holding them in the fume thereof. The remedy to help thoſe that have taken Henbane is to drink goat's milk, honeyed water, or pine kernels, with ſweet wine; or, in the abſence of theſe, Fennel-ſeed, Nettle-ſeed, the feed of Creffes, Muftard, or Raddifh; as alfo Onions or Garlick taken in wine, do all help to free them from danger, and reftore them to their due temper again.

Take notice, that this herb muft never be taken inwardly; outwardly, an oil, ointment, or plaifter of it, is moft admirable for the gout, to cool the venereal heat of the reins in the French-pox; to ftop the tooth-ach, being applied to the aking fide; to allay all inflammations, and to help the difeafes before premifed.

HEDGE HYSSOP.

Defcript.] DIVERS forts there are of this plant; the firft of which is an Italian by birth, and only nurfed up here in the gardens of the curious. Two or three forts are found commonly growing wild here, the defcription of two of which I fhall give you. The firft is a fmooth, low plant, not a foot high, very bitter in tafte, with many fquare ftalks, diverfely branched from the bottom to the top, with divers joints, and two fmall leaves at each joint, broader at the bottom than they are at the end, a little dented about the edges, of a fad green colour, and full of veins. The flowers ftand at the joints, being of a fair purple colour, with fome white fpots in them, in fafhion like thofe of dead nettles. The feed is fmall and yellow, and the roots fpread much under ground.

The fecond feldom groweth half a foot high, fending up many fmall branches, whereon grow many fmall leaves fet one againft the other, fomewhat broad, but very fhort. The flowers are like the flowers of the other in fafhion, but of a pale reddifh colour. The feeds are fmall and yellowifh. The root fpreadeth like the other, neither will it yield to its fellow one ace of bitternefs.

Place.] They grow in wet low grounds, and by the water-fides; the laft may be found among the bogs on Hamftead Heath.

Time.] They flower in June and July, and the feed is ripe prefently after.

Government and Virtues.] They are herbs of Mars, and as cholerick and churlifh as he is, being moft violent purges, efpecially of choler and phlegm. It is not fafe taking them inwardly, unlefs they be well rectified by the art of the

the alchymist, and only the purity of them given; so used they may be very helpful both for the dropsy, gout, and sciatica; outwardly used in ointments they kill worms, the belly anointed with it, and are excellent good to cleanse old and filthy ulcers.

Black Hellebore.

IT is also called Setter-wort, Setter-grass, Bears-foot, Christmas-herb, and Christmas-flower.

Descript.] It hath sundry fair green leaves rising from the root, each of them standing about an handful high from the earth; each leaf is divided into seven, eight, or nine parts, dented from the middle of the leaf to the point on both sides, abiding green all the Winter; about Christmas-time, if the weather be any thing temperate, the flowers appear upon foot-stalks, also consisting of five large, round, white leaves a-piece, which sometimes are purple towards the edges, with many pale yellow thumbs in the middle; the seeds are divided into several cells, like those of Columbines, save only that they are greater; the seeds are in colour black, and in form long and round. The root consisteth of numberless blackish strings all united into one head. There is another Black Hellebore, which grows up and down in the woods very like this, but only that the leaves are smaller and narrower, and perish in the Winter, which this doth not.

Place.] The first is maintained in gardens. The second is commonly found in the woods in Northamptonshire.

Time.] The first flowereth in December or January; the second in February or March.

Government and Virtues.] It is an herb of Saturn, and therefore no marvel if it hath some sullen conditions with it, and would be far safer, being purified by the art of the alchymist than given raw. If any have taken any harm by taking it, the common cure is to take goat's milk: If you cannot get goat's milk, you must make a shift with such as you can get. The roots are very effectual against all melancholy diseases, especially such as are of long standing, as quartan agues and madness; it helps the falling-sickness, the leprosy, both the yellow and black jaundice, the gout, sciatica, and convulsions; and this was found out by experience, that the root of that which groweth wild in our country, works not so churlishly as those do which are brought from beyond sea, as being maintained by a more temperate air. The root, used as a pessary, provokes the terms exceedingly; also being beaten into powder, and strewed upon foul ulcers, it consumes the dead flesh, and instantly heals them; nay, it will help gangreens in the beginning. Twenty grains taken inwardly is a sufficient dose for one time, and let that be corrected with half so much cinnamon; country people used to rowel their cattle with it. If a beast be troubled with a cough, or have taken any poison, they bore a hole through his ear, and put a piece of the root in it, this will help him in twenty-four hours time. Many other uses farriers put it to which I shall forbear.

HERB ROBERT.

Descript.] IT riseth up with a reddish stalk two feet high, having divers leaves thereon upon very long and reddish foot-stalks, divided at the ends into three or five divisions, each of them cut in on the edges, some deeper than others, and all dented likewise about the edges, which sometimes turn reddish. At the tops of the stalks come forth divers flowers made of five leaves, much larger than the doves foot, and of a more reddish colour; after which come black heads, as in others. The root is small and thready, and smelleth as the whole plant, very strong, almost stinking.

Place.] This groweth frequently every where by the way sides, upon ditch banks and waste grounds wheresoever one goeth.

Time.] It flowereth in June and July chiefly, and the seed is ripe shortly after.

Government and Virtues.] It is under the dominion of Venus. Herb Robert is commended not only against the stone, but to stay blood, where or howsoever flowing; it speedily healeth all green wounds, and is effectual in old ulcers in the privy parts, or elsewhere. You may persuade yourself this is true, and also conceive a good reason for it, do but consider it is an herb of Venus, for all it hath a man's name.

HERB TRUE-LOVE, or ONE-BERRY.

Descript.] ORDINARY Herb True-love hath a ſmall creeping root running under the uppermoſt cruſt of the ground, ſomewhat like couch graſs root, but not ſo white, ſhooting forth ſtalks with leaves, ſome whereof carry no berries, the others do; every ſtalk ſmooth without joints, and blackiſh green, riſing about half a foot high, if it bear berries, otherwiſe ſeldom ſo high, bearing at the top four leaves ſet directly one againſt another, in manner of a croſs or ribband tied (as it is called) in a true loves knot, which are each of them apart ſomewhat like unto a night-ſhade leaf, but ſomewhat broader, having ſometimes three leaves, ſometimes five, ſometimes ſix, and thoſe ſometimes greater than in others, in the middle of the four leaves riſeth up one ſmall ſlender ſtalk, about an inch high, bearing at the tops thereof one flower ſpread open like a ſtar, conſiſting of four ſmall and long narrow pointed leaves of a yellowiſh green colour, and four others lying between them leſſer than they; in the middle whereof ſtands a round dark purpliſh button or head, compaſſed about with eight ſmall yellow mealy threads with three colours, making it the more conſpicuous and lovely to behold. This button or head in the middle, when the other leaves are withered, becometh a blackiſh purple berry, full of juice, of the bigneſs of a reaſonable grape, having within it many white ſeeds. The whole plant is without any manifeſt taſte.

Place.] It groweth in woods and copſes, and ſometimes in the corners or borders of fields, and waſte grounds in very many places of this land, and abundantly in the woods, copſes, and other places about Chiſlehurſt and Maidſtone in Kent.

Time.] They ſpring up in the middle of April or May, and are in flower ſoon after. The berries are ripe in the end of May, and in ſome places in June.

Government and Virtues.] Venus owns it; the leaves or berries hereof are effectual to expel poiſon of all ſorts, eſpecially that of the aconites; as alſo, the plague, and other peſtilential diſorders: Matthiolus ſaith, that ſome that have lain long in a lingering ſickneſs, and others that

by

by witchcraft (as it was thought) were become half foolish, by taking a dram of the seeds or berries hereof in powder every day for twenty days together, were restored to their former health. The roots in powder taken in wine easeth the pains of the colick speedily. The leaves are very effectual as well for green wounds, as to cleanse and heal up filthy old sores and ulcers; and is very powerful to discuss all tumours and swellings in the cods, privy parts, the groin, or in any part of the body, and speedily to allay all inflammations. The juice of the leaves applied to felons, or those nails of the hands or toes that have imposthumes or sores gathered together at the roots of them, healeth them in a short space. The herb is not to be described for the premises, but is fit to be nourished in every good woman's garden.

HYSSOP.

HYSSOP is so well known to be an inhabitant in every garden, that it will save me labour in writing a description thereof. The virtues are as follow.

Temperature and Virtues.] The herb is Jupiter's, and the sign Cancer. It strengthens all the parts of the body under Cancer and Jupiter; which what they may be, is found amply discussed in my astrological judgement of diseases. Dioscorides saith, that Hyssop boiled with rue and honey, and drank, helpeth those that are troubled with coughs, shortness of breath, wheezing and rheumatic distillations upon the lungs; taken also with oxymel, it purgeth gross humours by stool; and with honey killeth worms in the belly; and with fresh and new figs bruised, helpeth to loosen the belly, and more forcibly if the root of Flower-de-luce and cresses be added thereto. It amendeth and cherisheth the native colour of the body, spoiled by the yellow jaundice; and being taken with figs and nitre, helpeth the dropsy and spleen; being boiled with wine, it is good to wash inflammations, and taketh away the black and blue spots and marks that come by strokes, bruises, or falls, being applied with warm water. It is an excellent medicine for the quinsy, or swelling in the throat to wash and gargle it, being boiled in figs; it helpeth the tooth-ach, being boiled in vinegar and gargled there-

therewith. The hot vapours of the decoction taken by a funnel in at the ears, eaſeth the inflammations and ſinging noiſe of them. Being bruiſed, and ſalt, honey, and cummin ſeed put to it, helpeth thoſe that are ſtung by ſerpents. The oil thereof (the head being anointed) killeth lice, and taketh away itcing of the head. It helpeth thoſe that have the falling ſickneſs, which way ſoever it be applied. It helpeth to expectorate tough phlegm and is effectual in all cold griefs or diſeaſes of the cheſts or lungs, being taken either in ſyrup or licking medicine. The green herb bruiſed and a little ſugar put thereto, doth quickly heal any cut or green wounds, being thereunto applied.

HOPS.

THESE are ſo well known that they need no deſcription; I mean the manured kind, which every good huſband or houſe-wife is acquainted with.

Deſcript.] The wild hop groweth up as the other doth, ramping upon trees or hedges, that ſtand next to them, with rough branches and leaves like the former, but it giveth ſmaller heads, and in far leſs plenty than it, ſo that there is ſcarce a head or two ſeen in a year on divers of this wild kind, wherein conſiſteth the chief difference.

Place.] They delight to grow in low moiſt grounds, and are found in all parts of this land.

Time.] They ſpring not up until April, and flower not until the latter end of June; the heads are not gathered until the middle or latter end of September.

Government and Virtues.] It is under the dominion of Mars. This, in phyſical operations, is to open obſtructions of the liver and ſpleen, to cleanſe the blood, to looſen the belly, to cleanſe the reins from gravel, and provoke urine. The decoction of the tops of Hops, as well of the tame as the wild, worketh the ſame effects. In cleanſing the blood they help to cure the French diſeaſe, and all manner of ſcabs, itch, and other breakings-out of the body; as alſo all tetters, ringworms, and ſpreading ſores, the morphew and all diſcolouring of the ſkin. The decoction of the flowers and tops, do help to expel poiſon that any one hath drank. Halp a dram of the ſeed in powder, taken

taken in drink, killeth worms in the body, bringeth down womens courses, and expelleth urine. A syrup made of the juice and sugar, cureth the yellow jaundice, easeth the head-ach that comes of heat, and tempereth the heat of the liver and stomach, and is profitably given in long and hot agues that rise in choler and blood. Both the wild and the manured are of one property, and alike effectual in all the aforesaid diseases. By all these testimonies beer appears to be better than ale.

Mars owns the plant, and then Dr Reason will tell you how it performs these actions.

HOREHOUND.

Descript.] COMMON Horehound groweth up with square hairy stalks, half a yard or two feet high, set at the joints with two round crumpled rough leaves of a sullen hoary green colour, of a reasonable good scent, but a very bitter taste. The flowers are small, white, and gaping, set in a rough, hard prickly husk round about the joints, with the leaves from the middle of the stalk upward, wherein afterward is found small round blackish seed. The root is blackish, hard and woody, with many strings, and abideth many years.

Place.] It is found in many parts of this land, in dry grounds, and waste green places.

Time.] It flowereth in July, and the seed is ripe in August.

Government and Virtues.] It is an herb of Mercury. A decoction of the dried herb, with the seed, or the juice of the green herb taken with honey, is a remedy for those that are short-winded, have a cough, or are fallen into a consumption, either through long sickness, or thin distillations of rheum upon the lungs. It helpeth to expectorate tough phlegm from the chest, being taken from the roots of Iris or Orris. It is given to women to bring down their courses, to expel their after-birth, and to them that have sore and long travails; as also to those that have taken poison, or are stung or bitten by venomous serpents. The leaves used with honey, purge foul ulcers, stay running or creeping sores, and the growing of the flesh over the nails. It also helpeth pains of the sides. The juice there-

thereof with wine and honey, helpeth to clear the eyesight, and ſnuffed up into the noſtrils, purgeth away the yellow jaundice, and with a little oil of roſes dropped into the ears, eaſeth the pains of them. Galen ſaith, it openeth obſtructions both of the liver and ſpleen, and purgeth the breaſt and lungs of phlegm; and uſed outwardly it both cleanſeth nnd digeſteth. A decoction of Horehound (ſaith Matthiolus) is available for thoſe that have hard livers, and for ſuch as have itches and running tetters. The powder hereof taken, or the decoction, killeth worms. The green leaves bruiſed, and boiled in old hog's-greaſe unto an ointment, healeth the biting of dogs, abateth the ſwellings and pains that come by any pricking of thorns, or ſuch like means; and uſed with vinegar, cleanſeth and healeth tetters. There is a ſyrup made of Horehound to be had at the apothecaries, very good for old coughs, to rid the tough phlegm; as alſo to void cold rheums from the lungs of old folks, and for thoſe that are aſthmatick or ſhort-winded.

HORSETAIL.

OF that there are many kinds, but I ſhall not trouble you nor myſelf with any large deſcription of them, which to do, were but as the proverb is, To find a knot in a ruſh, all the kinds thereof being nothing elſe but knotted ruſhes, ſome with leaves, and ſome without. Take the deſcription of the moſt eminent ſort as followeth.

Deſcript.] The great Horſetail at the firſt ſpringing hath heads ſomewhat like thoſe of aſparagus, and after grow to be hard, rough, hollow ſtalks, jointed at ſundry places up to the top, a foot high, ſo made as if the lower parts were put into the upper, where grow on each ſide a buſh of ſmall long ruſh-like hard leaves, each part reſembling a horſetail, from whence it is ſo called. At the tops of the ſtalks come forth ſmall catkins, like thoſe of trees. The root creepeth under ground, having joints at ſundry places.

Place.] This (as moſt of the other ſorts hereof) groweth in wet grounds.

Time.] They ſpring up in April, and their blooming catkins in July, ſeeding for the moſt part in Auguſt, and then

then perish down to the ground, rising afresh in the Spring.

Government and Virtues.] The herb belongs to Saturn, yet is very harmless, and excellent good for the things following: Horsetail, the smoother rather than the rough, and the leaved rather than the bare, is most physical. It is very powerful to stanch bleeding either inward or outward, the juice or the decoction thereof being drank, or the juice, decoction, or distilled water applied outwardly. It also stayeth all sorts of lasks and fluxes in man or woman, and the pissing of blood; and healeth also not only the inward ulcers, and the excoriation of the entrails, bladder, &c. but all other sorts of foul, moist and running ulcers, and soon sodereth together the tops of green wounds. It cureth all ruptures in children. The decoction thereof in wine being drank, provoketh urine, and helpeth the stone and stranguary; and the distilled water thereof drank two or three times in a day, and a small quantity at a time, also easeth the entrails or guts, and is effectual against a cough that comes by distillation from the head. The juice or distilled water being warmed, aud hot inflammations, pustles or red wheals, and other breakings-out in the skin, being bathed therewith, doth help them, and doth no less ease the swelling heat and inflammation of the fundament, or privy parts in men and women.

HOUSELEEK, or SENGREEN.

BOTH these are so well known to my countrymen, that I shall not need to write any description of them.

Place.] It groweth commonly upon walls and house-sides, and flowereth in July.

Government and Virtues.] It is an herb of Jupiter, and it is reported by Mezaldus, to preserve what it grows upon from fire and lightning. Our ordinary Houseleek is good for all inward heats as well as outward, and in the eyes or other parts of the body; a posset made with the juice of Houseleek, is singular good in all hot agues, for it cooleth and tempereth the blood and spirits, and quencheth the thirst; and also good to stay all hot defluctions or sharp and salt rheums in the eyes, the juice being dropped into them, or into the ears, helpeth them. It helpeth

helpeth alſo other fluxes of humours in the bowels, and the immoderate courſes of women. It cooleth and reſtraineth all other hot inflammations, St Anthony's fire, ſcaldings and burnings, the ſhingles, fretting ulcers, cankers, tetters, ringworms, and the like; and much eaſeth the pain of the gout proceeding from an hot cauſe. The juice alſo taketh away warts and corns in the hands or feet, being often bathed therewith, and the ſkin and leaves being laid on them afterwards. It eaſeth alſo the head-ach, and diſtempered heat of the brain in frenzies or thro' want of ſleep, being applied to the temples and forehead. The leaves bruiſed and laid upon the crown or ſeam of the head, ſtayeth bleeding at the noſe very quickly. The diſtilled water of the herb is profitable for all the purpoſes aforeſaid. The leaves being gently rubbed on any place ſtung with nettles or bees, doth quickly take away the pain.

HOUND'S TONGUE.

Deſcript.] THE [illegible]ary Hound's Tongue hath ma[illegible] ſomewhat narrow, ſoft, hairy, darkiſh green lea[illegible]ying on the ground, ſomewhat like unto Bugloſs leaves, from among which riſeth up a rough hairy ſtalk about two feet high, with ſome ſmaller leaves thereon and branched at the tops into divers parts, with a ſmall leaf at the foot of every branch, which is ſomewhat long with many flowers ſet along the ſame, which branch is crooked or turneth inwards before it flowereth, and openeth by degrees as the flowers doth blow, which conſiſt of ſmall purpliſh red leaves of a dead colour, riſing out of the huſks wherein they ſtand with ſome threads in the middle. It hath ſometimes a white flower. After the flowers are paſt, there cometh rough flat ſeed, with a ſmall pointle in the middle, eaſily cleaving to any garment that it toucheth, and not ſo eaſily pulled off again. The root is black, thick, and long, hard to break, and full of clammy juice, ſmelling ſomewhat ſtrong, of an evil ſcent, as the leaves alſo do.

Place.] It groweth in moiſt places of this land in waſte grounds, and untilled places, by highway ſides, lanes and hedge-ſides.

Time.] It flowereth about May or June, and the ſeed is ripe ſhortly after.

Government and Virtues.] It is a plant under the dominion of Mercury. The root is very effectual uſed in pills, as well as the decoction, or otherwiſe to ſtay all ſharp and thin defluctions of rheum from the head into the eyes or noſe, or upon the ſtomach or lungs, as alſo for coughs and ſhortneſs of breath. The leaves boiled in wine (ſaith Dioſcorides, but others do rather appoint it to be made with water, and to add thereto oil and ſalt) mollifieth or openeth the belly downwards. It alſo helpeth to cure the biting of a mad dog, ſome of the leaves being alſo applied to the wound: The leaves bruiſed, or the juice of them boiled in hog's lard, and applied, helpeth falling away of the hair, which cometh of hot and ſharp humours; as alſo for any place that is ſcalded or burnt; the leaves bruiſed or laid to any green wound doth heal it up quickly; the root baked under the embers, wrapped in paſte or wet paper, or in a wet double cloth, and thereof a ſuppoſitory made, and put up into or applied to the fundament, doth very effectually help the painful piles or hæmorrhoids. The diſtilled water of the herbs and roots is very good to all the purpoſes aforeſaid, to be uſed as well inwardly to drink, as outwardly to waſh any ſore place, for it healeth all manner of wounds and punctures, and thoſe foul ulcers that ariſe by the French pox. Mezaldus adds that the leaves laid under the feet, will keep the dogs from barking at you. It is called Hound's Tongue, becauſe it ties the tongues of hounds; whether true or not, I never tried, yet I cured the biting of a mad dog with this only medicine.

HOLLY, HOLM, or HULVER BUSH.

FOR to deſcribe a tree ſo well known is needleſs.

Govrnment and Virtues.] The tree is Saturnine. The berries expel wind, and therefore are held to be profitable in the colick. The berries have a ſtrong faculty with them; for if you eat a dozen of them in the morning faſting when they are ripe and not dried, they purge the body of groſs and clammy phlegm; but if you dry the berries, and beat them into powder, they bind the body,

and

and ſtop fluxes, bloody-fluxes, and the terms in women. The bark of the tree, and alſo the leaves, are excellent good, being uſed in fomentations for broken bones, and ſuch members as are out of joint. Pliny ſaith, the branches of the tree defend houſes from lightening, and men from witchcraft.

St John's Wort.

Deſcript.] COMMON St John's Wort ſhooteth forth browniſh, upright, hard, round ſtalks, two feet high, ſpreading many branches from the ſides up to the tops of them, with two ſmall leaves ſet one againſt another at every place, which are of a deep green colour, ſomewhat like the leaves of the leſſer Centaury, but narrow, and full of ſmall holes in every leaf, which cannot be ſo well percieved, as when they are held up to the light; at the tops of the ſtalks and branches ſtand yellow flowers of five leaves apiece, with many yellow threads in the middle, which being bruiſed do yield a reddiſh juice like blood; after which come ſmall round heads, wherein is contained ſmall blackiſh ſeed ſmelling like roſin. The root is hard and woody, with divers ſtrings and fibres at it, of a browniſh colour, which abideth in the ground many years, ſhooting anew every Spring.

Place.] This groweth in woods and copſes, as well thoſe that are ſhady, as open to the ſun.

Time.] They flower about Midſummer and July, and their ſeed is ripe in the latter end of July or Auguſt.

Government and Virtues.] It is under the celeſtial ſign Leo, and the dominion of the Sun. It may be if you meet a Papiſt, he will tell you, eſpecially if he be a lawyer, that St John made it over to him by a letter of attorney. It is a ſingular wound herb; boiled in wine and drank, it healeth inward hurts or bruiſes; made into an ointment, in opens obſtructions, diſſolves ſwellings, and cloſes up the lips of wounds. The decoction of the herb and flowers, eſpecially of the ſeed, being drank in wine, with the juice of knot-graſs, helpeth all manner of vomiting and ſpiting of blood, is good for thoſe that are bitten or ſtung by any venomous creature, and for thoſe that cannot make water. Two drams of the ſeed of St John's Wort made into powder and drank in a little broth, doth gently expel choler or congealed blood in the ſtomach. The decoction of the leaves and ſeeds drank ſomewhat warm before the fits of agues, whether they be tertians or quartans, alters the fits, and by often uſing, doth take them quite away. The ſeed is much commended, being drank for forty days together, to help the ſciatica, the falling ſickneſs and the palſy.

IVY.

IT is ſo well known, to every child almoſt, to grow in woods upon the trees, and upon the ſtone walls of churches, houſes, &c. and ſometimes to grow alone of itſelf, though but ſeldom.

Time.] It flowereth not until July, and the berries are not ripe till Chriſtmas, when they have felt winter froſts.

Government and Virtues.] It is under the dominion of Saturn. A pugil of the flowers, which may be about a dram (ſaith Dioſcorides), drank twice a day in red wine, helpeth the laſk and bloody-flux. It is an enemy to the nerves and ſinews, being much taken inwardly, but very helpful unto them, being outwardly applied. Pliny ſaith, the yellow berries are good againſt the jaundice; and taken before one be ſet to drink hard, preſerveth from drunkenneſs, and helpeth thoſe that ſpit blood; and that the white berries being taken inwardly, or applied outwardly, killeth the worms in the belly. The berries are a ſingular remedy to prevent the plague, as alſo to free them from it that have got it, by drinking the berries thereof made into a powder, for two or three days together. They being taken in wine, do certainly help to break the ſtone, provoke urine and womens courſes. The freſh leaves of Ivy, boiled in vinegar, and applied warm to the ſides of thoſe that are troubled with the ſpleen, ach, or ſtitch in the ſides, do give much eaſe: The ſame applied with ſome Roſewater, and oil of Roſes, to the temples and forehead, eaſeth the head-ach, though it be of long continuance. The freſh leaves boiled in wine, and old filthy ulcers hard to be cured waſhed therewith, do wonderfully help to cleanſe them. It alſo quickly health green wounds, and is effectual to heal all burnings and ſcaldings, and all kinds of exulcerations coming thereby or by ſalt

ſalt phlegm or humours in other parts of the body. The juice of the berries or leaves ſnuffed up into the noſe, purgeth the head and brain of thin rheum that maketh defluxions into the eyes and noſe, and curing the ulcers and ſtench therein; the ſame dropped into the ears, helpeth the old and running ſores of them; thoſe that are troubled with the ſpleen, ſhall find much eaſe by continual drinking out of a cup made of Ivy, ſo as the drink may ſtand ſome ſmall time therein before it be drank. Cato ſaith, That wine put into ſuch a cup, will ſoak through it, by reaſon of the antipathy that is between them.

There ſeems to be a very great antipathy between wine and Ivy; for if one hath got a ſurfeit by drinking of wine, his ſpeedieſt cure is to drink a draught of the ſame wine wherein a handful of Ivy leaves, being firſt bruiſed, have been boiled.

JUNIPER BUSH.

FOR to give a deſcription of a buſh ſo commonly known, is needleſs

Place.] They grow plentifully in divers woods in Kent, Warney Common near Brentwood in Eſſex, upon Finchley Common without Highgate; hard by the New-found Wells near Dulwich, upon a Common between Mitcham and Croydon, in the Highgate near Amerſham in Buckinghamſhire, and many other places.

Time.] The berries are not ripe the firſt year, but continue green two ſummers and one winter before they are ripe; at which time they are all of a black colour, and therefore you ſhall always find upon the buſh green berries; the berries are ripe about the fall of the leaf.

Government and Virtues.] This admirable ſolar ſhrub is ſcarce to be paralleled for its virtues. The berries are hot in the third degree, and dry but in the firſt, being a moſt admirable counter-poiſon, and as great a reſiſter of the peſtilence, as any grows; they are excellent good againſt the bitings of venomous beaſts, they provoke urine exceedingly, and therefore are very available to dyſuries and ſtranguries. It is ſo powerful a remedy againſt the dropſy, that the very lee made of the aſhes of the herb being drank, cures the diſeaſe. It provokes the terms, helps the fits of the mother, ſtrengthens the ſtomach exceedingly, and expels the wind. Indeed there is ſcarce a better remedy for wind in any part of the body, or the colic, than the chymical oil drawn from the berries; ſuch country people as know not how to draw the chymical oil, may content themſelves by eating ten or a dozen of the ripe berries every morning faſting. They are admirable good for a cough, ſhortneſs of breath, and conſumption, pains in the belly, ruptures, cramps, and convulſions. They give ſafe and ſpeedy delivery to women with child, they ſtrengthen the brain exceedingly, help the memory, and fortify the ſight by ſtrenthening the optic nerves; are excellent good in all ſorts of agues; help the gout and ſciatica, and ſtrengthen all the limbs of the body. The aſhes of the wood is a ſpeedy remedy to ſuch as have the ſcurvy, to rub their gums with. The berries ſtay all fluxes, help the hæmorrhoids or piles, and kill worms in children. A lee made of the aſhes of the wood, and the body bathed with it, cures the itch, ſcabs and leproſy. The berries break the ſtone, procure appetite when it is loſt, and are excellent good for all palſies, and falling-ſickneſs.

KIDNEYWORT, or WALL PENNYROYAL, or WALL PENNYWORT.

Deſcript.] IT hath many thick, flat, and round leaves growing from the root, every one having a long foot-ſtalk, faſtened underneath, about the middle of it, and a little unevenly weaved ſometimes about the edges, of a pale green colour, and ſomewhat yellow on the upper ſide like a ſaucer; from among which ariſe one or more tender, ſmooth, hollow ſtalks half a foot high, with two or three ſmall leaves thereon, uſually not round as thoſe below, but ſomewhat long and divided at the edges: the tops are ſomewhat divided into long branches, bearing a number of flowers, ſet round about a long ſpike one above another, which are hollow and like a little bell of a whitiſh green colour, after which come ſmall heads containing very ſmall browniſh ſeed, which falling on the ground, will plentifully ſpring up before winter, if it have moiſture. The root is round and moſt uſually ſmooth, greyiſh

greyish without, and white within, having small fibres at the head of the root, and bottom of the stalk.

Place.] It groweth very plentifully in many places of this land, but especially in all the west parts thereof, upon stone and mud walls, upon rocks also, and in stony places upon the ground, at the bottom of old trees, and sometimes on the bodies of them that are decayed and rotten.

Time.] It usually flowereth in the beginning of May, and the seed ripineth quickly after, sheddeth itself; so that about the end of May, usually the leaves and stalks are withered, dry, and gone until September, that the leaves spring up again, and so abide all winter.

Government and Virtues.] Venus challengeth the herb under Libra. The juice or the distilled water being drank, is very effectual for all inflammations and unnatural heats, to cool a fainting hot stomach, a hot liver, or the bowels; the herb, juice, or distilled water thereof, outwardly applied, healeth pimples, St Anthony's fire, and other outward heats. The said juice or water helpeth to heal sore kidneys, torn or fretted by the stone, or exulcerated within; it also provoketh urine, is available for the dropsy, and helpeth to break the stone. Being used as a bath, or made into an ointment, it cooleth the painful piles or hæmorrhoidal veins. It is no less effectual to give ease to pains of the hot gout, the sciatica, and the inflammations and swellings in the cods; it helpeth the kernels or knots in the neck or throat, called the king's evil; healing kibes and chilblains if they be bathed with the juice, or anointed with ointment made thereof, and some of the skin of the leaf upon them; it is also used in green wounds to stay the blood, and to heal them quickly.

KNAPWEED.

Descript.] THE common sort hereof hath many long and somewhat broad dark green leaves, rising from the root, dented about the edges, and sometimes a little rent or torn on both sides in two or three places, and somewhat hairy withal; amongst which ariseth a long round stalk, four or five feet high, divided into many branches, at the tops whereof stand great scaly green

green heads, and from the middle of them thrust forth a number of dark purplish red thrumbs or threads, which after they are withered and past, there are found divers black seeds, lying in a great deal of down, somewhat like unto Thistle-seed, but smaller; the root is white, hard and woody, and divers fibres annexed thereunto, which perisheth not, but abideth with leaves thereon all the winter, shooting out fresh every spring.

Place.] It groweth in most fields and meadows, and about their borders and hedges, and in many waste grounds also every where.

Time.] It usually flowereth in June and July, and the seed is ripe shortly after.

Government and Virtues.] Saturn challengeth the herb for his own. This Knapweed helpeth to stay fluxes, both of blood at the mouth or nose, or other outward parts, and those veins that are inwardly broken, or inward wounds, as also the fluxes of the belly; it stayeth distillations of thin and sharp humours from the head upon the stomach and lungs; it is good for those that are bruised by any fall, blows, or otherwise, and is profitable for those that are bursten, and have ruptures, by drinking the decoction of the herb and roots in wine, and applying the same outwardly to the place. It is singularly good in all running sores, cancerous and fistulous, drying up of the moisture, and healing them up gently, without sharpness; it doth the like to running sores or scabs of the head or other parts. It is of special use for the soreness of the throat, swelling of the uvula and jaws, and excellent good to stay bleeding, and heal up all green wounds.

KNOTGRASS.

IT is generally known so well that it needeth no description.

Place.] It groweth in every county of this land, by the highway-sides, and by foot-paths in fields; as also by the sides of old walls.

Time.] It springeth up late in the Spring, and abideth until the Winter, when all the branches perish.

Government and Virtues.] Saturn seems to me to own the herb, and yet some hold the sun; out of doubt 'tis Saturn.

Saturn. The juice of the common Knotgrafs is moft effectual to ftay bleeding of the mouth, being drank in fteeled or red wine; and the bleeding at the nofe, to be applied to the forehead or temples, or to be fquirted up into the noftrils. It is no lefs effectual to cool and temper the heat of the blood and ftomach, and to ftay any flux of the blood and humours, as lafks, bloody-flux, womens courfes, and running of the reins. It is fingular good to provoke urine, help the ftrangury, and allayeth the heat that cometh thereby; and is powerful by urine to expel the gravel or ftone in the kidneys and bladder, a dram of the powder of the herb being taken in wine for many days together: Being boiled in wine and drank, it is profitable to thofe that are ftung or bitten by venomous creatures, and very effectual to ftay all defluctions of rheumatick humours upon the ftomach, and killeth worms in the belly or ftomach, quieteth inward pains that arife from the heat, fharpnefs and corruption of blood and choler. The diftilled water hereof taken by itfelf or with the powder of the herb or feed, is very effectual to all the purpofes aforefaid, and is accounted one of the moft fovereign remedies to cool all manner of inflammations, breaking out through heat, hot fwellings and impofthumes, gangrene and fiftulous cankers, or foul filthy ulcers, being applied or put into them; but efpecially for all forts of ulcers and fores happening in the privy parts of men and women. It helpeth all frefh and green wounds, and fpeedily healeth them. The juice dropped into the ears, cleanfeth them being foul, and having running matter in them.

It is very prevalent for the premifes; as alfo for broken joints and ruptures.

Ladies-Mantle.

Defcript.] IT hath many leaves rifing from the root ftanding upon long hairy foot-ftalks, being almoft round, and a little cut on the edges, into eight or ten parts, making it feem like a ftar, with fo many corners and points, and dented round about, of a light green colour, fomewhat hard in handling, and as it were folded or plaited at firft, and then crumpled in divers places, and a little a little hairy, as the ſtalk is alſo, which riſeth up among them to the height of two or three feet; and being weak, is not able to ſtand upright, but bendeth to the ground, divided at the top into two or three ſmall branches, with ſmall yellowiſh green heads, and flowers of a whitiſh colour breaking out of them; which being paſt, there cometh a ſmall yellowiſh ſeed like a poppy ſeed: The root is ſomewhat long and black, with many ſtrings and fibres thereat.

Place.] It groweth naturally in many paſtures and wood-ſides in Hertfordſhire, Wiltſhire, and Kent, and other places of this land.

Time.] It flowereth in May and June, abideth after ſeed-time green all the winter.

Government and Virtues.] Venus claims the herb as her own. Ladies-Mantle is very proper for thoſe wounds that have inflammations, and is very effectual to ſtay bleeding, vomitings, fluxes of all ſorts, bruiſes by falls or otherwiſe, and helpeth ruptures; and ſuch women or maids as have over great flagging breaſts, cauſing them to grow leſs and hard, being both drank and outwardly applied; the diſtilled water drank for twenty days together helpeth conception, and to retain the birth; if the woman do ſometimes alſo ſit in a bath made of the decoction of the herb. It is one of the moſt ſingular wound herbs that is, and therefore highly prized and praiſed by the Germans, who uſe it in all wounds inward and outward, to drink a decoction thereof, and waſh the wounds therewith, or dip tents therein, and put them into the wounds, which wonderfully drieth up all humidity of the ſores, and abateth inflammations therein. It quickly healeth all green wounds, not ſuffering any corruption to remain behind, and cureth all old ſores, though fiſtulous and hollow.

LAVENDER.

BEING an inhabitant almoſt in every garden, it is ſo well known, that it needeth no deſcription.

Time.] It flowereth about the end of June, and beginning of July.

Government and Virtues.] Mercury owns the herb, and it carries his effects very potently. Lavender is of a ſpecial

cial good uſe for all the griefs and pains of the head and brain that proceed of a cold cauſe, as the apoplexy, falling-ſickneſs, the dropſy, or ſluggiſh malady, cramps, convulſions, palſies, and often faintings. It ſtrengthens the ſtomach, and freeth the liver and ſpleen from obſtructions, provoketh womens courſes, and expelleth the dead child and after-birth. The flowers of Lavender ſteeped in wine, helpeth them to make water that are ſtopped, or are troubled with the wind or colick, if the place be bathed therewith. A decoction made with the flowers of Lavender, Horehound, Fennel, and Aſparagus root, and a little Cinnamon, is very profitably uſed to help the falling-ſickneſs, and the giddineſs or turning of the brain; to gargle the mouth with the decoction thereof, is good againſt the tooth-ach. Two ſpoonfuls of the diſtilled water of the flowers taken, helpeth them that have loſt their voice, as alſo the tremblings and paſſions of the heart, and faintings and ſwooning, not only being drank, but applied to the temples, or noſtrils to be ſmelt unto; but it is not ſafe to uſe it where the body is replete with blood and humours, becauſe of the hot and ſubtil ſpirits wherewith it is poſſeſſed. The chymical oil drawn from Lavender, uſually called Oil of Spike, is of ſo fierce and piercing a quality, that it is cautiouſly to be uſed, ſome few drops being ſufficient, to be given with other things, either for inward or outward griefs.

LAVENDER-COTTON.

IT being a common garden herb, I ſhall forbear the deſcription; only take notice, that it flowereth in June and July.

Government and Virtues.] It is under the dominion of Mercury. It reſiſteth poiſon, putrefaction, and heals the bitings of venomous beaſts: A dram of the powder of the dried leaves taken every morning faſting, ſtops the running of the reins in men, and whites in women. The ſeed beaten into powder, and taken as worm-ſeed, kills the worms, not only in children, but alſo in people of riper years: the like doth the herb itſelf, being ſteeped in milk, and the milk drank; the body bathed with the decoction of it, helps ſcabs and itch.

LADIES-

LADIES-SMOCK, or CUCKOW-FLOWERS.

Descript.] THE root is composed of many small white threads, from whence spring up divers long stalks of winged leaves, consisting of round, tender, dark green leaves, set one against another upon a middle rib, the greatest being at the end, amongst which rise up divers tender, weak round, green stalks, somewhat streaked, with longer and smaller leaves upon them; on the tops of which stand flowers, almost like the Stock Gilliflowers, but rounder, and not so long, of a blushing white colour; the seed is reddish, and groweth to small bunches, being of a sharp biting taste, and so hath the herb.

Place.] They grow in moist places, and near to brooksides.

Time.] They flower in April and May, and the lower leaves continue green all the Winter.

Government and Virtues.] They are under the dominion of the Moon, and very little inferior to Water Cresses in all their operations; they are excellent good for the scurvy; they provoke urine, and break the stone, and excellently warm a cold and weak stomach, restoring lost appetite, and help digestion.

LETTUCE.

IT is so well known, being generally used as a Sallet-herb, that it is altogether needless to write any descip-tion thereof.

Government and Virtues.] The Moon owns them, and that is the reason they cool and moisten what heat and dryness Mars causeth, because Mars hath his fall in Cancer; and they cool the heat because the Sun rules it, between whom and the Moon is a reception in the generation of men, as you may see in my guide for women. The juice of Lettuce mixed or boiled with Oil of Roses, applied to the forehead and temples procureth sleep, and easeth the head-ach proceeding of an hot cause: Being eaten boiled, it helpeth to loosen the belly. It helpeth digestion, quencheth thirst, increaseth milk in nurses, easeth griping pains in the stomach or bowels, that come of choler. It abateth bodily lust, represseth venerous dreams,

being

being outwardly applied to the cods with a little camphire. Applied in the same manner to the region of the heart, liver or reins, or by bathing the said place with the juice of distilled water, wherein some white Sanders, or red roses are put; also it not only represseth the heat and inflammations therein, but comforts and strengthens those parts, and also tempereth the heat of urine. Galen adviseth old men to use it with spice; and where spices are wanting, to add mints, roches, and such like hot herbs, or else citron, lemon or orange seeds, to abate the cold of one, and heat of the other. The seed and distilled water of the Lettuce work the same effects in all things; but the use of Lettuce is chiefly forbidden to those that are short-winded, or have any imperfection in the lungs, or spit blood.

WATER LILY

OF these there are two principally noted kinds, viz. the White and the Yellow.

Descript.] The white Lily hath very large and thick dark green leaves lying on the water, sustained by long and thick foot-stalks, that rise from a great, thick, round, and long tuberous black root, spongy or loose, with many knobs thereon, like eyes, and whitish within; from amidst which rise other the like thick green stalks, sustaining one large great flower thereon, green on the outside, but as white as snow within, consisting of divers rows of long and somewhat thick and narrow leaves, smaller and thiner the more inward they be, encompassing a head with many yellow threads or thrums in the middle; where, after they are past, stand round Poppy like heads, full of broad oily and bitter seed.

The yellow kind is little different from the former, save only that it hath fewer leaves on the flowers, greater and more shining seed, and a whitish root, both within and without. The root of both is somewhat sweet in taste.

Place.] They are found growing in great pools, and standing waters, and sometimes in slow running rivers, and lesser ditches of water, in sundry places of this land.

Time.] They flower most commonly about the end of May, and their seed is ripe in August.

Government and Virtues.] The herb is under the dominion of the Moon, and therefore cools and moiſtens like the former. The leaves and flowers of the Water Lilies are cold and moiſt, but the roots and ſeeds are cold and dry; the leaves do cool all inflammations, both outward and inward heat of agues; and ſo doth the flowers alſo, either by the ſyrup or conſerve; the ſyrup helpeth much to procure reſt, and to ſettle the brain of frantick perſons, by cooling the hot diſtemperature of the head. The ſeed as well as the root is effectual to ſtay fluxes of blood or humours, either of wounds or of the belly; but the roots are moſt uſed, and more effectual to cool, bind, and reſtrain all fluxes in man or woman; alſo running of the reins, and paſſing away of the ſeed when one is aſleep; but the frequent uſe hereof extinguiſheth venereous actions. The root is likewiſe very good for thoſe whoſe urine is hot and ſharp, to be boiled in wine and water, and the decoction drank. The diſtilled water of the flowers is very effectual for all the diſeaſes aforeſaid, both inwardly taken, and outwardly applied; and is much commended to take away freckles, ſpots, ſunburn, and morphew from the face, or other parts of the body. The oil made of the flowers, as oil of roſes is made, is profitably uſed to cool hot tumours, and to eaſe the pains, and help the ſores.

Lily of the Valley.

Called alſo Conval Lily, Male Lily, and Lily Confancy.

Deſcript.] The root is ſmall, and creepeth far in the ground, as graſs roots do. The leaves are many, againſt which riſeth up a ſtalk half a foot high, with many white flowers, like little bells with turned edges, of a ſtrong, though pleaſing ſmell; the berries are red, not much unlike thoſe of Aſparagus.

Place.] They grow plentifully upon Hampſtead-Heath, and many other places in this nation,

Time.] They flower in May, and the ſeed is ripe in Semptember.

Temperature and Virtues.] It is under the dominion of Mercury, and therefore it ſtrengthens the brain, recruits a weak a weak memory, and makes it ſtrong again: The diſtill-water dropped into the eyes, helps inflammations there; as alſo that infirmity which they call a pin and web. The ſpirit of the flowers diſtilled in wine, reſtoreth loſt ſpeech helps the palſy, and is exceeding good in the apoplexy, comforteth the heart and vital ſpirits. Gerrard ſaith, that the flowers being cloſe ſtopped up in a glaſs, put into an ant-hill, and taken away again a month after, ye ſhall find a liquor in the glaſs, which, being outwardly applied, helps the gout.

White Lilies.

IT were in vain to deſcribe a plant ſo commonly known in every one's garden; therefore I ſhall not tell you what they are, but what they are good for.

Government and Virtues.] They are under the dominion of the Moon, and by antipathy to Mars expel poiſon; they are excellent good in peſtilential fevers, the roots being bruiſed and boiled in wine, and the decoction drank; for it expels the venom to the exterior parts of the body: The juice of it being tempered with barley-meal, baked, and ſo eaten for ordinary bread, is an excellent cure for the dropſy: An ointment made of the root and hog's greaſe, is excellent good for ſcald heads, unites the ſinews when they are cut, and cleanſes ulcers. The root boiled in any convenient decoction, gives ſpeedy delivery to women in travail, and expels the after-birth. The root roaſted, and mixed with a little hog's greaſe, makes a gallant poultice to ripen and break plague ſores. The ointment is excellent good for ſwellings in the privities, and will cure burnings and ſcaldings without a ſcar, and trimly deck a blank place with hair.

Liquorice.

Deſcript.] OUR Engliſh Liquorice riſeth up with divers woody ſtalks, whereon are ſet at ſeveral diſtances, many narrow, long, green leaves, ſet together on both ſides of the ſtalk, and an odd one at the end, very well reſembling a young aſh tree, ſprung up from the ſeed. This by many years continuance in a place without removing, and not elſe, will bring forth flowers, many ſtanding together ſpike faſhion, one above another upon the ſtalk, of the form of peaſe bloſſoms, but of a very pale blue colour, which turn into long, ſomewhat flat and ſmooth cods, wherein is contained a ſmall, round, hard ſeed: The roots run down exceeding deep into the ground, with divers other ſmall roots and fibres growing with them, and ſhoot out ſuckers from the main roots all about, whereby it is much increaſed, of a browniſh colour on the outſide, and yellow within.

Place.] It is planted in fields and gardens, in divers places of this land, and thereof good profit is made.

Government and Virtues.] It is under the dominion of Mercury. Liquorice boiled in fair water, with ſome Maiden-Hair and figs, maketh a good drink for thoſe that have a dry cough or hoarſeneſs, wheezing or ſhortneſs of breath, and for all the griefs of the breaſts and lungs, phthyſick or conſumptions cauſed by the diſtillation of ſalt humours on them. It is alſo good in all pains of the reins, the ſtrangury, and heat of urine: The fine powder of Liquorice blown through a quill into the eyes that have a pin and web (as they call it) or rheumatick diſtillations in them, doth cleanſe and help them: The juice of Liquorice is as effectual in all the diſeaſes of the breaſt and lungs, the reins and the bladder, as the decoction. The juice diſtilled in Roſe-water, with ſome gum tragacanth, is a fine licking medicine for hoarſeneſs, wheezing, &c.

Liverwort.

Deſcript.] Common Liverwort groweth cloſe, and ſpreadeth much upon the ground in moiſt and ſhady places, with many ſmall green leaves, or rather (as it were) ſticking flat to one another, very unevenly cut in on the edges, and crumpled; from among which ariſe ſmall ſlender ſtalks, an inch or two high at moſt, bearing ſmall ſtar-like flowers at the top; the roots are very fine and ſmall.

Government and Virtues.] It is under the dominion of Jupiter, and under the ſign Cancer. It is a ſingular good herb for all the diſeaſes of the liver, both to cool and cleanſe it, and helpeth the inflammations in any part, and the yellow jaundice likewiſe: Being bruiſed and boiled in ſmall

ſmall beer, and drank, it cooleth the heat of the liver and kidneys, and helpeth the running of the reins in men, and the whites in women; it is a ſingular remedy to ſtay the ſpreading of tetters, ringworms, and other fretting and running ſores and ſcabs, and is an excellent remedy for ſuch whoſe livers are corrupted by ſurfeits, which cauſe their bodies to break out, for it fortifieth the liver exceedingly, and makes it impregnable.

LOOSESTRIFE or WILLOWHERB.

Deſcript.] COMMON yellow Looſeſtrife groweth to be four or five feet high, or more, with great round ſtalks a little creſted, diverſly branched from the middle of them to the tops into great and long branches, on all which at the joints there grow long and narrow leaves, but broader below, and uſually two at a joint, yet ſometimes three or four, ſomewhat like willow leaves, ſmooth on the edges, and of a fair green colour from the upper joints of the branches, and at the tops of them alſo ſtand many yellow flowers of five leaves a-piece, with divers yellow threads in the middle, which turn into ſmall round heads, containing ſmall cornered ſeeds; the root creepeth under ground, almoſt like cough-graſs, but greater, and ſhooteth up every Spring browniſh heads, which afterwards grow up into ſtalks. It hath no ſcent or taſte, but only aſtringent.

Place.] It groweth in many places of this land in moiſt meadows, and by water-ſides.

Time.] It flowereth from June to Auguſt.

Government and Virtues.] This herb is good for all manner of bleeding at the mouth, noſe, or wounds and all fluxes of the belly, and the bloody-flux, given either to drink or taken by clyſter; it ſtayeth alſo the abundance of women's courſes, it is a ſingular good wound herb for green wounds, to ſtay the bleeding, and quickly cloſe together the lips of the wound, if the herb be bruiſed, and the juice only applied. It is often uſed in gargles for ſore mouths, as alſo for the ſecret parts. The ſmoak hereof being burned, driveth away flies and gnats, which in the night time moleſt people inhabiting near marſhes, and in the fenny countries.

LOOSESTRIFE, with spiked heads of Flowers.

Descript.] THIS groweth with many woody square stalks, full of joints, about three feet high at least; at every one whereof stand two long leaves, shorter, narrower, and a larger green colour than the former, and some brownish. The stalks are branched into many long stems of spiked flowers, half a foot long, growing in bundels one above another, out of small husks, very like the spiked heads of lavender, each of which flowers have five round pointed leaves of a purple violet colour, or somewhat inclining to redness; in which husks stand small round heads after the flowers are fallen, wherein is contained small seed. The root creepeth under ground like unto the yellow, but is greater than it, and so are the heads of the leaves when they first appear out of the ground, and more brown than the other.

Place.] It groweth usually by rivers, and ditch-sides in wet ground, as about the ditches at and near Lambeth, and in many other places of this land.

Time.] It flowereth in the months of June and July.

Government and Virtues.] It is an herb of the Moon, and under the sign Cancer; neither do I know a better preserver of the sight when 'tis well, nor a better cure of sore eyes than Eyebright, taken inwardly, and this used outwardly; 'tis cold in quality. This herb is no whit inferior unto the former, it having not only all the virtues which the former hath, but some peculiar virtues of its own, found out by experience; as namely, The distilled water is a present remedy for hurts and blows on the eyes, and for blindness, so as the Crystalline humour be not perished or hurt; and this hath been sufficiently proved true by the experience of a man of judgment, who kept it long to himself as a great secret. It cleareth the eyes of dust, or any thing gotten into them, and preserveth the sight. It is also very available against wounds and thrusts, being made into an ointment in this manner: To every ounce of the water, add two drams of May butter without salt, and of sugar and wax, of each as much also; let them boil gently together. Let tents dipped into the liquor that remaineth after it is cold, be put into the wounds, and the place covered with a linnen cloth doubled and anointed with the ointment; and this is also an approved medicine. It likewise cleanseth and healeth all foul ulcers, and sores whatsoever, and stayeth their inflammations by washing them with the water, and laying on them a green leaf or two in the Summer, or dry leaves in the Winter. This water gargled warm in the mouth, and sometimes drank also, doth cure the quinsy, or king's evil, in the throat. The said water applied warm, taketh away all spots, marks, and scabs in the skin; and a little of it drank, quencheth thirst when it is extraordinary.

LOVAGE.

Descript.] IT hath many long and great stalks, of large winged leaves, divided into many parts, like Smallage, but much larger and greater, every leaf being cut about the edges, broadest forward, and smallest at the stalk, of a sad green colour, smooth and shining; from among which rise up sundry strong, hollow green stalks, five or six, sometimes seven or eight feet high, full of joints but lesser leaves set on them than grow below; and with them towards the tops come forth large branches, bearing at their tops large umbels of yellow flowers, and after them flat brownish seed. The root groweth thick, great and deep, spreading much, and enduring long, of a brownish colour on the outside, and whitish within. The whole plant and every part of it smelling strong, and aromatically, and is of a hot, sharp, biting taste.

Place.] It is usually planted in gardens, where, if it be suffered, it groweth huge and great.

Time.] It flowereth in the end of July, and seedeth in August.

Government and Virtues.] It is an herb of the Sun, under the sign Taurus. If Saturn offend the throat (as he always doth if he be occasioner of the malady, and in Taurus is the Genesis) this is your cure. It openeth, cureth and digesteth humours, and mightily provoketh womens courses and urine. Half a dram at a time of the dried root in powder taken in wine, doth wonderfully warm a cold stomach, helpeth digestion, and consumeth all raw and superfluous moisture therein; easeth all inward gripings and pains, dissolveth wind and resisteth poison

son and infection. It is a known and much praised remedy to drink the decoction of the herb for any sort of ague, and to help the pains and torments of the body and bowels coming of cold. The seed is effectual to all the purposes aforesaid (except the last) and worketh more powerfully. The distilled water of the herb helpeth the quinsy in the throat, if the mouth and throat be gargled and washed therewith, and helpeth the pleurisy, being drank three or four times. Being dropped into the eyes, it taketh away the redness or dimness of them; it likewise taketh away spots or freckles in the face. The leaves bruised, and fried with a little hog's lard, and laid hot to any blotch or boil, will quickly break it.

LUNGWORT.

Descript.] THIS is a kind of moss that groweth on sundry sorts of trees, especially oaks and beeches, with broad, greyish, tough leaves diversly folded, crumpled, and gashed in on the edges, and some spotted also with many small spots on the upper side. It was never seen to bear any stalk or flower at any time.

Government and Virtues.] Jupiter seems to own this herb. It is of great use to physicians to help the diseases of the lungs, and for coughs, wheezings, and shortness of breath, which it cureth both in man and beast. It is very profitable to put into lotions that are taken to stay the moist humours that flow to ulcers, and hinder their healing, as also to wash all other ulcers in the privy parts of a man or woman. It is an excellent remedy boiled in beer for broken-winded horses.

MADDER.

Descript.] GARDEN Madder shooteth forth many very long, weak, four-square, reddish stalks, trailing on the ground a great way, very rough or hairy, and full of joints: At every one of these joints come forth divers long and narrow leaves, standing like a star about the stalks, rough also and hairy, towards the tops whereof come forth many small pale yellow flowers, after which come small round heads, green at first, and reddish afterwards, but black when they are ripe, wherein is contained ed the seed. The root is not very great, but exceeding long, running down half a man's length into the ground, red and very clear while it is fresh, spreading divers ways.

Place.] It is only manured in gardens, or larger fields, for the profit that is made thereof.

Time.] It flowereth towards the end of Summer, and the seed is ripe quickly after.

Government and Virtues.] It is an herb of Mars. It hath an opening quality, and afterward to bind and strengthen. It is a sure remedy for the yellow jaundice, by opening the obstructions of the liver and gall, and cleansing those parts; it openeth also the obstructions of the spleen, and diminisheth the melancholy humour: It is available for the palsy and sciatica, and effectual for bruises inward and outward, and is therefore much used in vulnerary drinks. The root for all those aforesaid purposes, is to be boiled in wine or water, as the cause requireth, and some honey and sugar put thereunto afterwards. The seed hereof taken in vinegar and honey, helpeth the swelling and hardness of the spleen. The decoction of the leaves and branches is a good fomentation for women to sit over that have not their courses. The leaves and roots beaten and applied to any part that is discoloured with freckles, morphew, the white scurf, or any such deformity of the skin, cleanseth thoroughly, and taketh them away.

MAIDEN-HAIR.

Descript.] OUR common Maiden-Hair doth, from a number of hard black fibres, send forth a great many blackish shining brittle stalks, hardly a span long, in many not half so long, on each side set very thick with small, round, dark, green leaves, and spitted on the back of them like a fern.

Place.] It groweth upon old stone walls in the West parts, in Kent, and divers other places of this land; it delighteth likewise to grow by springs, wells, and rocky moist and shady places, and is always green.

WALL RUE, or, White Maiden-Hair.

Descript.] THIS hath very fine pale, green stalks, almost as fine as hairs, set confusedly with divers

divers pale green leaves on very ſhort foot-ſtalks, ſomewhat near unto the colour of garden Rue, and not much differing in form, but more diverſly cut in on the edges, and thicker, ſmooth on the upper part, and ſpotted finely underneath.

Place.] It groweth in many places of this land, at Dartford, and the bridge at Aſhford in Kent, at Beaconsfield in Buckinghamſhire, at Wolly in Huntingtonſhire on Framingham Caſtle in Suffolk, on the church walls at Mayfield in Suſſex, in Somerſetſhire, and divers other places of this land; and is green in Winter as well as Summer.

Government and Virtues.] Both this and the former are under the dominion of Mercury, and ſo is that alſo which followeth after, and the virtue of both theſe are ſo near alike, that though I have deſcribed them and their places of growing ſeverally, yet I ſhall, in writing the virtues of them, join them both together as followeth:

The decoction of the herb Maiden-Hair being drank, helpeth thoſe that are troubled with the cough, ſhortneſs of breath, the yellow jaundice, diſeaſes of the ſpleen ſtopping of the urine, and helpeth exceedingly to break the ſtone in the kidneys, (in all which diſeaſes the Wall Rue is alſo very effectual.) It provoketh womens courſes, and ſtays both bleedings and fluxes of the ſtomach and belly, eſpecially when the herb is dry; for being green it looſeneth the belly, and voideth choler and phlegm from the ſtomach and liver; it cleanſeth the lungs, and by rectifying the blood, cauſeth a good colour to the whole body. The herb boiled in oil of camomile, diſſolveth knots, allayeth ſwellings, and drieth up moiſt ulcers. The lee made thereof is ſingular good to cleanſe the head from ſcurf, and from dry and running ſores, ſtayeth the falling or ſhedding of the hair, and cauſeth it to grow thick, fair, and well coloured; for which purpoſe ſome boil it in wine, putting ſome Smallage ſeed thereto, and afterwards ſome oil. The Wall Rue is as effectual as Maiden-Hair, in all diſeaſes of the head, or falling and recovering of the hair again, and generally for all the aforementioned diſeaſes: And beſides, the powder of it taken in drink for forty days together, helpeth the burſtings in children.

GOLDEN

Golden Maiden-Hair.

TO the former give me leave to add this, and I ſhall no more but only deſcribe it unto you, and for the virtues refer you to the former, ſince whatſoever is ſaid of them, may be alſo ſaid of this.

Deſcript.] It hath many ſmall, browniſh, red hairs to make up the form of leaves growing about the ground from the root; and in the middle of them, in Summer, riſe ſmall ſtalks of the ſame colour, ſet with very fine yelloviſh green hairs on them, and bearing a ſmall gold, yellow head, leſſer than a wheat corn, ſtanding in a great huſk. The root is very ſmall and thready.

Place.] It groweth in bogs and mooriſh places, and alſo on dry ſhady places, as Hampſtead Heath, and elſewhere.

Mallows and Marshmallows.

COMMON Mallows are generally ſo well known that they need no deſcription.

Our common Marſhmallow have divers ſoft hairy white ſtalks, riſing to be three or four feet high, ſpreading forth many branches, the leaves whereof are ſoft and hairy, ſomewhat leſſer than the other Mallow leaves, but longer pointed, cut (for the moſt part) into ſome few diviſions, but deep. The flowers are many, but ſmaller alſo than the other Mallows, and white, or tending to a blueiſh colour. After which come ſuch long, round caſes and ſeeds, as in the other Mallows. The roots are many and long, ſhooting from one head, of the bigneſs of a thumb or finger, very pliant, tough, and being like liquorice, of a whitiſh yellow colour on the outſide, and more white whithin, full of a ſlimy juice, which being laid in water, will thicken, as if it were a jelly.

Place.] The common Mallows grow in every county of this land. The common Marſhmallows in moſt of the ſalt marſhes, from Woolwich down to the ſea, both on the Kentiſh and Eſſex ſhores, and in divers other places of this land.

Time.] They flower all the Summer months, even until the Winter do pull them down.

Government and Virtues.] Venus owns them both. The leaves

leaves of either of the ſorts before ſpecified, and the roots alſo boiled in wine or water, or in broth with parſley or fennel roots, do help to open the body, and are very convenient in hot agues, or other diſtempers of the body, to apply the leaves ſo boiled warm to the belly. It not only voideth hot cholerick, and other offenſive humours, but eaſeth the pains and torments of the belly coming thereby; and are therefore uſed in all clyſters conducing to thoſe purpoſes. The ſame uſed by nurſes, procureth them ſtore of milk. The decoction of the ſeed of any of the common Mallows made in milk or wine, doth marvellouſly help excoriations, the phthiſic, pleuriſy, and other diſeaſes of the cheſt and lungs, that proceed of hot cauſes, if it be continued taking for ſome time together. The leaves and roots work the ſame effects. They help much alſo in the excoriations of the guts and bowels, and hardneſs of the mother, and in all hot and ſharp diſeaſes thereof. The juice drank in wine, or the decoction of them therein, doth help women to a ſpeedy and eaſy delivery. Pliny ſaith, that whoſoever ſhall take a ſpoonful of any of the Mallows, ſhall that day be free from all diſeaſes that may come unto him; and that it is ſpecial good for the falling-ſickneſs. The ſyrup alſo and conſerve made of the flowers, are very effectual for the ſame diſeaſes, and to open the body, being coſtive. The leaves bruiſed, and laid to the eyes with a little honey, take away the impoſthumations of them. The leaves bruiſed or rubbed upon any place ſtung with bees, waſps, or the like, preſently take away the pains, redneſs, and ſwelling that riſe thereupon. And Dioſcrides ſaith, The decoction of the roots and leaves helpeth all ſorts of poiſon, ſo as the poiſon be preſently voided by vomit. A poultice made of the leaves boiled and bruiſed, with ſome bean or barley flower, and oil of roſes added, is an eſpecial remedy againſt all hard tumours and inflammations, or impoſthumes, or ſwellings of the cods, and other parts, and eaſeth the pains of them; as alſo againſt the hardneſs of the liver or ſpleen, being applied to the places. The juice of Mallows boiled in old oil and applied, taketh away all roughneſs of the ſkin, as alſo the ſcurf, dandriff, or dry ſcabs in the head, or other parts, if they be anointed therewith,

with, or washed with the decoction, and preserveth the hair from falling off. It is also effectual against scaldings and burnings, St Anthony's fire, and all other hot, red and painful swellings in any part of the body. The flowers boiled in oil or water (as every one is disposed) whereunto a little honey and alum is put, is an excellent gargle to wash, cleanse or heal any sore mouth or throat in a short space. If the feet be bathed or washed with the decoction of the leaves, roots and flowers, it helpeth much the defluctions of rheum from the head; if the head be washed therewith, it stayeth the falling and shedding of the hair. The green leaves (saith Pliny) beaten with nitre, and applied, draw out thorns or prickles in the flesh.

The Marshmallows are more effectual in all the diseases before mentioned: The leaves are likewise used to loosen the belly gently, and in decoctions for clysters to ease all pains of the body, opening the strait passages, and making them slippery, whereby the stone may descend the more easily, and without pain, out of the reins, kidneys and bladder, and to ease the torturing pains thereof. But the roots are of more special use for those purposes, as well for coughs, hoarseness, shortness of breath and wheezings, being boiled in wine, or honeyed water and drank. The roots and seeds hereof being boiled in wine or water, are with good success used by them that have excoriations in the guts, or the bloody flux, by qualifying the violence of sharp fretting humours, easing the pains, and healing the soreness. It is profitably taken of them that are troubled with ruptures, cramps, or convulsions of the sinews, and boiled in white wine, for the imposthumes of the throat, commonly called the king's evil, and of those kernels that rise behind the ears, and inflammations or swellings in womens breasts. The dried roots boiled in milk and drank, is special good for the chin-cough. Hippocrates used to give the decoction of the roots, or the juice thereof, to drink, to those that are wounded, and ready to faint thro' loss of blood, and applied the same mixed with honey and rosin to the wounds. As also, the roots boiled in wine to those that have recieved any hurt by bruises, falls, or blows, or had any bone or member out of joint, or any swelling pain, or ach in the muscles, sinews or arteries. The mucilage of the roots, and of linseed and fenugreek put together, is much used in poultices, ointments, and plaisters, to mollify and digest all hard swellings, and the inflammation of them, and to ease pains in any part of the body. The seed either green or dry, mixed with vinegar, cleanseth the skin of morphew, and all other discolourings, being boiled therewith in the Sun.

You may remember, that not long since there was a raging disease called the bloody-flux; the collge of physicians not knowing what to make of it, called it the plague of the guts, for their wits were at *Ne plus ultra* about it. My son was taken with the same disease, and the excoriation of his bowels was exceeding great; myself being in the country, was sent for up; the only thing I gave him was Mallows bruised and boiled both in milk and drink, in two days (the blessing of God being upon it) it cured him. And I here, to shew my thankfulness to God, in communicating it to his creatures, leave it to posterity.

MAPLE TREE.

Government and Virtues.] IT is under the dominion of Jupiter. The decoction either of the leaves or bark, must needs strengthen the liver much, and so you shall find it to do, if you use it. It is excellent good to open obstructions both of the liver and spleen, and easeth pains of the sides thence proceeding.

WILD MARJORAM.

CALLED also Origane, Origanum, Eastward Marjoram, wild Marjoram, and Grove Marjoram.

Descript.] Wild or field Marjoram hath a root which creepeth much under ground, which continueth a long time, sending up sundry brownish, hard, square stalks with small dark green leaves, very like those of sweet Marjoram, but harder, and somewhat broader; at the top of the stalks stand tufts of flowers, of a deep purplish red colour. The seed is small and something blacker than that of sweet Marjoram.

Place.] It groweth plentifully in the borders of corn-fields, and in some copses.

Time,

Time.] It flowereth towards the latter end of Summer.

Government and Virtues.] This is also under the dominion of Mercury. It strengthens the stomach and head much, there being scarce a better remedy growing for such as are troubled with a sour humour in the stomach; it restores the appetite being lost; helps the cough, and consumption of the lungs; it cleanseth the body of choler, expelleth poison, and remedieth the infirmities of the spleen; helps the bitings of venomous beasts, and helps such as have poisoned themselves by eating hemlock, henbane, or opium. It provoketh urine and the terms in women, helps the dropsy, and the scurvy, scabs, itch, and yellow jaundice. The juice being dropped into the ears, helps deafness, pain and noise in the ears. And thus much for this herb, between which and adders, there is a deadly antipathy.

SWEET MARJORAM.

SWEET Marjoram is so well known, being an inhabitant in every garden, that it is needless to write any description thereof, neither of the Winter Sweet Marjoram, or Pot Marjoram.

Place.] They grow commonly in gardens; some sort there are that grow wild in the borders of corn fields and pastures, in sundry places of this land; but it is not my purpose to insist upon them. The garden kinds being most used and useful.

Time.] They flower in the end of Summer.

Government and Virtues.] It is an herb of Mercury, and under Aries, and therefore is an excellent remedy for the brain and other parts of the body and mind, under the dominion of the same planet. Our common Sweet Marjoram is warming and comfortable in cold diseases of the head, stomach, sinews, and other parts, taken inwardly or outwardly applied. The decoction thereof being drank, helpeth all diseases of the chest which hinder the freeness of breathing, and is also profitable for the obstructions of the liver and spleen. It helpeth the cold griefs of the womb, and the windiness thereof, and the loss of speech, by resolution of the tongue. The decoction thereof made with some pellitory of Spain, and long pepper, or with a little acorns or origanum, being drank, is good for those that are beginning to fall into a dropsy, for those that cannot make water, and against pains and torments in the belly; it provoketh womens courses, if it be put up as a pessary. Being made into powder, and mixed with honey, it taketh away the black marks of blows, and bruises, being thereunto applied; it is good for the inflammations and watering of the eyes, being mixed with fine flour, and laid unto them. The juice dropped into the ears, easeth the pains and singing noise in them. It is profitably put into those ointments and salves that are warm, and comfort the outward parts, as the joints and sinews; for swellings also, and places out of joint. The powder thereof snuffed up into the nose provoketh sneezing, and thereby purgeth the brain; and chewed in the mouth, draweth forth much phlegm. The oil made thereof, is very warm and comfortable to the joints that are stiff, and the sinews that are hard, to mollify and supple them. Marjoram is much used in all odoriferous waters, powders, &c. that are for ornament or delight.

MARIGOLDS.

THESE being so plentiful in every garden, are so well known that they need no description.

Time.] They flower all the Summer long, and sometimes in Winter, if it be mild.

Government and Virtues.] It is an herb of the Sun, and under Leo. They strengthen the heart exceedingly, and are very expulsive, and little less effectual in the small-pox and measles than saffron. The juice of Marigold leaves mixed with vinegar, and any hot swellings bathed with it, instantly giveth ease, and assuageth it. The flowers, either green or dried, are much used in possets, broths, and drink, as a comforter of the heart and spirits, and to expel any malignant or pestilential quality which might annoy them. A plaister made with the dry flowers in powder, hog's-grease, turpentine, and rosin, applied to the breast, strengthens and succours the heart infinitely in fevers, whether pestilential or not pestilential.

MASTERWORT.

Descript.] COMMON Masterwort hath divers stalks of winged leaves divided into sundry parts, three for the most part standing together at a small foot-stalk on both sides of the greater, and three likewise at the end of the stalk, somewhat broad, and cut in on the edges into three or more divisions, all of them dented about the brims, of a dark green colour, somewhat resembling the leaves of Angelica, but that these grow lower to the ground, and on lesser stalks; among which rise up two or three short stalks about two feet high, and slender, with such like leaves at the joints which grow below, but with lesser and fewer divisions, bearing umbels of white flowers, and after them, thin, flat blackish seeds, bigger than Dill seeds. The root is somewhat greater and growing rather side-ways than down deep in the ground, shooting forth sundry heads, which taste sharp, biting on the tongue, and is the hottest and sharpest part of the plant, and the seed next unto it being somewhat blackish on the outside, and smelling well.

Place.] It is usually kept in gardens with us in England.

Time.] It flowereth and seedeth about the end of August.

Government and Virtues.] It is an herb of Mars. The root of Masterwort is hotter than pepper, and very available in cold griefs and diseases both of the stomach and body, dissolving very powerfully upwards and downwards. It is also used in a decoction with wine against all cold rheums, distillation upon the lungs, or shortness of breath, to be taken morning and evening. It also provoketh urine, and helpeth to break the stone, and expel the gravel from the kidneys; provoketh womens courses, and expelleth the dead-birth. Is singular good for strangling of the mother, and other such like feminine diseases. It is effectual also against the dropsy, cramps, and falling-sickness; for the decoction in wine being gargled in the mouth, draweth down much water and phlegm, from the brain, purging and easing it of what oppresseth it. It is of a rare quality against all sorts of cold poison, to be taken as there is cause; it provoketh sweat. But lest the taste hereof, or of the seed (which worketh to the like effect, tho' not so powerfully) should be too offensive, the best way is to take the water distilled both from the herb and root. The juice hereof dropped, or tents dipped therein, and applied either to green wounds or filthy rotten ulcers, and those that come by envenomed weapons, doth soon cleanse and heal them. The same is also very good to help the gout coming of a cold cause.

SWEET MAUDLIN.

Descript.] COMMON Maudlin hath somewhat long and narrow leaves, snipped about the edges. The stalks are two feet high, bearing at the tops many yellow flowers set round together, and all of an equal height, in umbels or tufts like unto Tansy; after which followeth small whitish seed, almost as big as worm-seed.

Place and Time.] It groweth in gardens, and flowereth in June and July.

Government and Virtues.] The virtues hereof being the same with Costmary or Alecost, I shall not make any repetition thereof, lest my book grow too big; but rather refer you unto Costmary for satisfaction.

The MEDLAR.

Descript.] THE Tree groweth near the bigness of the Quince Tree, spreading branches reasonably large, with longer and narrower leaves than either the apple or quince, and not dented about the edges. At the end of the sprigs stand the flowers, made of five white, great broad pointed leaves, nicked in the middle with some white threads also; after which cometh the fruit, of a brownish green colour being ripe, bearing a crown as it were on the top, which were the five green leaves; and being rubbed off, or fallen away, the head of the fruit is seen to be somewhat hollow. The fruit is very harsh before it is mellowed, and hath usually five hard kernels within it. There is another kind hereof nothing differing from the former, but that it hath some thorns on it in several places, which the other hath not; and usually the fruit is small, and not so pleasant.

Time and Place.] They grow in this land, and flower

in

in May for the most part, and bear fruit in September and October.

Government and Virtues.] The fruit is old Saturn's, and sure a better medicine he hardly hath to strengthen the retentive faculty; therefore it stays womens longings: The good old man cannot endure womens minds should run a gadding. Also a plaister made of the fruit dried before they are rotten, and other convenient things, and applied to the reins of the back, stops miscarriage in women with child. They are very powerful to stay fluxes of blood or humours in men or women; the leaves also have this quality. The fruit eaten by women with child, stayeth their longing after unusual meats, and is very effectual for them that are apt to miscarry, and be delivered before their time, to help that malady, and make them joyful mothers. The decoction of them is good to gargle and wash the mouth, throat and teeth, when there is any defluxions of blood to stay it, or of humours, which causeth the pains and swellings. It is a good bath for women to sit over, that have their courses flow too abundant; or for the piles when they bleed too much. If a poultice or plaister be made with dried medlars beaten and mixed with the juice of red roses, whereunto a few cloves and nutmegs may be added, and a little red coral also, and applied to the stomach, that is given to casting or loathing of meat, it effectually helpeth. The dried leaves in powder strewed on fresh bleeding wounds restraineth the blood, and healeth up the wound quickly. The Medlar-stones made into powder, and drank in wine, wherein some Parsley-roots have lain infused all night, or a little boiled, do break the stone in the kidneys, helping to expel it.

MELLILOT, or KING'S CLOVER.

Descript.] THIS hath many green stalks, two or three feet high, rising from a tough, long, white root, which dieth not every year, set round about at the joints with small and somewhat long, well smelling leaves, set three together unevenly dented about the edge. The flowers are yellow, and well smelling also, made like other trefoil, but small, standing in long spikes one above another,

another, for an hand-breadth long or better, which afterwards turn into long crooked cods, wherein is contained flat feed, fomewhat brown.

Place] It groweth plentifully in many places of this land, as in the edge of Suffolk, and in Effex, as alfo in Huntingtonfhire, and in other places, but moft ufually in corn-fields, in corners of meadows.

Time.] It flowereth in June and July, and is ripe quickly after.

Government and Virtues.] Mellilot, boiled in wine, and applied, mollifieth all hard tumours and inflammations that happen in the eyes, or other parts of the body, as the fundament, or privy parts of men or women; and fometimes the yolk of a roafted egg, or fine flour, or poppy feed, or endive, is added unto it. It helpeth the fpreading ulcers in the head, it being wafhed with a lee made thereof. It helpeth the pains of the ftomach, being applied frefh; or boiled with any of the aforenamed things: Alfo, the pains of the ears, being dropped into them; and fteeped in vinegar, or rofe water, it mitigateth the head-ach. The flowers of Mellilot or camomile are much ufed to be put together in clyfters to expel wind, and eafe pains; and alfo in poultices for the fame purpofe, and to affuage fwelling tumours in the fpleen or other parts, and helpeth inflammations in any part of the body. The juice dropped into the eyes, is a fingular good medicine to take away the film or fkin that cloudeth or dimneth the eyefight. The head often wafhed with the diftilled water of the herb and flower, or a lee made therewith, is effectual for thofe that fuddenly lofe their fenfes; as alfo to ftrengthen the memory, to comfort the head and brain, and to preferve them from pain, and the apoplexy.

FRENCH and DOGS MERCURY.

Defcript.] THIS rifeth up with a fquare green ftalk full of joints, two feet high, or thereabouts, with two leaves at every joint, and the branches likewife from both fides of the ftalk, fet with frefh green leaves, fomewhat broad and long, about the bignefs of the leaves of Bafil, finely dented about the edges; towards the tops of the ftalks and branches, come forth at every joint

joint in the male Mercury two ſmall, round green heads, ſtanding together upon a ſhort foot-ſtalk, which growing ripe, are ſeeds, not having flowers. The female ſtalk is longer, ſpike-faſhion, ſet round about with ſmall green huſks, which are the flowers, made like ſmall bunches of grapes, which give no ſeed, but abide long upon the ſtalks without ſhedding. The root is compoſed of many ſmall fibres, which periſheth every year at the firſt approach of Winter, and riſeth again of its own ſowing; and if once it is ſuffered to ſow itſelf, the ground will never want afterwards, even both ſorts of it.

Dog Mercury.

Having deſcribed unto you that which is called French Mercury, I come now to ſhew you a deſcription of this kind alſo.

Deſcript.] This is likewiſe of two kinds, male and female, having many ſtalks ſlender and lower than Mercury, without any branches at all upon them, the root is ſet with two leaves at every joint, ſomewhat greater than the female, but more pointed and full of veins, and ſomewhat harder in handling; of a dark green colour, and leſs dented or ſnipp'd about the edges. At the joints with the leaves come forth longer ſtalks than the former, with two hairy round ſeeds upon them, twice as big as thoſe of the former Mercury. The taſte hereof is herby, and the ſmell ſomewhat ſtrong and virulent. The female has much harder leaves ſtanding upon longer foot-ſtalks, and the ſtalks are alſo longer; from the joints come forth ſpikes of flowers like the French Female Mercury. The roots of them both are many, and full of ſmall fibres which run under ground, and mat themſelves very much, not periſhing as the former Mercuries do, but abiding the winter, and ſhoot forth new branches every year, for the old lie down to the ground.

Plac.] The male and female French Mercury are found wild in divers places of this land, as by a village called Brookland in Rumney Marſh in Kent.

The Dog Mercury in ſundry places of Kent alſo, and elſewhere; but the female more ſeldom than the male.

Time.

Time.] They flower in the Summer months, and therein give their seed.

Government and Virtues.] Mercury, they say, owns the herb, but I rather think it is Venus's, and I am partly confident of it too, for I never heard that Mercury ever midded womens business so much: I believe he minds his study more. The decoction of the leaves of Mercury, or the juice thereof in broth, or drank with a little sugar put to it, purgeth cholerick and waterish humours. Hippocrates commended it wonderfully for womens diseases, and applied to the secret parts to ease the pains of the mother; and used the decoction of it, both to procure womens courses and to expel the after-birth; and gave the decoction thereof with myrrh or pepper, or used to apply the leaves outwardly against the strangury and diseases of the reins and bladder. He used it also for sore and watering eyes, and for the deafness and pains in the ears, by dropping the juice thereof into them, and bathing them afterwards in white wine. The decoction thereof made with water and a cock chicken, is a most safe medicine against the hot fits of agues. It also cleanseth the breast and lungs of phlegm, but a little offendeth the stomach. The juice or distilled water snuffed up into the nostrils, purgeth the head and eyes of catarrhs and rheums. Some use to drink two or three ounces of the distilled water, with a little sugar put to it, in the morning fasting, to open and purge the body of gross, viscous, and melancholy humours. It is wonderful (if it be not fabulous) which Dioscorides and Theophrastes do relate of it, viz. That if a woman use these herbs either inwardly or outwardly, for three days together after conception, and their courses be past, they shall bring forth male or female children, according to that kind of herb they use. Matthiolus saith, that the seed both of the male and female Mercury boiled with wormwood and drank, cureth the yellow jaundice in a speedy manner. The leaves or the juice rubbed upon warts, taketh them away. The juice mingled with some vinegar, helpeth all running scabs, tetters, ringworms, and the itch. Galen saith, that being applied in manner of a poultice to any swelling or inflammation, it digesteth the swelling, and allayeth the inflammation,

mation, and is therefore given in clysters to evacuate from the belly offensive humours. The Dog Mercury, although it be less used, yet may serve in the same manner, to the same purpose, to purge waterish and melancholy humours.

MINT.

OF all the kinds of Mint, the Spear Mint, or Heart Mint, being most usual, I shall only describe as follows:

Descript.] Spear Mint hath divers round stalks, and long but narrowish leaves set thereon, of a dark green colour. The flowers stand in spiked heads at the tops of the branches, being of a pale blue colour. The smell or scent thereof is somewhat near unto Basil; it increaseth by the root under ground as all the others do.

Place.] It is an usual inhabitant in gardens: And because it seldom giveth any good seed, the effects is recompensed by the plentiful increase of the root, which being once planted in a garden, will hardly be rid out again.

Time.] It flowereth not until the beginning of August, for the most part.

Government and Virtues.] It is an herb of Venus. Dioscorides saith it hath a heating, binding and drying quality, and therefore the juice taken in vinegar, stayeth bleeding: It stirreth up venery, or bodily lust; two or three branches thereof taken in the juice of four pomegranates, stayeth the hiccough, vomiting, and allayeth the choler. It dissolveth imposthumes being laid to with barley-meal. It is good to repress the milk in womens breasts, and for such as have swollen, flagging, or great breasts. Applied with salt, it helpeth the biting of a mad dog; with mead and honied water, it easeth the pains of the ears, and taketh away the roughness of the tongue, being rubbed thereupon. It suffereth not milk to curdle in the stomach, if the leaves thereof be steeped or boiled in it before you drink it: Briefly it is very profitable to the stomach. The often use hereof is a very powerful medicine to stay womens courses and the whites. Applied to the forehead and temples, it easeth the pains in the head, and is good to wash the heads of young children therewith, against all manner

manner of breakings-out, sores or scabs therein, and healeth the chops of the fundament. It is also profitable against the poison of venomous creatures. The distilled water of mint is available to all the purposes aforesaid, yet more weakly. But if a spirit thereof be rightly and chymically drawn, it is much more powerful than the herb itself. Simeon Sethi saith, it helpeth a cold liver, strengtheneth the belly, causeth digestion, stayeth vomits and the hiccough; it is good against the gnawing of the heart, provoketh appetite, taketh away obstructions of the liver, and stirreth up bodily lust; but therefore too much must not be taken, because it maketh the blood thin and wheyish, and turneth it into choler, and therefore cholerick persons must abstain from it. It is a safe medicine for the biting of a mad dog, being bruised with salt, and laid thereon. The powder of it being dried and taken after meat, helpeth digestion, and those that are splenetick. Taken with wine, it helpeth women in their sore travail in child-bearing. It is good against the gravel and stone in the kidneys, and the strangury. Being smelled unto, it is comfortable for the head and memory. The decoction hereof gargled in the mouth, cureth the gums and mouth that is sore, and mendeth an ill-favoured breath; as also the rue and coriander, causeth the palate of the mouth to turn to its place, the decoction being gargled and held in the mouth.

The virtues of the Wild or Horse Mint, such as grow in ditches (whose description I purposely omitted, in regard they are well enough known) are especially to dissolve wind in the stomach, to help the colick, and those that are short-winded, and are an especial remedy for those that have venereal dreams and pollutions in the night, being outwardly applied to the testicles or cods. The juice dropped into the ears easeth the pains of them, and destroyeth the worms that breed therein. They are good against the venomous biting of serpents. The juice laid on warm, helpeth the king's evil, or kernels in the throat. The decoction or distilled water helpeth a stinking breath, proceeding from corruption of the teeth, and snuffed up the nose, purgeth the head. Pliny saith, that eating of the leaves hath been found by experience to cure the le-

prosy,

profy, applying fome of them to the face, and to help the fcurf or dandriff of the head ufed with vinegar. They are extreme bad for wounded people; and they fay a wounded man that eats Mint, his wound will never be cured, and that is a long day.

MISSELTO.

Defcript.] THIS rifeth up from the branch or arm of the tree whereon it groweth, with a woody ftem, putting itfelf into fundry branches, and they again divided into many other fmaller twigs, interlacing themfelves one within another, very much covered with a greyifh green bark, having two leaves fet at every joint, and at the end likewife, which are fomewhat long and narrow, fmall at the bottom, but broader towards the end. At the knots or joints of the boughs and branches grow fmall yellow flowers, which run into fmall, round, white, tranfparent berries, three or four together, full of a glutinous moifture, with a blackifh feed in each of them, which was never yet known to fpring, being put into the ground, or any where elfe to grow.

Place.] It groweth very rarely on oaks with us; but upon fundry other, as well timber as fruit trees, plentifully in woody groves, and the like, through all this land.

Time.] It flowereth in the Spring-time, but the berries are not ripe until October, and abideth on the branches all the Winter, unlefs the blackbirds, and other birds, do devour them.

Government and Virtues.] This is under the dominion of the Sun, I do not queftion; and can alfo take for granted, that that which grows upon oaks, participates fomething of the nature of Jupiter, becaufe an oak is one of his trees; as alfo that which grows upon pear trees, and apple trees, participates fomething of his nature, becaufe he rules the tree it grows upon, having no root of its own. But why that fhould have moft virtues that grows upon oaks I know not, unlefs becaufe it is rareft and hardeft to come by; and our college's opinion is in this contrary to fcripture, which faith, *God's tender mercies are over all his works;* and fo it is, let the college of phyficians walk as contrary to him as they pleafe, and that is as contrary as the east to the west. Clusius affirms that which grows upon pear trees to be as prevalent, and gives order, that it should not touch the ground after it is gathered; and also saith, that, being hung about the neck, it remedies witchcraft. Both the leaves and berries of Misselto do heat and dry, and are of subtil parts; the birdlime doth mollify hard knots, tumours, and imposthumes; ripeneth and discusseth them, and draweth forth thick as well as thin humours from the remote parts of the body, digesting and separating them. And being mixed with equal parts of rosin and wax, doth mollify the hardness of the spleen, and helpeth old ulcers and sores. Being mixed with sandarick and orpiment, it helpeth to draw off foul nails; and if quick-lime and wine lees be added thereunto, it worketh the stronger. The Misselto itself of the oak (as the best) made into powder, and given in drink to those that have the falling-sickness, doth assuredly heal them, as Matthiolus saith; but it is fit to use it for forty days together. Some have so highly esteemed it for the virtues thereof, that they have called it *Lignum Sanctæ Crucis*, Wood of the Holy Cross, believing it helps the falling-sickness, apoplexy and palsy very speedily, not only to be inwardly taken, but to be hung at their neck. Tragus saith, that the fresh wood of any Misselto bruised, and the juice drawn forth and dropped in the ears that have imposthumes in them, doth help and ease them within a few days.

MONEYWORT, OR HERB TWOPENCE.

Descript.] THE common Moneywort sendeth forth from a small thready root divers long, weak, and slender branches, lying and running upon the ground two or three feet long or more, set with leaves two at a joint one against another at equal distances, which are almost round, but pointed at the ends, smooth, and of a good green colour. At the joints with the leaves from the middle forward come forth at every point sometimes one yellow flower, and sometimes two, standing each on a small foot-stalk, and made of five leaves, narrow-pointed at the end, with some yellow threads in the middle, which being past, there stand in their places small round heads of seed.

Place.] It groweth plentifully in almost all places of this land, commonly in moist grounds by hedge-sides, and in the middle of grassy fields.

Time.] They flower in June and July, and their seed is ripe quickly after.

Government and Virtues.] Venus owns it. Moneywort is singular good to stay all fluxes in man or woman, whether they be lasks, bloody-fluxes, the flowering of womens courses. Bleeding inwardly or outwardly, and the weakness of the stomach that is given to casting. It is very good also for the ulcers or excoriations of the lungs, or other inward parts. It is exceeding good for all wounds, either fresh or green, to heal them speedily, and for all old ulcers that are of spreading natures. For all which purposes the juice of the herb, or the powder drank in water wherein hot steel hath been often quenched; or the decoction of the green herb in wine or water drank, or used to the outward place, to wash or bathe them, or to have tents dipped therein and put into them, are effectual.

MOONWORT.

Descript.] IT riseth up usually but with one dark, green, thick and flat leaf, standing upon a short foot-stalk, not above two fingers breadth; but when it flowers it may be said to bear a small slender stalk about four or five inches high, having but one leaf in the middle thereof, which is much divided on both sides into sometimes five or seven parts on a side, sometimes more; each of which parts is small like the middle rib, but broad forwards, pointed and round, resembling therein a half-moon, from whence it took the name; the uppermost parts or divisions being bigger than the lowest. The stalks rise above this leaf two or three inches, bearing many branches of small long tongues, every one like the spiky head of the adder's tongue, of a brownish colour, (which whether I shall call them flowers, or the seed, I well know not) which, after they have continued a while, resolve into a mealy dust. The root is small and fibrous. This hath sometimes divers such like leaves as are before described, with so many branches or tops rising from one stalk, each divided from the other.

Place.] It groweth on hills and heaths, yet where there is much graſs, for therein it delighteth to grow.

Time.] It is to be found only in April and May; for in June, when any hot weather cometh, for the moſt part it is withered and gone.

Government and Virtues.] The Moon owns the herb. Moonwort is cold, and drying more than adder's tongue, and is therefore held to be more available for all wounds both inward and outward. The leaves boiled in red wine, and drank, ſtay the immoderate flux of womens courſes, and the whites. It alſo ſtayeth bleeding, vomiting, and other fluxes. It helpeth all blows and bruiſes, and to conſolidate all fractures and diſlocations. It is good for ruptures, but it is chiefly uſed by moſt with other herbs to make oils or balſams to heal freſh or green wounds (as I ſaid before) either inward or outward, for which it is excellent good.

Moonwort is an herb which (they ſay) will open locks, and unſhoe ſuch horſes as tread upon it: This ſome laugh to ſcorn, and thoſe no ſmall fools neither; but country people that I know, call it Unſhoe the Horſe. Beſides I have heard commanders ſay, that on White Down in Devonſhire, near Tiverton, there were found thirty Horſeſhoes, pulled off from the feet of the Earl of Eſſex's horſes, being there drawn up in a body, many of them being but newly ſhod, and no reaſon known, which cauſed much admiration, and the herb deſcribed uſually grows upon heaths.

MOSSES.

I Shall not trouble the reader with a deſcription of theſe, ſince my intent is to ſpeak only of two kinds, as the moſt principal, viz. Ground Moſs and Tree Moſs, both which are very well known.

Place.] The Ground Moſs groweth in our moiſt woods, and in the bottom of hills, in boggy grounds, and in ſhadowy ditches, and many other ſuch like places. The tree Moſs groweth only on trees.

Government and Virtues.] All ſorts of Moſſes are under the dominion of Saturn. The Ground Moſs is held to be ſingular good to break the ſtone, and to expel and drive

it

it forth by urine, being boiled in wine and drank. The herb, being bruiſed and boiled in water, and applied, eaſeth all inflammations and pains coming from an hot cauſe; and is therefore uſed to eaſe the pains of the gout.

The tree Moſſes are cooling and binding, and partake of a digeſting and mollifying quality withal, as Galen ſaith. But each Moſs doth partake of the nature of the tree from whence it is taken; therefore that of the oak is more binding, and is of good effect to ſtay fluxes in man or woman; as alſo vomiting or bleeding, the powder thereof being taken in wine. The decoction thereof in wine is very good for women to be bathed, or to ſit in, that are troubled with the overflowing of their courſes. The ſame being drank, ſtayeth the ſtomach that is troubled with caſting, or the hiccough; and, as Avicena ſaith, it comforteth the heart. The powder thereof taken in drink for ſome time together, is thought available for the dropſy. The oil that has had freſh Moſs ſteeped therein for a time, and afterwards boiled and applied to the temples and forehead, doth marvellouſly eaſe the head-ach coming of a hot cauſe; as alſo the diſtillations of hot rheums or humours in the eyes, or other parts. The ancients much uſed it in their ointments and other medicines againſt the laſſitude, and to ſtrengthen and comfort the ſinews: For which, if it was good then, I know no reaſon but it may be found ſo ſtill.

MOTHERWORT.

Deſcript.] THIS hath a hard, ſquare, browniſh, rough, ſtrong ſtalk, riſing three or four feet high at leaſt, ſpreading into many branches, whereon grow leaves on each ſide, with long foot-ſtalks, two at every joint, which are ſomewhat broad and long, as if it were rough or coupled, with many great veins therein of a ſad green colour, and deeply dented about the edges, and almoſt divided. From the middle of the branches up to the tops of them (which are long and ſmall) grow the flowers round them at diſtances, in ſharp pointed, rough, hard huſks, of a more red or purple colour than balm or horehound, but in the ſame manner or form as the horehounds, after which come ſmall, round, blackiſh ſeeds in great plenty. The root ſendeth forth a number of long ſtrings and ſmall fibres, taking ſtrong hold in the ground, of a dark yellowiſh or browniſh colour, and abideth as the horehound doth; the ſmell of this not much differeth from that.

Place.] It groweth only in gardens with us in England.

Government and Virtues.] Venus owns the herb, and it is under Leo. There is no better herb to take melancholy vapours from the heart, to ſtrengthen it, and make a merry, chearful, blithe ſoul than this herb. It may be kept in a ſyrup or conſerve; therefore the Latins called it Cardiaca. Beſides, it makes women joyful mothers of children, and ſettles their wombs as they ſhould be, therefore we call it Motherwort. It is held to be of much uſe for the trembling of the heart, and faintings and ſwoonings; from whence it took the name Cardiaca. The powder thereof to the quantity of a ſpoonful, drank in wine, is a wonderful help to women in their ſore travail, as alſo for the ſuffocating or riſings of the mother, and for theſe effects, it is likely it took the name of Motherwort with us. It alſo provoketh urine and womens courſes, cleanſeth the cheſt of cold phlegm, oppreſſing it, killeth worms in the belly. It is of good uſe to warm and dry up the cold humours, to digeſt and diſperſe them that are ſettled in the veins, joints and ſinews of the body, and to help cramps and convulſions.

MOUSE-EAR.

Deſcript.] MOUSE-EAR is a low herb, creeping upon the ground by ſmall ſtrings, like the ſtrawberry plant, whereby it ſhooteth forth ſmall roots, whereat grow upon the ground many ſmall and ſomewhat ſhort leaves, ſet in a round form together, and very hairy, which being broken do give a whitiſh milk: From among theſe leaves ſpring up two or three ſmall hoary ſtalks about a ſpan high, with a few ſmaller leaves thereon; at the tops whereof ſtandeth uſually but one flower, conſiſting of many pale yellow leaves, broad at the point, and a little dented in, ſet in three or four rows (the greater uppermoſt) very like a dandelion flower, and a little reddiſh underneath about the edges, eſpecially if it grow

in

in a dry ground; which after they have ſtood long in flower do turn into down, which, with the ſeed, is carried away with the wind.

Place.] It groweth on ditch banks, and ſometimes in ditches, if they be dry, and in ſandy grounds.

Time.] It flowereth about June or July, and abideth green all the Winter.

Government and Virtues.] The Moon owns this herb alſo; and though authors cry out upon Alchymiſts, for attempting to fix quickſilver by this herb and Moonwort, a Roman would not have judged a thing by the ſucceſs; if it be to be fixed at all, it is by lunar influence. The juice thereof taken in wine, or the decoction thereof drank, doth help the jaundice, although of long continuance, to drink thereof morning and evening, and abſtain from other drink two or three hours after. It is a ſpecial remedy againſt the ſtone, and the tormenting pains thereof; as alſo other tortures and gripping pains of the bowels. The decoction thereof with ſuccory and centaury is held very effectual to help the dropſy, and them that are inclining thereunto, and the diſeaſes of the ſpleen. It ſtayeth the fluxes of blood, either at the mouth or noſe, and inward bleeding alſo, for it is a ſingular wound herb for wounds both inward and outward: It helpeth the bloody-flux, and helpeth the abundance of womens courſes. There is a ſyrup made of the juice hereof, and ſugar, by the apothicaries of Italy, and other places, which is of much account with them, to be given to thoſe that are troubled with the cough or phthiſick. The ſame alſo is ſingular good for ruptures or burſtings. The green herb bruiſed and preſently bound to any cut or wound, doth quickly ſolder the lips thereof. And the juice, decoction, or powder of the dried herb is moſt ſingular to ſtay the malignity of ſpreading and fretting cankers and ulcers whatſoever, yea in the mouth and ſecret parts. The diſtilled water of the plant is available in all the diſeaſes aforeſaid, and to waſh outward wounds and ſores, and apply tents of cloths wet therein.

MUGWORT.

Descript.] COMMON Mugwort hath divers leaves lying upon the ground, very much divided, or cut deeply in about the brims, somewhat like wormwood, but much larger, of a dark green colour on the upper side, and very hoary white underneath. The stalks rise to be four or five feet high, having on it such like leaves as those below, but somewhat smaller, branching forth very much towards the top, whereon are set very small, pale, yellowish flowers like buttons, which fall away, and after them come small seeds inclosed in round heads. The root is long and hard, with many small fibres growing from it, whereby it taketh strong hold on the ground; but both stalks and leaf do lie down every year, and the root shooteth a-new in the Spring. The whole plant is of a reasonable scent, and is more easily propagated by the slips than the seed.

Place.] It groweth plentifully in many places of this land, by the water-sides; as also by small water courses, and in divers others places.

Time.] It flowereth and seedeth in the end of Summer.

Government and Virtues.] This is an herb of Venus, therefore maintaineth the parts of the body she rules, remedies the diseases of the parts that are under her signs Taurus and Libra. Mugwort is with good success put among other herbs that are boiled for women to sit over the hot decoction to draw down their courses, to help the delivery of their birth, and expel the after-birth. As also for the obstructions and inflammations of the mother. It breaketh the stone, and causeth one to make water where it is stopped. The juice thereof made up with myrrh, and put under as a pessary, worketh the same effects, and so doth the root also. Being made up with hog's grease into an ointment, it taketh away wens and hard knots and kernels that grow about the neck more effectually, if some field Daisies be put with it. The herb itself being fresh, or the juice thereof taken, is a special remedy upon the overmuch taking of opium. Three drams of the powder of the dried leaves taken in wine, is a speedy and the best certain help for the sciatica. A decoction thereof

thereof made with camomile and agrimony, and the place bathed therewith while it is warm, taketh away the pains of the ſinews, and the cramp.

The MULBERRY-TREE.

THIS is ſo well known where it groweth, that it needeth no deſcription.

Time] It beareth fruit in the months of July and Auguſt

Government and Virtues.] Mercury rules the Tree, therefore are its effects variable as his are. The Mulberry is of different parts; the ripe berries, by reaſon of their ſweetneſs and ſlippery moiſture, opening the body, and the unripe binding it, eſpecially when they are dried, and then they are good to ſtay fluxes, laſks, and the abundance of womens courſes. The bark of the root killeth the broad worms in the body. The juice or the ſyrup made of the juice of the berries, helpeth all inflammations or ſores in the mouth or throat, and palate of the mouth when it is fallen down. The juice of the leaves is a remedy againſt the biting of ſerpents, and for thoſe that have taken aconite. The leaves beaten with vinegar, are good to lay on any place that is burnt with fire. A decoction made of the bark and leaves is good to waſh the mouth and teeth when they ache. If the root be a little ſlit or cut, and a ſmall hole made in the ground next thereunto, in the Harveſt-time, it will give out a certain juice, which being hardened the next day, is of good uſe to help the tooth-ach, to diſſolve knots and purge the belly. The leaves of Mulberries are ſaid to ſtay bleeding at the mouth or noſe, or the bleeding of the piles, or of a wound, being bound unto the places. A branch of the tree taken when the moon is at the full, and bound to the wriſt of a woman's arm, whoſe courſes come down too much, doth ſtay them in a ſhort ſpace.

MULLEIN.

Deſcript.] COMMON White Mullein hath many fair, large, woolly white leaves, lying next the ground, ſomewhat larger than broad, pointed at the end, and as it were dented about the edges. The ſtalk riſeth up to be four or five feet high, covered over with ſuch like

like leaves, but lesser, so that no stalk can be seen for the multitude of leaves thereon up to the flowers, which come forth on all sides of the stalk, without any branches for the most part, and are many set together in a long spike, in some of a yellow colour, in others more pale, consisting of five round pointed leaves, which afterwards have small round heads, wherein is small brownish seed contained. The root is long, white, and woody, perishing after it hath borne seed.

Place.] It groweth by way-sides and lanes, in many places of this land.

Time.] It flowereth in July, or thereabouts.

Government and Virtues.] It is under the dominion of Saturn. A small quantity of the root given in wine, is commended by Dioscorides, against lasks and fluxes of the belly. The decoction hereof drank, is profitable for those that are burster, and for cramps and convulsions, and for those that are troubled with an old cough. The decoction thereof gargled, easeth the pains of the tooth-ach. And the oil made by the often infusion of the flowers, is of very good effect for the piles. The decoction of the root in red wine or water, (if there be an ague) wherein red-hot steel hath been often quenched, doth stay the bloody-flux. The same also openeth obstructions of the bladder and reins when one cannot make water. A decoction of the leaves hereof, and of sage, marjoram, and camomile flowers, and the places bathed therewith, that have sinews stiff with cold or cramps, doth bring them much ease and comfort. Three ounces of the distilled water of the flowers drank morning and evening for some days together, is said to be the most excellent remedy for the gout. The juice of the leaves and flowers being laid upon rough warts, as also the powder of the dried roots rubbed on, doth easily take them away, but doth no good to smooth warts. The powder of the dried flowers is an especial remedy for those that are troubled with the belly-ach, or the pains of the colick. The decoction of the root, and so likewise of the leaves, is of great effect to dissolve the tumours, swellings, or inflammations of the throat. The seed and leaves boiled in wine, and applied, draw forth speedily thorns or splinters gotten into the flesh,

flesh, ease the pains, and heal them also. The leaves bruised and wrapped in double papers, and covered with hot ashes and embers to bake a while, and then taken forth and laid warm on any blotch or boil happening in the groin or share, doth dissolve and heal them. The seed bruised and boiled in wine, and laid on any member that hath been out of joint, and newly set again, taketh away all swelling and pain thereof.

MUSTARD.

Descript.] OUR common Mustard hath large and broad rough leaves, very much jagged with uneven and unorderly gashes, somewhat like turnip leaves, but lesser and rougher. The stalk riseth to be more than a foot high, and sometimes two feet high, being round, rough, and branched at the top, bearing such like leaves thereon as grow below, but lesser, and less divided, and divers yellow flowers one above another at the tops, after which come small rough pods, with small, lank, flat ends, wherein is contained round yellowish seed, sharp, hot, and biting upon the tongue. The root is small, long, and woody, when it beareth stalks, and perisheth every year.

Place] This groweth with us in gardens only, and other manured places.

Time.] It is an annual plant, flowering in July, and the seed is ripe in August.

Government and Virtues.] It is an excellent sauce for such whose blood wants clarifying, and for weak stomachs, being an herb of Mars, but nought for cholerick people, though as good for such as are aged, or troubled with cold diseases. Aries claims something to do with it, therefore it strengthens the heart and resisteth poison. Let such whose stomachs are so weak they cannot digest their meat, or appetite it, take of Mustard-seed a dram, cinnamon as much, and having beaten them to powder, and half as much mastick in powder, and with gum-arabick dissolved in rose-water, make it up into troches, of which they may take one of about half a dram weight an hour or two before meals; let old men and women make much of this medicine, and they will either give me thanks,

or

or shew manifest ingratitude. Mustard-seed hath the virtue of heat, discussing, ratifying, and drawing out splinters of bones, and other things of the flesh. It is of good effect to bring down womens courses, for the falling-sickness or lethargy, drowsy forgetful evil, to use it both inwardly and outwardly, to rub the nostrils, forehead, and temples, to warm and quicken the spirits; for by the fierce sharpness it purgeth the brain by sneezing, and drawing down rheum and other viscous humours, which by their distillations upon the lungs and chest, procure coughing, and therefore, with some honey added thereto, doth much good therein. The decoction of the seed made in wine, and drank, provoketh urine, resisteth the force of poison, the malignity of mushrooms, and venom of scorpions, or other venomous creatures, if it be taken in time; and taken before the cold fits of agues, altereth, lesseneth, and cureth them. The seed taken either by itself, or with other things, either in an electuary or drink, doth mightily stir up bodily lust, and helpeth the spleen and pains in the sides, and gnawings in the bowels; and used as a gargle draweth up the palate of the mouth, being fallen down; and also it dissolveth the swellings about the throat, if it be outwardly applied. Being chewed in the mouth it oftentimes helpeth the tooth-ach. The outward application hereof upon the pained place of the sciatica, discusseth the humours, and easeth the pains, as also the gout, and other joint-achs; and is much and often used to ease pains in the sides or loins, the shoulders, or other parts of the body, upon the plying thereof to raise blisters, and cureth the disease by drawing it to the outward parts of the body. It is also used to help the falling off the hair. The seed bruised, mixed with honey, and applied, or made up with wax, taketh away the marks and black and blue spots of bruises, or the like, the roughness or scabbiness of the skin, as also the leprosy, and lousy evil. It helpeth also the crick in the neck. The distilled water of the herb, when it is in the flower, is much used to drink inwardly to help in any of the diseases aforesaid, or to wash the mouth when the palate is down, and for the diseases of the throat to gargle, but outwardly also for scabs, itch, or other the like infirmities, and cleanseth the face from morphew, spots, freckles, and other deformities.

The

The HEDGE-MUSTARD.

Descript.] THIS groweth up usually but with one blackish green stalk, tough, easy to bend, but not to break, branched into divers parts, and sometimes with divers stalks, set full of branches, whereon grow long, rough, or hard rugged leaves, very much tore or cut on the edges in many parts, some bigger, and some lesser, of a dirty green colour. The flowers are small and yellow, that grow on the tops of the branches in long spikes, flowering by degrees; so that continuing long in flower, the stalk will have small round cods at the bottom growing upright and close to the stalk, while the top flowers yet shew themselves, in which are contained small yellow seed, sharp and strong, as the herb is also. The root groweth down slender and woody, yet abiding and springing again every year.

Place.] This groweth frequently in this land, by the ways and hedge-sides, and sometimes in the open fields.

Time.] It flowereth most usually about July.

Government and Virtues.] Mars owns this herb also. It is singular good in all the diseases of the chest and lungs, hoarseness of voice; and by the use of the decoction thereof for a little space, those have been recovered who had utterly lost their voice, and almost their spirits also. The juice thereof made into a syrup, or licking medicine, with honey or sugar, is no less effectual for the same purpose, and for all other coughs, wheezing, and shortness of breath. The same is also profitable for those that have the jaundice, pleurisy, pains in the back and loins, and for torments in the belly, or colick, being also used in clysters. The seed is held to be a special remedy against poison and venom. It is singular good for the sciatica, and in joint-aches, ulcers and cankers in the mouth, throat, or behind the ears, and no less for the hardness and swelling of the testicles, or of womens breasts.

NAILWORT, or WHITLOWGRASS.

Descript.] THIS very small and common herb hath no roots, save only a few strings: neither doth it ever grow to be above a hand's breadth high, the leaves are very ſmall, and ſomething long, not much unlike thoſe of chickweed, among which riſe up divers ſlender ſtalks, bearing many white flowers one above another, which are exceeding ſmall; after which come ſmall flat pouches containing the ſeed, which is very ſmall, but of a ſharp taſte.

Place.] It grows commonly upon old ſtone and brick walls, and ſometimes in dry gravelly grounds, eſpecially if there be graſs or moſs near to ſhadow it.

Time.] They flower very early in the year, ſometimes in January, and in February; for before the end of April they are not to be found.

Government and Virtues.] It is held to be exceeding good for thoſe impoſthumes in the joints, and under the nails, which they call Whitlows, Felons, Andicons and Nailwheals. Such as would be knowing phyſicians, let them read thoſe books of mine, of the laſt edition, viz. Reverius, Riolanus, Johnſon, Veſtingus, Sennertus.

NEP, or CATMINT.

Deſcript.] COMMON Garden Nep ſhooteth forth hard four-ſquare ſtalks, with a hoarineſs on them, a yard high or more, full of branches, bearing at every joint two broad leaves like balm, but longer pointed, ſofter, white, and more hoary, nicked about the edges, and of a ſtrong ſweet ſcent. The flowers grow in large tufts at the tops of the branches, and underneath them likewiſe on the ſtalks many together, of a whitiſh purple colour. The roots are compoſed of many long ſtrings or fibres, faſtening themſelves ſtronger in the ground, and abide with green leaves thereon all the winter.

Place.] It is only nurſed up in our gardens.

Time.] And it flowereth in July, or thereabouts.

Government and Virtues.] It is an herb of Venus. Nep is generally uſed for women to procure their courſes, being taken inwardly or outwardly, either alone, or with other convenient herbs in a decoction to bathe them, or ſit over the hot fumes thereof; and by the frequent uſe thereof, it takes away barrenneſs, and the wind, and pains of the mother. It is alſo uſed in pains of the head coming of any cold cauſe, catarrhs, rheums, and for ſwimming

and

and giddineſs thereof, and is of ſpecial uſe for the windineſs of the ſtomach and belly. It is effectual for any cramp or cold aches, to diſſolve cold and wind that afflicteth the place, and is uſed for colds, coughs, and ſhortneſs of breath. The juice thereof drank in wine, is profitable for thoſe that are bruiſed by an accident. The green herb bruiſed and applied to the fundament, and lying there two or three hours, eaſeth the pains of the piles; the juice alſo being made up into an ointment, is effectual for the ſame purpoſe. The head waſhed with a decoction thereof, it taketh away ſcabs, and may be effectual for other parts of the body alſo.

NETTLES.

NETTLES are ſo well known, that they need no deſcription; they may be found by feeling, in the darkeſt night.

Government and Virtues.] This is alſo an herb Mars claims dominion over. You know Mars is hot and dry, and you know as well that Winter is cold and moiſt; then you may know as well the reaſon why Nettle Tops eaten in the Spring conſumeth the phlegmatick ſuperfluities in the body of man, that the coldneſs and moiſtneſs of winter hath left behind. The roots or leaves boiled, or the juice of either of them, or both made into an electuary with honey and ſugar, is a ſafe and ſure medicine to open the pipes and paſſages of the lungs, which is the cauſe of wheezing and ſhortneſs of breath, and helpeth to expectorate tough phlegm, as alſo to raiſe the impoſthumed pleuriſy; and ſpend it by ſpitting; the ſame helpeth the ſwelling of the almonds of the throat, the mouth and throat being gargled therewith. The juice is alſo effectual to ſettle the palate of the mouth in its place, and to heal and temper the inflammations and ſoreneſs of the mouth and throat. The decoction of the leaves in wine, being drank, is ſingular good to provoke womens courſes, and ſettle the ſuffocation, ſtrangling of the mother, and all other diſeaſes thereof; as alſo applied outwardly with a little myrrh. The ſame alſo, or the ſeed, provoketh urine, and expelleth the gravel and ſtone in the reins or bladder, often proved to be effectual in many that have taken it. The same killeth the worms in children, easeth pains in the sides, and dissolveth the windiness in the spleen, as also in the body, although others think it only powerful to provoke venery. The juice of the leaves taken two or three days together, stayeth bleeding at the mouth. The seed being drank, is a remedy against the stinging of venomous creatures, the biting of mad dogs, the poisonful qualities of hemlock, henbane, nightshade, mandrake, or other such like herbs that stupify or dull the senses; as also the lethargy, especially to use it outwardly, to rub the forehead or temples in the lethargy, and the places stung or bitten with beasts, with a little salt. The distilled water of the herb is also effectual (though not so powerful) for the diseases aforesaid; as for outward wounds and sores to wash them, and to cleanse the skin from morphew, leprosy, and other discolourings thereof. The seed or leaves bruised and put into the nostrils, stayeth the bleeding of them, and taketh away the flesh growing in them called polypus. The juice of the leaves, or the decoction of them, or of the root, is singular good to wash either old, rotten, or stinking sores or fistulas, and gangrenes, and such as fretting, eating, or corroding scabs, manginess, and itch, in any part of the body, as also green wounds, by washing them therewith, or applying the green herb bruised thereunto, yea, although the flesh were separated from the bones; the same applied to our wearied members, refresh them, or to place those that have been out of joint, being first set up again, strengtheneth, drieth, and comforteth them, as also those places troubled with aches and gouts, and the defluction of humours upon the joints or sinews; it easeth the pains, and drieth or dissolveth the defluctions. An ointment made of the juice, oil, and a little wax, is singular good to rub cold and benummed members. An handful of the leaves of green nettles, and another of wallwort, or deanwort, bruised and applied simply themselves to the gout, sciatica, or joint aches in any part, hath been found to be an admirable help thereunto.

NIGHT-

NIGHTSHADE.

Descript.] COMMON Nightshade hath an upright, round, green, hollow ſtalk, about a foot or half a yard high, buſhing forth in many branches whereon grow many green leaves, ſomewhat broad, and pointed at the ends, ſoft and full of juice, ſomewhat like unto Baſil, but longer and a little unevenly dented about the edges: At the tops of the ſtalks and branches come forth three or four more white flowers made of five ſmall pointed leaves a-piece, ſtanding on a ſtalk together, one above another, with yellow pointels in the middle, compoſed of four or five yellow threads ſet together, which afterwards run into ſo many pendulous green berries, of the bigneſs of ſmall peaſe, full of green juice, and ſmall whitiſh round flat ſeed lying within it. The root is white, and a little woody when it hath given flower and fruit, with many ſmall fibres at it: The whole plant is of a wateriſh inſipid taſte, but the juice within the berries is ſomewhat viſcous, and of a cooling and binding quality.

Place.] It groweth wild with us under our walls, and in rubbiſh, the common paths, and ſides of hedges and fields, as alſo in our gardens here in England, without any planting.

Time.] It lieth down every year, and riſeth again of its own ſowing, but ſpringeth not until the latter end of April at the ſooneſt.

Government and Virtues.] It is a cold Saturnine plant. The common Nightſhade is wholly uſed to cool hot inflammations either inwardly or outwardly, being no ways dangerous to any that uſe it, as moſt of the reſt of the Nightſhades are; yet it muſt be uſed moderately. The diſtilled water only of the whole herb is fitteſt and ſafeſt to be taken inwardly: The juice alſo clarified and taken, being mingled with a little vinegar, is good to waſh the mouth and throat that is inflamed: But outwardly the juice of the herbs or berries, with oil of roſes and a little vinegar and ceruſe laboured together in a leaden mortar, is very good to anoint all hot inflammations in the eyes. It alſo doth much good for the ſhingles, ringworms, and in all running, fretting, and corroding ulcers, applied thereunto. A peſſary dipped in the juice, and dropped into the matrix, ſtayeth the immoderate flux of womens courſes; a cloth wet therein, and applied to the teſticles or cods, upon any ſwelling therein, giveth much eaſe, alſo to the gout that cometh of hot and ſharp humours. The juice dropped into the ears, eaſeth pains thereof that ariſe of heat or inflammations. And Pliny ſaith, it is good for hot ſwellings under the throat. Have a care you miſtake not the deadly nightſhade for this; if you know it not, you may let them both alone, and take no harm, having other medicines ſufficient in the book.

The OAK.

IT is ſo well known (the timber thereof being the glory and ſaftety of this nation by ſea) that it needeth no deſcription.

Government and Virtues.] Jupiter owns the tree. The leaves and bark of the Oak, and the acorn cups, do bind and dry very much. The inner bark of the Tree, and the thin ſkin that covereth the acorn, are moſt uſed to ſtay the ſpitting of blood, and the bloody-flux. The decoction of that bark, and the powder of the cups, do ſtay vomitings, ſpitting of blood, bleeding at the mouth, or other flux of blood in men or women; laſks alſo, and the involuntary flux of natural ſeed. The acorn in powder taken in wine, provoketh urine, and reſiſteth the poiſon of venomous creatures. The decoction of acorns and the bark made in milk and taken, reſiſteth the force of poiſonous herbs and medicines, as alſo the virulency of cantharides, when one by eating them hath his bladder exulcerated, and piſſeth blood. Hippocrates ſaith, he uſed the fumes of Oak leaves to women that were troubled with the ſtrangling of the mother; and Galen applied them, being bruiſed, to cure green wounds. The diſtilled water of the Oaken bud, before they break out into leaves, is good to be uſed either inwardly or outwardly, to aſſuage inflammations, and to ſtop all manner of fluxes in man or woman. The ſame is ſingular good in peſtilential and hot burning fevers; for it reſiſteth the force of the infection, and allayeth the heat: It cooleth the heat of the liver, breaketh the ſtone in the kidneys, and ſtayeth

ſtayeth womens courſes. The decoction of the leaves worketh the ſame effects. The water that is found in the hollow places of old Oaks, is very effectual againſt any foul or ſpreading ſcabs. The diſtilled water (or concoction, which is better) of the leaves, is one of the beſt remedies that I know of for the whites in women.

OATS

ARE ſo well known that they need no deſcription.

Government and Virtues.] Oats fried with bay ſalt, and applied to the ſides, take away the pains of ſtitches and wind in the ſides of the belly. A poultice made of meal of Oats, and ſome oil of bays put thereunto, helpeth the itch and the leproſy, as alſo the fiſtulas of the fundament, and diſſolveth hard impoſthumes. The meal of Oats boiled with vinegar, and applied, taketh away freckles and ſpots in the face, and other parts of the body.

ONE BLADE.

Deſcript.] THIS ſmall plant never beareth more than one leaf, but only when it riſeth up with his ſtalk, which thereon beareth another, and ſeldom more which are of a blueiſh green colour, pointed, with many ribs or veins therein, like plantain. At the top of the ſtalk grow many ſmall white flowers, ſtar faſhion, ſmelling ſomewhat ſweet; after which come ſmall red berries, when they are ripe. The root is ſmall, of the bigneſs of a ruſh, lying and creeping under the upper cruſt of the earth, ſhooting forth in divers places.

Place.] It groweth in moiſt, ſhadowy, and graſſy places of woods, in many places of this land.

Time.] It flowereth about May, and the berries are ripe in June, and then quickly periſheth, until the next year it ſpringeth from the ſame root again.

Government and Virtues.] It is a precious herb of the Sun. Half a dram, or a dram at moſt, in powder of the roots hereof taken in wine and vinegar, of each equal parts, and the party laid preſently to ſweat thereupon, is held to be a ſovereign remedy for thoſe that are infected with the plague, and have a ſore upon them, by expelling the poiſon and infection, and defending the heart and

ſpirits

ſpirits from danger. It is a ſingular good wound herb, and is thereupon uſed with others of the like effects in many compound balms for curing of wounds, be they freſh and green, or old and malignant, and eſpecially if the ſinews be burnt.

ORCHIS.

IT hath gotten almoſt as many ſeveral names attributed to the ſeveral ſorts of it, as would almoſt fill a ſheet of paper; as dog-ſtones, goat-ſtones, fool-ſtones, fox-ſtones, ſatirion, cullians, together with many others too tedious to rehearſe.

Deſcript.] To deſcribe all the ſeveral ſorts of it were an endleſs piece of work; therefore I ſhall only deſcribe the roots, becauſe they are to be uſed with ſome diſcretion. They have each of them a double root within, ſome of them are round, in others like a hand; theſe roots alter every year by courſe, when the one riſeth and waxeth full, the other waxeth lank, and periſheth: Now, it is that which is full which is to be uſed in medicines, the other being either of no uſe at all, or elſe, according to the humour of ſome, it deſtroys and diſannuls the virtue of the other, quite undoing what that doth.

Time.] One or other of them may be found in flower from the beginning of April to the latter end of Auguſt.

Temperature and Virtues.] They are hot and moiſt in operation, under the dominion of Dame Venus, and provoke luſt exceedingly, which, they ſay, the dried and withered roots do reſtrain. They are held to kill worms in children; as alſo, being bruiſed and applied to the place, to heal the king's evil.

ONIONS.

THEY are ſo well known, that I need not ſpend time about writing a deſcription of them.

Government and Virtues.] Mars owns them, and they have gotten this quality, to draw any corruption to them, for if you peel one, and lay it upon a dunghill, you ſhall find him rotten in half a day, by drawing putrefaction to it; then being bruiſed and applied to a plague ſore, it is very probable it will do the like. Onions are flatulent,

or

or windy; yet they do somewhat provoke appetite, increase thirst, ease the belly and bowels, provoke womens courses, help the biting of a mad dog, and of other venomous creatures, to be used with honey and rue, increase sperm, especially the seed of them. They also kill worms in children if they drink the water fasting wherein they have been steeped all night. Being roasted under the embers, and eaten with honey or sugar and oil, they much conduce to help an inveterate cough, and expectorate the tough phlegm. The juice being snuffed up in the nostrils, purgeth the head, and helpeth the lethargy, (yet the often eating them is said to procure pains in the head.) It hath been held by divers country people a great preservative against infection, to eat Onions fasting with bread and salt: As also to make a great Onion hollow, filling the place with good treacle, and after to roast it well under the embers, which, after taking away the outermost skin thereof, being beaten together, is a sovereign salve for either plague or sores, or any other putrefied ulcer. The juice of Onions is good for either scalding or burning by fire, water, or gunpowder, and used with vinegar, taketh away all blemishes, spots and marks in the skin; and dropped in the ears, easeth the pains and noise of them. Applied also with figs beaten together, helpeth to ripen and break imposthumes, and other sores.

Leeks are as like them in quality, as the pome-water is like an apple: They are a remedy against a surfeit of mushrooms, being baked under the embers and taken; and being boiled and applied very warm, help the piles. In other things they have the same property as the Onions although not so effectual.

ORPINE.

Descript.] COMMON Orpine riseth up with divers round brittle stalks, thick set with flat and fleshy leaves, without any order, and little or nothing dented about the edges, of a green colour: The flowers are white, or whitish, growing in tufts, after which come small chaffy husks, with seeds like dust in them. The roots are divers thick, round, white tuberous clogs; and the plant

plant groweth not so big in some places as in others where it is found.

Place.] It is frequent in almost every county of this land, and is cherished in gardens with us, where it groweth greater than that which is wild, and groweth in shadowy sides of fields and woods.

Time.] It flowereth about July, and the seed is ripe in August.

Government and Virtues.] The Moon owns the herb, and he that knows but her exaltation, knows what I say is true. Orpine is seldom used in inward medicines with us, altho' Tragus saith from experience in Germany, that the distilled water thereof is profitable for gnawings or excoriations in the stomach or bowels, or for ulcers in the lungs, liver, or other inward parts, as also in the matrix, and helpeth all those diseases, being drank for certain days together. It stayeth the sharpness of humours in the bloody-flux, and other fluxes in the body or in wounds. The root thereof also performeth the like effect. It is used outwardly to cool any heat or inflammation upon any hurt or wound, and easeth the pains of them; as also, to heal scaldings or burnings, the juice thereof being beaten with some green sallad oil, and anointed. The leaf bruised, and laid to any green wound in the hands or legs, doth heal them quickly; and being bound to the throat, much helpeth the quinsy; it helpeth also ruptures and burstenness. If you please to make the juice thereof into a syrup with honey or sugar, you may safely take a spoonful or two at a time, (let my author say what he will) for a quinsy, and you shall find the medicine more pleasant, and the cure more speedy, than if you had taken a dog's turd, which is the vulgar cure.

PARSLEY.

THIS is so well known, that it needs no description.

Government and Virtues.] It is under the dominion of Mercury; is very comfortable to the stomach; helpeth to provoke urine and womens courses, to break wind both in the stomach and bowels, and doth a little open the body, but the root much more. It openeth obstructions both of liver and spleen, and is therefore accounted one of the

five

five opening roots. Galen commended it against the falling-sickness, and to provoke urine mightily, especially if the roots be boiled, and eaten like parsnips. The seed is effectual to provoke urine and womens courses, to expel wind, to break the stone, and easeth the pains and torments thereof; it is also effectual against the venom of any poisonous creature, and the danger that cometh to them that have the lethargy, and is as good against the cough. The distilled water of Parsley is a familiar medicine with nurses to give their children when they are troubled with wind in the stomach or belly, which they call the frets; and is also much available to them that are of great years. The leaves of Parsley laid to the eyes that are inflamed with heat, or swollen, doth much help them, if it be used with bread or meal; and being fried with butter, and applied to womens breasts that are hard through the curdling of their milk, it abateth the hardness quickly, and also it taketh away black and blue marks coming of bruises or falls. The juice thereof dropped into the ears with a little wine, easeth the pains. Tragus setteth down an excellent medicine to help the jaundice and falling-sickness, the dropsy, and stone in the kidneys in this manner: Take of the seed of Parsley, Fennel, Annise, and Carraways, of each an ounce; of the roots of Parsley, Burnet, Saxifrage, and Carraways, of each an ounce and an half; let the seeds be bruised, and the roots washed and cut small; let them lie all night and steep in a bottle of white wine, and in the morning be boiled in a close earthen vessel until a third part or more be wasted; which being strained and cleared, take four ounces thereof morning and evening first and last, abstaining from drink after it for three hours. This openeth obstructions of the liver and spleen, and expelleth the dropsy and jaundice by urine.

PARSLEY PIERT, or PARSLEY BREAKSTONE.

Descript.] THE root, although it be very small and thready, yet it continues many years, from whence arise many leaves lying along on the ground, each standing upon a long small foot-stalk, the leaves as broad as a man's nail, very deeply dented on the edges, somewhat like a Parsley-leaf, but of a very dusky green colour.

The

The ſtalks are very weak and ſlender, about three or four fingers in length, ſet ſo full of leaves that they can hardly be ſeen, either having no foot-ſtalk at all, or but very ſhort; the flowers are ſo ſmall they can hardly be ſeen, and the ſeed as ſmall as may be.

Place.] It is a common herb throughout the nation, and rejoiceth in barren, ſandy, moiſt places. It may be found plentifully about Hampſtead-Heath, Hyde-Park, and in Tothill-fields.

Time.] It may be found all the Summer-time, even from the beginning of April, to the end of October.

Government and Virtues.] Its operation is very prevalent, to provoke urine, and to break the ſtone. It is a very good ſallad herb. It were good the gentry would pickle it up as they pickle up ſamphire for their uſe all the winter. I cannot teach them how to do it; yet this I can tell them, it is a very wholeſome herb. They may alſo keep the herb dry, or in a ſyrup, if they pleaſe. You may take a dram of the powder of it in white wine; it would bring away gravel from the kidneys inſenſibly, and without pain. It alſo helps the ſtrangury.

PARSNIP.

THE garden kind thereof is ſo well known (the root being commonly eaten) that I ſhall not trouble you with any deſcription of it. But the wild kind being of more phyſical uſe, I ſhall in this place deſcribe it unto you.

Deſcript.] The wild Parſnip differeth little from the garden, but groweth not ſo fair and large, nor hath ſo many leaves, and the root is ſhorter, more woody, and not ſo fit to be eaten, and therefore more medicinal.

Place.] The name of the firſt ſheweth the place of its growth. The other groweth wild in divers places, as in the marſhes by Rocheſter, and elſewhere, and flowereth in July; the ſeed being ripe about the beginning of Auguſt, the ſecond year after the ſowing; for if they do flower the firſt year, the country people call them Madneps.

Government and Virtues.] The garden Parſnips are under Venus. The garden Parſnip nouriſheth much, and is is good and wholeſome nouriſhment, but a little windy, whereby it is thought to procure bodily luſt; but it fatteneth the body much, if much uſed. It is conduicible to the ſtomach and reins, and provoketh urine. But the wild Parſnip hath a cutting, attenuating, cleanſing, and opening quality therein. It reſiſteth and helpeth the bitings of ſerpents, eaſeth the pains and ſtitches in the ſides, and diſſolveth wind both in the ſtomach and bowels, which is the colick, and provoketh urine. The root is often uſed, but the ſeed much more. The wild being better than the tame, ſhews Dame Nature to be the beſt phyſician.

COW PARSNIP.

Deſcript.] THIS groweth with three or four large, ſpread winged, rough leaves, lying often on the ground, or elſe raiſed a little from it, with long, round, hairy foot-ſtalks under them, parted uſually into five diviſions, the two couples ſtanding each againſt the other; and one at the end, and each leaf being almoſt round, yet ſomewhat deeply cut in on the edges in ſome leaves, and not ſo deep in others, of a whitiſh green colour, ſmelling ſomewhat ſtrongly; among which riſeth up a round, creſted, hairy ſtalk, two or three feet high, with a few joints and leaves thereon, and branched at the top, where ſtand large umbels of white, and ſometimes reddiſh flowers, and after them flat, whitiſh, thin, winged ſeed, two always joined together. The root is long and white, with two or three long ſtrings growing down into the ground, ſmelling likewiſe ſtrongly and unpleaſant.

Place.] It groweth in moiſt meadows, and the borders and corners of fields, and near ditches, through this land.

Time.] It flowereth in July, and ſeedeth in Auguſt.

Government and Virtues.] Mercury hath the dominion over them. The ſeed thereof, as Galen ſaith, is of a ſharp and cutting quality, and therefore is a fit medicine for a cough and ſhortneſs of breath, the falling-ſickneſs and jaundice. The root is available to all the purpoſes aforeſaid, and is alſo of great uſe to take away the hard ſkin that groweth on a fiſtula, if it be but ſcraped upon it. The ſeed hereof being drank, cleanſeth the belly from tough phlegmatick matter therein, easeth them that are liver grown, womens passions of the mother, as well being drank as the smoke thereof received underneath, and likewise raiseth such as are fallen into a deep sleep, or have the lethargy, by burning it under their nose. The seed and root boiled in oil, and the head rubbed therewith, helpeth not only those that are fallen into a frenzy, but also the lethargy or drowsy evil, and those that have been long troubled with the head-ach, if it be likewise used with rue. It helpeth also the running scab and the shingles. The juice of the flowers dropped into the ears that run and are full of matter, cleanseth and healeth them.

The PEACH TREE.

Descript.] A Peach Tree groweth not so great as the Apricot Tree, yet spreadeth branches reasonable well, from whence spring smaller reddish twigs, whereon are set long and narrow green leaves dented about the edges. The blossoms are greater than the plumb, and of a light purple colour; the fruit round, and sometimes as big as a reasonable pippin, others smaller, as also differing in colour and taste, as russet, red, or yellow, waterish or firm, with a frize or cotton all over, with a cleft therein like an apricot, and a rugged, furrowed, great stone within it, and a bitter kernel within the stone. It sooner waxeth old, and decayeth, than the apricot, by much.

Place.] They are nursed in gardens and orchards through this land.

Time.] They flower in the spring, and fructify in Autumn.

Government and Virtues.] Lady Venus owns this Tree, and by it opposeth the ill effects of Mars, and indeed for children and young people, nothing is better to purge choler and the jaundice, than the leaves or flowers of this Tree, being made into a syrup or conserve; let such as delight to please their lust regard the fruit; but such as have lost their health, and their childrens, let them regard what I say, they may safely give two spoonfuls of the syrup at a time; it is as gentle as Venus herself. The leaves of peaches bruised and laid on the belly, kill worms; and

and ſo they do alſo being boiled in ale and drank, and open the belly likewiſe; and being dried is a ſafer medicine to diſcuſs humours. The powder of them ſtrewed upon freſh bleeding wounds ſtayeth their bleeding, and cloſeth them up. The flowers ſteeped all night in a little wine ſtanding warm, ſtrained forth in the morning, and drank faſting, doth gently open the belly, and move it downward. A ſyrup made of them, as the ſyrup of roſes is made, worketh more forcibly than that of roſes, for it provoketh vomiting, and ſpendeth wateriſh and hydropick humours by the continuance thereof. The flowers made into a conſerve, worketh the ſame effect. The liquor that droppeth from the tree, being wounded, is given in the decoction of Coltsfoot, to thoſe that are troubled with the cough or ſhortneſs of breath, by adding thereunto ſome ſweet wine, and putting ſome ſaffron alſo therein. It is good for thoſe that are hoarſe, or have loſt their voice; helpeth all defects of the lungs, and thoſe that vomit and ſpit blood. Two drams hereof given in the juice of lemons, or of radiſh, is good for them that are troubled with the ſtone. The kernels of the ſtones do wonderfully eaſe the pains and wringings of the belly, through wind or ſharp humours, and help to make an excellent medicine for the ſtone upon all occaſions, in this manner: *I take fifty kernels of peach-ſtones, and one hundred of the kernels of cherry-ſtones, a handful of elder flowers freſh or dried, and three pints of muſcadel; ſet them in a cloſe pot into a bed of horſe dung for ten days, after which diſtil in a glaſs with a gentle fire*, and keep it for your uſe: You may drink upon occaſion three or four ounces at a time. The milk or cream of theſe kernels being drawn forth with ſome vervain water, and applied to the forehead and temples, doth much help to procure reſt and ſleep to ſick perſons wanting it. The oil drawn from the kernels, the temples being therewith anointed, doth the like. The ſaid oil put into clyſters, eaſeth the pains of the wind colick: and anointed on the lower part of the belly, doth the like, and dropped into the ears, eaſeth pains in them; the juice of the leaves doth the like. Being alſo anointed on the forehead and temples, it helpeth the megrim, and all other parts in the head.

If the kernels be bruised and boiled in vinegar, until they become thick, and applied to the head, it marvellously procures the hair to grow again upon bald places, or where it is too thin.

The Pear Tree.

PEAR Trees are so well known, that they need no description.

Government and Virtues.] The Tree belongs to Venus, and so doth the apple tree. For their physical use they are best discerned by their taste. All the sweet and luscious sorts, whether manured or wild, do help to move the belly downwards, more or less. Those that are hard and sour, do, on the contrary, bind the belly as much, and the leaves do so also: Those that are moist do in some sort cool, but harsh or wild sorts much more, and are very good in repelling medicines; and if the wild sort be boiled with mushrooms, it makes them less dangerous. The said Pears boiled with a little honey, help much the oppressed stomach, as all sorts of them do, some more some less; but the harsher sorts do more cool and bind, serving well to be bound to green wounds, to cool and stay the blood, and to heal up the wound without farther trouble, or inflammation, as Galen saith he hath found by experience. The wild pears do sooner close up the lips of green wounds than others.

Schola Salerni adviseth to drink much wine after pears, or else (say they) they are as bad as poison; nay, and they curse the tree for it too; but if a poor man find his stomach oppressed by eating pears, it is but working hard, and it will do as well as drinking wine.

Pellitory of Spain.

COMMON Pellitory of Spain, if it be planted in our gardens, it will prosper very well; yet there is one sort growing ordinarily here wild, which I esteem to be little inferior to the other, if at all. I shall not deny you the description of them both.

Descript.] Common Pellitory is a very common plant, and will not be kept in our gardens without diligent looking to. The root goes down right into the ground bear-

ing

ing leaves, being long and finely cut upon the ſtalk, lying on the ground, much larger than the leaves of the camomile are. At the top it bears one ſingle large flower at a place, having a border of many leaves, white on the upper ſide, and reddiſh underneath, with a yellow thrumb in the middle, not ſtanding ſo cloſe as that of camomile doth.

The other common Pellitory which groweth here, hath a root of a ſharp biting taſte, ſcarce diſcernable by the taſte from that before deſcribed, from whence ariſe divers brittle ſtalks, a yard high and more, with narrow long leaves finely dented about the edges, ſtanding one above another up to the tops. The flowers are many and white, ſtanding in tufts like thoſe of yarrow, with a ſmall, yellowiſh thrum in the middle. The ſeed is very ſmall.

Place.] The laſt groweth in fields by the hedge-ſides and paths, almoſt every where.

Time.] It flowereth at the latter end of June and July.

Government and Virtues.] It is under the government of Mercury, and I am perſuaded it is one of the beſt purgers of the brain that grows. An ounce of the juice taken in a draught of muſkadel an hour before the fit of the ague comes, it will aſſuredly drive away the ague at the ſecond or third time taking at the fartheſt. Either the herb or root dried and chewed in the mouth, purgeth the brain of phlegmatic humours; thereby not only eaſing pains in the head and teeth, but alſo hindereth the diſtilling of the brain upon the lungs and eyes, thereby preventing coughs, phthiſicks and conſumption, the apoplexy and falling-ſickneſs. It is an excellent approved remedy in the lethargy. The powder of the herb or root being ſnuffed up the noſtrils, procureth ſneezing, and eaſeth the head-ach; being made into an ointment with hog's greaſe, it takes away black and blue ſpots, occaſioned by blows or falls, and helps both the gout and ſciatica.

PELLITORY of the WALL.

Deſcript.] IT riſeth with browniſh, red, tender, weak, clear, and almoſt tranſparent ſtalks, about two feet high, upon which grow at the joints two leaves ſomewhat broad and long, of a dark green colour, which afterwards turn brownish, smooth on the edges, but rough and hairy, as the stalks are also. At the joints with the leaves from the middle of the stalk upwards, where it spreadeth into branches, stand many small, pale, purplish flowers in hairy rough heads, or husks, after which come small, black, rough seed, which will stick to any cloth or garment that shall touch it. The root is somewhat long, with small fibres thereat, of a dark reddish colour, which abideth the winter, altho' the stalks and leaves perish and spring every year.

Place.] It groweth wild generally through the land, about the borders of fields, and by the sides of walls, and among rubbish. It will endure well being brought up in gardens, and planted on the shady side, where it will spring of its own sowing.

Time.] It flowereth in June and July, and the seed is ripe soon after.

Government and Virtues.] It is under the dominion of Mercury. The dried herb Pellitory made up into an electuary with honey, or the juice of the herb, or the decoction thereof made up with sugar or honey, is a singular remedy for an old or dry cough, the shortness of breath, and wheezing in the throat. Three ounces of the juice thereof taken at a time, doth wonderfully help stopping of the urine, and to expel the stone or gravel in the kidneys or bladder, and is therefore usually put among other herbs used in clysters to mitigate pains in the back, sides, or bowels, proceeding of wind, stopping of urine, the gravel or stone, as aforesaid. If the bruised herb, sprinkled with some muskadel, be warmed upon a tile, or in a dish upon a few quick coals in a chasing-dish, and applied to the belly, it worketh the same effect. The decoction of the herb, being drank, easeth pains of the mother, and bringeth down womens courses: It also easeth those griefs that arise from obstructions of the liver, spleen, and reins. The same decoction, with a little honey added thereto, is good to gargle a sore throat. The juice held a while in the mouth, easeth pains in the teeth. The distilled water of the herb drank with some sugar, worketh the same effects, and cleanseth the skin from spots, freckles, purples, wheals, sun-burn, morphew, &c. The juice dropped

ped into the ears, easeth the noise in them, and taketh away the pricking and shooting pains therein: The same, or the distilled water, assuageth hot and swelling imposthumes, burnings, and scaldings by fire or water; as also all other hot tumours and inflammations, or breakings-out of heat, being bathed often with wet cloths dipped therein: The said juice made into a liniment with ceruse, and oil of roses, and anointed therewith, cleanseth foul rotten ulcers, and stayeth spreading or creeping ulcers, and running scabs or sores in childrens heads; and helpeth to stay the hair from falling off the head. The said ointment, or the herb applied to the fundament, openeth the piles, and easeth their pains; and being mixed with goats tallow, helpeth the gout: The juice is very effectual to cleanse fistulas, and to heal them up safely; or the herb itself bruised and applied with a little salt. It is likewise also effectual to heal any green wound; if it be bruised and bound thereto for three days, you shall need no other medicine to heal it further. A poultice made hereof with mallows, and boiled in wine and wheat bran and bean flower, and some oil put thereto, and applied warm to any bruised sinews, tendon, or muscle, doth in a very short time restore them to their strength, taking away the pains of the bruises, and dissolveth the congealed blood coming of blows, or falls from high places.

The juice of Pellitory of the Wall clarified and boiled in a syrup with honey, and a spoonful of it drank every morning by such as are subject to the dropsy; if continuing that course, though but once a week, if ever they have the dropsy, let them come but to me, and I will cure them *gratis*.

PENNYROYAL.

PENNYROYAL is so well known unto all, I mean the common kind, that it needeth no description.

There is a greater kind than the ordinary sort found wild with us, which so abideth being brought into gardens, and differeth not from it, but only in the largeness of the leaves and stalks, in rising higher, and not creeping upon the ground so much. The flowers whereof are purple, growing in rundles about the stalks like the other.

Place.

Place.] The first, which is common in gardens, groweth also in many moist and watery places of this land.

The second is found wild in effect in divers places by the high-ways from London to Colchester, and thereabouts, more abundantly than in any other countries, and is also planted in their gardens in Essex.

Time.] They flower in the latter end of Summer, about August.

Government and Virtues.] The herb is under Venus. Dioscorides saith, that Pennyroyal maketh thin tough, phlegm, warmeth the coldness of any part whereto it is applied, and digesteth raw or corrupt matter: Being boiled and drank, it provoketh womens courses, and expelleth the dead child and after-birth, and stayeth the disposition to vomit being taken in water and vinegar mingled together. And being mingled with honey and salt, it voideth phlegm out of the lungs, and purgeth melancholy by the stool. Drank with wine, it helpeth such as are bitten and stung with venomous beasts, and applied to the nostrils with vinegar, reviveth those that are fainting and swooning. Being dried and burnt, it strengtheneth the gums: It is helpful to those that are troubled with the gout, being applied of itself to the place until it was red, and applied in a plaister, it takes away spots or marks in the face, applied with salt, it profiteth those that are splenetick, or liver-grown. The decoction doth help the itch, if washed therewith; being put into baths for women to sit therein, it helpeth the swellings and hardness of the mother. The green herb bruised and put into vinegar, cleanseth foul ulcers, and taketh away the marks of bruises and blows about the eyes, and all discolourings of the face by fire, yea, and the leprosy, being drank and outwardly applied: Boiled in wine with honey and salt, it helpeth the tooth-ach. It helpeth the cold griefs of the joints, taking away the pains, and warmeth the cold part, being fast bound to the place, after a bathing or sweating in an hot house. Pliny addeth, that Pennyroyal and mints together, help faintings, being put into vinegar, and smelled unto, or put into the nostrils or mouth. It easeth head-achs, pains of the breast and belly, and gnawing of the stomach; applied with honey, salt, and vinegar, it help-

eth

eth cramps or convulsions of the sinews: Boiled in milk, and drank, it is effectual for the cough, and for ulcers and sores in the mouth; drank in wine it provoketh womens courses, and expelleth the dead child, and after-birth. Matthiolus saith, The decoction thereof being drank, helpeth the jaundice and dropsy, all pains of the head and sinews that come of a cold cause, and cleareth the eye-sight. It helpeth the lethargy, and applied with barley-meal, helpeth burnings; and put into the ears easeth the pains of them.

MALE and FEMALE PEONY.

Descript.] MALE Peony riseth up with brownish stalks, whereon grow green and reddish leaves, upon a stalk without any particular division in the leaf at all. The flowers stand at the top of the stalks, consisting of five or six broad leaves, of a fair purplish red colour, with many yellow threads in the middle, standing about the head, which after riseth up to be the seed vessels, divided into two, three, or four crooked pods like horns, which being full ripe, open and turn themselves down backward, shewing within them divers round, black, shining seeds, having also many crimson grains, intermixed with black, whereby it maketh a very pretty shew. The roots are great, thick, and long, spreading and running down deep in the ground.

The ordinary Female Peony hath as many stalks, and more leaves on them than the Male; the leaves not so large but nicked on the edges, some with great and deep, others with smaller cuts and divisions, of a dead green colour. The flowers are of a strong heady scent, usually smaller, and of a more purple colour than the Male, with yellow thrums about the head, as the Male hath. The seed vessels are like horns, as in the Male, but smaller, the seed is black, but less shining. The roots consist of many short tuberous clogs, fastened at the end of long strings, and all from the heads of the roots, which is thick and short, and of the like scent with the Male.

Place and Time.] They grow in gardens, and flower usually about May.

Government and Virtues.] It is an herb of the Sun, and under

under the Lion. Physicians say, Male Peony roots are best; but Dr Reason told me Male Peony was best for men, and Female Peony for women, and he desires to be judged by his brother Dr Experience. The roots are held to be of more virtue than the seed; next the flowers, and last of all the leaves. The root of the Male Peony, fresh gathered, having been found by experience to cure the falling-sickness; but the surest way is, besides hanging it about the neck, by which children have been cured, to take the root of the Male Peony washed clean, and stamped somewhat small, and laid to infuse in sack for twenty-four hours at the least, afterwards strain it, and take it first and last morning and evening, a good draught for sundry days together, before and after a full moon, and this will also cure older persons, if the disease be not grown too old, and past cure, especially if there be a due and orderly preparation of the body with posset drink made of betony, &c. The root is also effectual for women that are not sufficiently cleansed after child-birth, and such as are troubled with the mother; for which likewise the black seed beaten to powder, and given in wine, is also available. The black seed also taken before bed-time, and in the morning, is very effectual for such as in their sleep are troubled with the disease called Ephialtes, or Incubus, but we do commonly call it the Night-mare; a disease which melancholy persons are subject unto: It is also good against melancholy dreams. The distilled water or syrup made of the flowers, worketh the same effects that the root and seed do, although more weakly. The Female is often used for the purposes aforesaid, by reason the Male is so scarce a plant, that it is possessed by few, and those great lovers of rarities in this kind.

PEPPERWORT, OR DITTANDER.

Descript.] OUR common Pepperwort sendeth forth somewhat long and broad leaves, of a light blueish greenish colour, finely dented about the edges, and pointed at the ends, standing upon round hard stalks, three or four feet high, spreading many branches on all sides, and having many small white flowers at the tops of them, after which follow small seeds in small heads.

heads. The root is slender, running much under ground, and shooting up again in many places, and both leaves and roots are very hot and sharp of taste, like pepper, for which cause it took the name.

Place.] It groweth naturally in many places of this land, as at Clare in Essex; also near unto Exeter in Devonshire; upon Rochester Common in Kent; in Lancashire, and divers other places; but usually kept in gardens.

Time.] It flowereth in the end of June, and in July.

Government and Virtues.] Here is another martial herb for you, make much of it. Pliny and Paulus Ægineta say, that Pepperwort is very successful for the sciatica, or any other gout or pain in the joints, or any other inveterate grief: The leaves hereof to be bruised, and mixed with old hog's grease, and applied to the place, and to continue thereon four hours in men, and two hours in women, the place being afterwards bathed with wine and oil mixed together, and then wrapt up with wool or skins, after they have sweat a little. It also amendeth the deformities or discolourings of the skin, and helpeth to take away marks, scars, and scabs, or the foul marks of burning with fire or iron. The juice hereof is by some used to be given in ale to drink to women with child, to procure them a speedy delivery in travail.

PERIWINKLE.

Descript.] THE common sort hereof hath many branches trailing or running upon the ground, shooting out small fibres at the joints as it runneth, taking thereby hold in the ground, and rooteth in divers places. At the joints of these branches stand two small, dark, green, shining leaves, somewhat like bay-leaves, but smaller, and with them come forth also the flowers (one at a joint) standing upon a tender foot-stalk, being somewhat long and hollow, parted at the brims, sometimes into four, sometimes into five leaves: The most ordinary sorts are of a pale blue colour; some are pure white, and some of a dark reddish purple colour. The root is little bigger than a rush, bushing in the ground and creeping with his branches far about, whereby it quickly possesseth a great compass, and

and is therefore most usually planted under hedges where it may have room to run.

Place.] Those with the pale blue, and those with the white flowers, grow in woods and orchards, by the hedge-sides, in divers places of this land; but those with the purple flowers in gardens only.

Time.] They flower in March and April.

Temperature and Virtues.] Venus owns this herb, and saith, That the leaves eaten by man and wife together, cause love between them. The Periwinkle is a great binder, stayeth bleeding both at mouth and nose, if some of the leaves be chewed. The French used it to stay womens courses. Dioscorides, Galen, and Ægineta, commend it against the lasks and fluxes of the belly to be drank in wine.

St Peter's Wort.

If Superstition had not been the fater of Tradition, as well as Ignorance the mother of Devotion, this herb, (as well as St John's Wort) had found some other name to be known by; but we may say of our forefathers, as St Paul of the Athenians, "I perceive in many things "you are too superstitious." Yet seeing it is come to pass, That custom having got in possession, pleads prescription for the name, I shall let it pass, and come to the description of the herb, which take as followeth.

Descript.] It riseth up with square upright stalks for the most part, some greater and higher than St John's Wort (and good reason too, St Peter being the greater apostle, (ask the Pope else;) for though God would have the saints equal, the Pope is of another opinion) but brown in the same manner, having two leaves at every joint, somewhat like, but larger than St John's Wort, and a little rounder pointed, with few or no holes to be seen thereon, and having sometimes some smaller leaves rising from the bosom of the greater, and sometimes a little hairy also. At the tops of the two stalks stand many star-like flowers, with yellow threads in the middle, very like those of St John's Wort, insomuch that this is hardly discerned from it, but only by the largeness and height, the seed being alike also

in

in both. The root abideth long, sending forth new shoots every year.

Place.] It groweth in many groves, and small low woods, in divers places of this land, as in Kent, Huntingdon, Cambridge, and Northamptonshire; as also near water-courses in other places.

Time.] It flowereth in June and July, and the seed is ripe in August.

Government and Virtues.] There is not a straw to choose between this and St John's wort, only St Peter must have it, lest he should want pot herbs: It is of the same property of St John's Wort, but somewhat weak, and therefore more seldom used. Two drams of the seed taken at a time in honied water, purgeth cholerick humours (as saith Dioscorides, Pliny, and Galen) and thereby helpeth those that are troubled wi h the sciatica. The leaves are used as St John's Wort, to help those places of the body that have been burnt with fire.

PIMPERNEL.

Descript.] COMMON Pimpernel hath divers weak square stalks lying on the ground, beset all with two small and almost round leaves at every joint, one against another, very like chickweed, but hath no footstalks; for the leaves, as it were, compass the stalk. The flowers stand singly each by themselves at them and the stalk, consisting of five small round-pointed leaves, of a pale red colour, tending to an orange, with so many threads in the middle, in whose places succeed smooth round heads, wherein is contained small seed. The root is small and fibrous, perishing every year.

Place.] It groweth almost every where, as well in the meadows and corn-fields, as by the way-sides, and in gardens, arising of itself.

Time.] It flowereth from May until April, and the seed ripeneth in the mean time, and falleth.

Government and Virtues.] It is a gallant solar herb, of a cleansing attractive quality, whereby it draweth forth thorns or splinters, or other such like things gotten into the flesh; and put up into the nostrils, purgeth the head: and Galen saith also, they have a drying faculty, whereby

X they

they are good to ſolder the lips of wounds, and to cleanſe foul ulcers. The diſtilled water or juice is much eſteemed by French Dames to cleanſe the ſkin from any roughneſs, deformity, or diſcolouring thereof; being boiled in wine and given to drink, it is a good remedy againſt the plague, and other peſtilential fevers, if the party after taking it be warm in his bed, and ſweat for two hours after, and uſe the ſame for twice at leaſt. It helpeth alſo all ſtingings and bitings of venomous beaſts, or mad dogs, being uſed inwardly, and applied outwardly. The ſame alſo openeth obſtructions of the liver, and is very available againſt the infirmities of the reins: It provoketh urine, and helpeth to expel the ſtone and gravel out of the kidneys and bladder, and helpeth much in all inward pains and ulcers. The decoction, or diſtilled water, is no leſs effectual to be applied to all wounds that are freſh and green, or old, filthy, fretting, and running ulcers, which it very effectually cureth in a ſhort ſpace. A little mixed with the juice, and dropped into the eyes, cleanſeth them from cloudy miſts, or thick films which grow over them, and hinder the ſight. It helpeth the tooth-ach, being dropped into the ear on the contrary ſide of the pain. It is alſo effectual to eaſe the pains of the hæmorrhoids or piles.

GROUND PINE, or CHAMEPITYS.

Deſcript.] OUR common Ground Pine groweth low, ſeldom riſing above an hand's breadth high, ſhooting forth divers ſmall branches ſet with ſlender, ſmall, long, narrow, greyiſh, or whitiſh leaves, ſomewhat hairy, and divided into three parts, many buſhing together at a joint, ſome growing ſcatteringly upon the ſtalks, ſmelling ſomewhat ſtrong like unto roſin: The flowers are ſmall, and of a pale yellow colour, growing from the joint of the ſtalk all along among the leaves; after which come ſmall and round huſks. The root is ſmall and woody, periſhing every year.

Place.] It groweth more plentifully in Kent than any other county of this land; as, namely, in many places on this ſide Dartford, along to Southfleet, Chatham, and Rocheſter, and upon Chatham Down, hard by the Beacon, and half a mile from Rocheſter, in a field nigh a houſe called Seleſys.

Time.] It flowereth and giveth seed in the Summer months.

Government and Virtues.] Mars owns the herb. The decoction of Ground Pine drank, doth wonderfully prevail against the strangury, or any inward pains arising from the diseases of the reins and urine, and is special good for all obstructions of the liver and spleen, and gently openeth the body; for which purpose they were wont in former times to make pills with the powder thereof, and the pulp of figs. It marvellously helpeth all the diseases of the mother, inwardly or outwardly applied, procuring womens courses, and expelling the dead child and after-birth; yea, it is so powerful upon those feminine parts, that it is utterly forbidden for women with child, for it will cause abortion or delivery before the time. The decoction of the herb in wine taken inwardly, or applied outwardly, or both, for some time together, is also effectual in all pains and diseases of the joints, as gouts, cramps, palsies, sciatica, and aches; for which purpose the pills made with powder of Ground Pine, and of hermodactyls with Venice turpentine are very effectual. The pills also continued for some time, are special good for those that have the dropsy, jaundice, and for gripping pains of the joints, belly, or inward parts. It helpeth also all diseases of the brain, proceeding of cold and phlegmatick humours and distillations, as also for the falling-sickness. It is a special remedy for the poison of the aconites, and other poisonable herbs, as also against the stinging of any venomous creature. It is a good remedy for a cold cough, especially in the beginning. For all the purposes aforesaid, the herb being tunned up in new drink and drank, is almost as effectual, but far more acceptable to weak and dainty stomachs. The distilled water of the herb hath the same effects, but more weakly. The conserve of the flowers doth the like, which Matthiolus much commendeth against the palsy. The green herb, or the decoction thereof, being applied, dissolveth the hardness of womens breasts, and all other hard swellings in any other part of the body. The green herb also applied, or the juice thereof with some honey, not only cleanseth putrid, stinking, foul, and malignant ulcers and sores of all sorts,

 but

but healeth and foldereth up the lips of green wounds in any part alfo. Let women forbear, if they be with child, for it works violently upon the feminine part.

PLANTAIN.

THIS groweth ufually in meadows and fields, and by path-fides, and is fo well known, that it needeth no defcription.

Time.] It is in its beauty about June, and the feed ripeneth fhortly after.

Government and Virtues.] It is true, Mizaldus and others, yea, almoft all aftrology-phyficians hold this to be an herb of Mars, becaufe it cures the difeafes of the head and privities, which are under the houfes of Mars, Aries, and Scorpio: The truth is, it is under the command of Venus, and cures the head by antipathy to Mars, and the privities by fympathy to Venus; neither is there hardly a martial difeafe but it cures.

The juice of Plantain clarified and drank for divers days together, either of itfelf, or in other drink, prevaileth wonderfully againft all torments or excoriations in the guts or bowels, helpeth the diftillations of rheum from the head, and ftayeth all manner of fluxes, even womens courfes, when they flow too abundantly. It is good to ftay fpitting of blood and other bleedings at the mouth, or the making of foul and bloody water, by reafon of any ulcer in the reins or bladder, and alfo ftayeth the too free bleeding of wounds. It is held an efpecial remedy for thofe that are troubled with the phthfiic, or confumption of the lungs, or ulcers of the lungs, or coughs that come of heat. The decoction or powder of the roots or feeds, is much more binding for all the purpofes aforefaid than the leaves. Diofcorides faith, that three roots boiled in wine and taken, helpeth the tertian ague, and for the quartan ague, (but letting the number pafs as fabulous) I conceive the decoction of divers roots may be effectual. The herb (but efpecially the feed) is held to be profitable againft the dropfy, the falling-ficknefs, the yellow jaundice, and ftoppings of the liver and reins. The roots of Plantain, and Pellitory of Spain, beaten into powder, and put into the hollow teeth, taketh away the pains of them.

The

The clarified juice, or distilled water, dropped into the eyes, cooleth the inflammations in them, and taketh away the pin and web; and dropped into the ears, easeth the pains in them, and helpeth and removeth the heat. The same also with the juice of houseleek is profitable against all inflammations and breakings out of the skin, and against burnings and scaldings by fire and water. The juice or decoction made either of itself, or other things of the like nature, is of much use and good effect for old and hollow ulcers that are hard to be cured, and for cankers and sores in the mouth or privy parts of man or woman; and helpeth also the pains of the piles in the fundament. The juice mixed with oil of roses, and the temples and forehead anointed therewith, easeth the pains of the head proceeding from heat, and helpeth lunatick and frantick persons very much; as also the biting of serpents, or a mad dog. The same also is profitably applied to all hot gouts in the feet or hands, especially in the beginning. It is also good to be applied where any bone is out of joint, to hinder inflammations, swellings, and pains that presently rise thereupon. The powder of the dried leaves taken in drink, killeth worms of the belly; and boiled in wine, killeth worms that breed in old and foul ulcers. One part of Plantain water, and two parts of the brine of powdered beef, boiled together and clarified, is a most sure remedy to heal all spreading scabs or itch in the head and body, all manner of tetters, ringworms, the shingles, and all other running and fretting sores. Briefly, the Plantains are singular good wound herbs to heal fresh or old wounds or sores, either inward or outward.

PLUMBS

ARE so well known, that they need no description.

Government and Virtues.] All Plumbs are under Venus, and are like women, some better, some worse. As there is great diversity of kinds, so there is in the operation of Plumbs, for some that are sweet moisten the stomach, and make the belly soluble; those that are sour quench thirst more, and bind the belly; the moist and waterish do sooner corrupt in the stomach, but the firm do nourish more, and offend less. The dried fruit sold by the grocers under the name of Damaſk Prunes, do ſomewhat looſen the belly, and being ſtewed, are often uſed, both in health and ſickneſs, to reliſh the mouth and ſtomach, to procure appetite, and a little to open the body, allay choler, and cool the ſtomach. Plumb-tree leaves boiled in wine, are good to waſh and gargle the mouth and throat, to dry the flux of rheum coming to the palate, gums, or almonds of the ears. The gum of the tree is good to break the ſtone. The gum or leaves boiled in vinegar, and applied, kills tetters and ringworms. Matthiolus ſaith, The oil preſſed out of the kernels of the ſtones, as oil of almonds is made, is good againſt the inflamed piles, the tumours or ſwellings of ulcers, hoarſeneſs of the voice, roughneſs of the tongue and throat, and likewiſe the pains in the ears. And that five ounces of the ſaid oil taken with one ounce of muſkadel, driveth forth the ſtone, and helpeth the colick.

POLYPODY of the OAK.

Deſcript.] THIS is a ſmall herb conſiſting of nothing but roots and leaves, bearing neither ſtalk, flower, nor ſeed, as it is thought. It hath three or four leaves riſing from the root, every one ſingle by itſelf, of about a hand length, are winged, conſiſting of many ſmall narrow leaves, cut into the middle rib, ſtanding on each ſide of the ſtalk, large below, and ſmaller up to the top, not dented nor notched at the edges at all, as the male fern hath, of ſad green colour, and ſmooth on the upper ſide, but on the other ſide ſomewhat rough, by reaſon of ſome yellowiſh ſpots ſet thereon. The root is ſmaller than one's little finger, lying aſlope, or creeping along under the upper cruſt of the earth, browniſh on the outſide and greeniſh within, of a ſweetiſh harſhneſs in taſte, ſet with certain rough knags on each ſide thereof, having alſo much moſſineſs or yellow hairineſs upon it, and ſome fibres underneath it, whereby it is nouriſhed.

Place.] It groweth as well upon old rotten ſtumps, or trunks of trees, as oak, beech, hazel, willow, or any other, as in the woods under them, and upon old mud walls, as alſo in moſſy, ſtoney, and gravelly places near unto wood. That which groweth upon oak is accounted the beſt

beſt; but the quantity thereof is ſcarce ſufficient for the common uſe.

Time.] It being always green, may be gathered for uſe at any time.

Government and Virtues.] And why, I pray, muſt Polypodium of the Oak only be uſed, gentle college of phyſicians? Can you give me but a glimpſe of reaſon for it? It is only becauſe it is deareſt. Will you never leave your covetouſneſs till your lives leave you? The truth is, that which grows upon the earth is beſt ('tis an herb of Saturn, and he ſeldom climbs trees) to purge melancholy; if the humour be otherwiſe, chuſe you Polypodium accordingly. Meuſe (who is called the phyſicans Evangeliſt for the certainty of his medicines, and the truth of his opinion) ſaith, That it drieth up thin humours, digeſteth thick and tough, and purgeth burnt choler, and eſpecially tough and thick phlegm, and thin phlegm alſo, even from the joints, and therefore good for thoſe that are troubled with melancholy, or quartan agues, eſpecially if it be taken in whey or honied water, or in barley-water, or the broth of a chicken with epithymum, or with beets and mallows. It is good for the hardneſs of the ſpleen, and for prickings or ſtitches in the ſides, as alſo for the colick: Some uſe to put to it ſome fennel ſeeds, or anniſe ſeeds, or ginger, to correct that loathing it bringeth to the ſtomach, which is more than needeth, it being a ſafe and gentle medicine, fit for all perſons, which daily experience confirmeth; and an ounce of it may be given at a time in a decoction, if there be not ſena, or ſome other ſtrong purger put with it. A dram or two of the powder of the dried roots taken faſting in a cup of honied water, worketh gently, and for the purpoſes aforeſaid. The diſtilled water, both of roots and leaves, is much commended for the quartan ague, to be taken for many days together, as alſo againſt melancholy, or fearful and troubleſome ſleeps or dreams; and with ſome ſugar-candy diſſolved therein, is good againſt the cough, ſhortneſs of breath, and wheezings, and thoſe diſtillations of thin rheum upon the lungs, which cauſe phthiſics, and often times conſumptions. The freſh roots beaten ſmall, or the powder of the dried roots mixed with honey, and ap-

plied

plied to the member that is out of joint, doth much help it; and applied also to the nose, cureth the disease called Polypus, which is a piece of flesh growing therein, which in time stoppeth the passage of breath thro' that nostril; and it helpeth those clefts or chops that come between the fingers or toes

The Poplar Tree.

THERE are two sorts of Poplars, which are most familiar with us, *viz.* the Black and White, both which I shall here describe unto you.

Descript.] The White Poplar groweth great, and reasonably high, covered with thick, smooth, white bark, especially the branches, having long leaves cut into several divisions almost like a vine leaf, but not of so deep a green on the upper side, and hoary white underneath, of a reasonable good scent, the whole form representing the form of Coltsfoot. The catkins which it bringeth forth before the leaves, are long, and of a faint reddish colour, which fall away, bearing seldom good seed with them. The wood hereof is smooth, soft, and white, very finely waved, whereby it is much esteemed.

The Black Poplar groweth higher and straiter than the White, with a greyish bark, bearing broad green leaves, somewhat like ivy leaves, not cut in on the edges like the White, but whole and dented, ending in a point, and not white underneath, hanging by slender long foot-stalks, which with the air are continually shaken like as the aspen leaves are. The catkins hereof are greater than those of the White, composed of many round green berries, as if they were set together in a long cluster, containing much downy matter, which being ripe, is blown away with the wind. The clammy buds hereof, before they spread into leaves, are gathered to make Unguentum Populneum, and are of a yellowish green colour, and small, somewhat sweet, but strong. The wood is smooth, tough and white, and easy to be cloven: On both these trees groweth a sweet kind of musk, which in former times was used to put into sweet ointments.

Place.] They grow in moist woods, and by water-sides in sundry places of this land; yet the White is not so frequent as the other.

Time.

Time.] Their time is likewiſe expreſſed before: The catkins coming forth before the leaves in the end of Summer.

Government and Virtues.] Saturn hath dominion over both. White Poplar, ſaith Galen, is of a cleanſing property: The weight of one ounce in powder of the bark thereof being drank, ſaith Dioſcorides, is a remedy for thoſe that are troubled with the ſciatica, or the ſtrangury. The juice of the leaves dropped warm into the ears, eaſeth the pains in them. The young clammy buds or eyes, before they break out into leaves, bruiſed, and a little honey put to them, is a good medicine for a dull ſight. The Black Poplar is held to be more cooling than the White, and therefore the leaves bruiſed with vinegar and applied, help the gout. The ſeed drank in vinegar, is held good againſt the falling-ſickneſs. The water that droppeth from the hollow places of this tree, taketh away warts, puſhes, wheals, and other the like breakings out of the body. The young Black Poplar buds, ſaith Matthiolus, are much uſed by women to beautify their hair, bruiſing them with freſh butter, ſtraining them after they have been kept for ſome time in the Sun. The ointment called Populneon, which is made of this Poplar, is ſingular good for all heat and inflammations in any part of the body, and tempereth the heat of wounds. It is much uſed to dry up the milk of womens breaſts, when they have weaned their children.

POPPY.

OF this I ſhall deſcribe three kinds, *viz.* the White and black of the garden, and the Erratick Wild Poppy, or Corn Roſe.

Deſcript.] The White Poppy hath at firſt four or five whitiſh green leaves lying upon the ground, which riſe with the ſtalk, compaſſing it at the bottom of them, and are very large, much cut or torn on the edges, and dented alſo beſides: The ſtalk, which is uſually four or five feet high, hath ſometimes no branches at the top, and uſually but two or three at moſt, bearing every one but one head wrapped up in a thin ſkin, which boweth down before it is ready to blow, and then riſing, and being broken, the flower

flower within it ſpreading itſelf open, and conſiſting of four very large, white round leaves, with many whitiſh round threads in the middle, ſet about a ſmall, round, green head, having a crown, or ſtar-like cover at the head thereof, which growing ripe, becomes as large as a great apple, wherein are contained a great number of ſmall round ſeeds in ſeveral partitions or diviſions next unto the ſhell, the middle thereof remaining hollow, and empty. The whole plant, both leaves, ſtalks and heads, while they are freſh, young, and green, yield a milk when they are broken, of an unpleaſant bitter taſte, almoſt ready to provoke caſting, and of a ſtrong heady ſmell, which being condenſate, is called Opium. The root is white and woody, periſhing as ſoon as it hath given ripe ſeed.

The Black Poppy little differeth from the former, until it beareth its flower, which is ſomewhat leſs, and of a black purpliſh colour, but without any purple ſpots in the bottom of the leaf. The head of the ſeed is much leſs than the former, and openeth itſelf a little round about the top, under the crown, ſo that the ſeed, which is very black, will fall out, if one turn the head thereof downward.

The Wild Poppy, or Corn Roſe, hath long and narrow leaves, very much cut in on the edges into many diviſions, of a light green colour, ſometimes hairy withal: The ſtalk is blackiſh and hairy alſo, but not ſo tall as the garden-kind, having ſome ſuch like leaves thereon as grow below, parted into three or four branches ſometimes, whereon grow ſmall hairy heads bowing down before the ſkin break, wherein the flower is incloſed, which when it is full blown open, is of a fair yellowiſh red or crimſon colour, and in ſome much paler, without any ſpot in the bottom of the leaves, having many black ſoft threads in the middle, compaſſing a ſmall green head, which when it is ripe, is not bigger than one's little fingers end, wherein is contained much black ſeed, ſmaller by half than that of the garden. The root periſheth every year, and ſpringeth again of its own ſowing. Of this kind there is one leſſer in all the parts thereof, and differeth in nothing elſe.

Place.] The garden kinds do not naturally grow wild in any place, but are all ſown in gardens where they grow.

The

The wild Poppy or Corn Rose, is plentifully enough, and many times too much in the corn fields of all counties through this land, and also upon ditch-banks, and by hedge-sides. The smaller wild kind is also found in corn fields, and also in some other places, but not so plentifully as the former.

Time.] The garden kinds are usually sown in the spring, which then flower about the end of May, and somewhat earlier, if they spring of their own sowing.

The Wild kind flower usually from May until July, and the seed of them is ripe soon after the flowering.

Government and Virtues.] The herb is Lunar, and of the juice of it is made Opium; only for lucre of money they cheat you, and tell you it is a kind of tear, or some such like thing, that drops from poppies when they weep, and that is somewhere beyond the seas, I know not where beyond the Moon. The garden poppy heads with seeds made into a syrup, is frequently, and to good effect used to procure rest, and sleep, in the sick and weak, and to stay catarrhs and defluctions of thin rheums from the head into the stomach and lungs, causing a continual cough, the fore-runner of a consumption; it helpeth also hoarseness of the throat, and when one hath lost their voice, which the oil of the seed doth likewise. The black seed boiled in wine, and drank, is said also to stay the flux of the belly, and womens courses. The empty shells, or poppy heads, are usually boiled in water, and given to procure rest and sleep: So do the leaves in the same manner; as also if the head and temples be bathed with the decoction warm, or with the oil of poppies, the green leaves or heads bruised, and applied with a little vinegar, or made into a poultice with barley-meal or hog's-grease, cooleth and tempereth all inflammations, as also the disease called St Anthony's fire. It is generally used in treacle and mithridate, and in all other medicines that are made to procure rest and sleep, and to ease pains in the head as well as in other parts. It is also used to cool inflammations, agues, or frenzies, or to stay defluctions which cause a cough, or consumption, and also other fluxes of the belly, or womens courses; it is also put into to hollow teeth, to eaſe the pain, and hath been found by experience to eaſe the pains of the gout.

The Wild Poppy, or Corn Roſe (as Matthiolus ſaith) is good to prevent the falling-ſickneſs. The ſyrup made with the flower, is with good effect given to thoſe that have the pleuriſy; and the dried flowers alſo, either boiled in water, or made into powder and drank, either in the diſtilled water of them, or ſome other drink, worketh the like effect. The diſtilled water of the flowers is held to be of much good uſe againſt ſurfeits, being drank evening and morning: It is alſo more cooling than any of the other poppies, and therefore cannot but be as effectual in hot agues, frenzies, and other inflammations either inward or outward. Galen ſaith, The ſeed is dangerous to be uſed inwardly.

PURSLANE.

GARDEN Purſlane (being uſed as a ſallad herb) is ſo well known that it needeth no deſcription; I ſhall therefore only ſpeak of its virtues as followeth.

Government and Virtues.] 'Tis an herb of the Moon. It is good to cool any heat in the liver, blood, reins, and ſtomach, and in hot agues nothing better: It ſtayeth hot and cholerick fluxes of the belly, womens courſes, the whites, and gonorrhæa, or running of the reins, the diſtillation from the head, and pains therein proceeding from heat, want of ſleep or the frenzy. The ſeed is more effectual than the herb, and is of ſingular good uſe to cool the heat and ſharpneſs of urine, and the outrageous luſt of the body, venereous dreams, and the like: Inſomuch that the over frequent uſe hereof extinguiſheth the heat and virtue of natural procreation. The ſeed bruiſed and boiled in wine, and given to children, expelleth the worms. The juice of the herb is held as effectual to all the purpoſes aforeſaid; as alſo to ſtay vomitings, and taken with ſome ſugar or honey, helpeth an old and dry cough, ſhortneſs of breath, and the phthiſick, and ſtayeth immoderate thirſt. The diſtilled water of the herb is uſed by many (as the more pleaſing) with a little ſugar to work the ſame effects. The juice alſo is ſingular good in the inflammations and ulcers in the ſecret parts of man or woman,

woman, as alſo the bowels and hæmorrhoids, when they are ulcerous, or excoriations in them: The herb bruiſed and applied to the forehead and temples, allays exceſſive heat therein, that hinders reſt and ſleep; and applied to the eyes, taketh away the redneſs and inflammation in them, and thoſe other parts where puſhes, wheals, pimples, St Anthony's fire, and the like, break forth; if a little vinegar be put to it, and laid to the neck, with as much of galls and linſeed together, it taketh away the pains therein, and the crick in the neck. The juice is uſed with oil of roſes for the ſame cauſes, or for blaſting by lightening, and burnings by gunpowder, or for womens ſore breaſts, and to allay the heat in all other ſores or hurts; applied alſo to the navels of children that ſtick forth, it helpeth them; it is alſo good for ſore mouths and gums that are ſwollen, and to faſten looſe teeth. Camerarius ſaith, that the diſtilled water uſed by ſome, took away the pain of their teeth, when all other remedies failed, and the thickened juice made into pills with the powder of gum, tragacanth, and arabick, being taken, prevaileth much to help thoſe that make bloody water. Applied to the gout it eaſeth pains thereof, and helpeth the hardneſs of the ſinews, if it come not of the cramp, or a cold cauſe.

PRIMROSES.

THEY are ſo well known, that they need no deſcription. Of the leaves of Primroſes is made as fine a ſalve to heal wounds as any that I know; you ſhall be taught to make ſalves of any herb at the latter end of the book: make this as you are taught there, and do not (you that have any ingenuity in you) ſee your poor neighbours go with wounded limbs when an halfpenny coſt will heal them.

PRIVET.

Deſcript.] OUR common Privet is carried up with many ſlender branches to a reaſonable height and breadth, to cover arbours, bowers and banquetting houſes, and brought, wrought, and cut into ſo many forms, of men, horſes, birds, &c. which though at

 firſt

first supported, groweth afterwards strong of itself. It beareth long and narrow green leaves by the couples, and sweet smelling white flowers in tufts at the end of the branches, which turn into small black berries that have a purplish juice with them, and some seeds that are flat on the one side, with a hole or dent therein.

Place.] It groweth in this land, in divers woods.

Time.] Our Privet flowereth in June and July, the berries are ripe in August and September.

Government and Virtues.] The Moon is lady of this. It is little used in physick with us in these times, more than in lotions to wash sores, and sore mouths, and to cool inflammations, and dry up fluxes. Yet Matthiolus saith, it serveth to all the uses for the which cypress, or the East Privet, is appointed by Dioscorides and Galen. He farther saith, That the oil that is made of the flowers of Privet infused therein, and set in the Sun, is singular good for the inflammations of wounds and for the head-ach, coming of an hot cause. There is a sweet water also distilled from the flowers, that is good for all those diseases that need cooling and drying, and therefore helpeth all fluxes of the belly or stomach, bloody-fluxes, and womens courses, being either drank or applied; as all those that void blood at the mouth, or any other place, and for distillations of rheum in the eyes, especially if it be used with tutia.

QUEEN of the MEADOWS, MEADOW SWEET, or MEAD SWEET.

Descript.] THE stalks of this are reddish, rising to be three feet high, sometimes four or five feet, having at the joints thereof large winged leaves, standing one above another at distances, consisting of many and somewhat broad leaves, set on each side of a middle rib, being hard, rough, or rugged, crumpled much like unto elm leaves, having also some smaller leaves with them (as agrimony hath) somewhat deeply dented about the edges, of a sad green colour on the upper side, and greyish underneath, of a pretty sharp scent and taste, somewhat like unto the burnet, and a leaf hereof put into a cup of claret wine, giveth also a fine relish to it. At the tops

tops of the ſtalks and branches ſtand many tufts of ſmall white flowers thruſt thick together, which ſmell much ſweeter than the leaves; and in their places, being fallen, ſome crooked and cornered ſeed. The root is ſomewhat woody, and blackiſh on the outſide, and browniſh within, with divers great ſtrings, and leſſer fibres ſet thereat, of a ſtrong ſcent, but nothing ſo pleaſant as the flowers and leaves, and periſheth not, but abideth many years, ſhooting forth a-new every ſpring.

Place.] It groweth in moiſt meadows that lie much wet, or near the courſes of water.

Time.] It flowereth in ſome places or other all the three Summer months, that is, June, July, and Auguſt, and the ſeed is ripe ſoon after.

Government and Virtues.] Venus claims dominion over the herb. It is uſed to ſtay all manner of bleedings, fluxes, vomitings, and womens courſes, as alſo their whites: It is ſaid to alter and take away the fits of the quartan agues, and to make a merry heart, for which purpoſe ſome uſe the flowers, and ſome the leaves. It helpeth ſpeedily thoſe that are troubled with the colick; being boiled in wine, and with a little honey taken warm, it openeth the belly, but boiled in red wine, and drank, it ſtayeth the flux of the belly. Outwardly applied, it helpeth old ulcers that are cankerous, or hollow and fiſtulous, for which it is by many much commended, as alſo for the ſores in the mouth or ſecret parts. The leaves, when they are full grown, being laid on the ſkin, will, in a ſhort time, raiſe bliſters thereon, as Tragus ſaith. The water thereof helpeth the heat and inflammation in the eyes.

The QUINCE TREE.

Deſcript.] THE ordinary Quince Tree groweth often to the height and bigneſs of a reaſonable apple tree, but more uſually lower, and crooked, with a rough bark, ſpreading arms and branches far abroad. The leaves are ſomewhat like thoſe of the apple tree, but thicker, broader, and fuller of veins, and whiter on the under ſide, not dented at all about the edges. The flowers are large and white, ſometimes daſhed over with a bluſh. The fruit that followeth is yellow, being near ripe, and covered with a white freeze, or cotton; thick ſet on the younger, and growing leſs as they grow to be thorough ripe, bunched out oftentimes in ſome places, ſome being like an apple, and ſome a pear, of a ſtrong heady ſcent, and not durable to keep, and is ſour, harſh, and of an unpleaſant taſte to eat freſh; but being ſcalded, roaſted, baked, or preſerved, becometh more pleaſant.

Place and Time.] It beſt likes to grow near ponds and water ſides, and is frequent through this land; and flowereth not until the leaves be come forth. The fruit is ripe in September or October.

Government and Virtues.] Old Saturn owns the Tree, Quinces when they are green, help all ſorts of fluxes in men or women, and cholerick laſks, caſting and whatever needeth aſtriction, more than any way prepared by fire; yet the ſyrup of the juice, or the conſerve, are much conducible, much of the binding quality being conſumed by the fire; if a little vinegar be added, it ſtirreth up the languiſhing appetite, and the ſtomach given to caſting; ſome ſpices being added, comforteth and ſtrengtheneth the decaying and fainting ſpirits, and helpeth the liver oppreſſed, that it cannot perfect the digeſtion, or correcteth choler and phlegm. If you would have them purging, put honey to them inſtead of ſugar; and if more laxative, for choler, rhubarb; for phlegm, turbith; for watery humours, ſcammony; but if more forcibly to bind, uſe the unripe Quinces, with roſes and acacia, hypociſtis, and ſome torrified rhubarb. To take the crude juice of Quinces, is held a preſervative againſt the force of deadly poiſon; for it hath been found moſt certainly true, that the very ſmell of a Quince hath taken away all the ſtrength of the poiſon of white hellibore. If there be need of any outwardly binding and cooling of hot fluxes, the oil of Quinces, or other medicines that may be made thereof, are very available to anoint the belly or other parts therewith; it likewiſe ſtrengtheneth the ſtomach and belly, and the ſinews that are looſened by ſharp humours falling on them, and reſtraineth immoderate ſweatings. The mucilage taken from the ſeeds of Quinces, and boiled in a little water, is very good to cool the heat, and heal the ſore breaſts of women. The ſame with a little

little sugar, is good to lenify the harshness and hoarseness of the throat, and roughness of the tongue. The cotton or down of Quinces boiled and applied to plague sores, healeth them up; and laid as a plaister, made up with wax, it bringeth hair to them that are bald, and keepeth it from falling, if it be ready to shed.

Raddish, or Horse-Raddish.

THE garden Raddish is so well known, that it needeth no description.

Descript.] The Horse Raddish hath its first leaves that rise before Winter, about a foot and a half long, very much cut in or torn on the edges into many parts, of a dark green colour, with a great rib in the middle; after these have been up a while, others follow, which are greater, rougher, broader and longer, whole and not divided at first, but only somewhat rougher dented about the edges; the stalks when it beareth flowers (which is seldom) is great, rising up with some few lesser leaves thereon, to three or four feet high, spreading at the top many small branches of whitish flowers, made of four leaves a-piece; after which come small pods, like those of shepherd's purse, but seldom with any seed in them. The root is great, long, white and rugged, shooting up divers heads of leaves, which may be parted for increase, but it doth not creep in the ground, nor run above ground, and is of a strong, sharp and bitter taste, almost like mustard.

Place.] It is found wild in some places, but is chiefly planted in gardens, and joyeth in moist and shadowy places.

Time.] It seldom flowereth, but when it doth, it is in July.

Government and Virtues.] They are both under Mars. The juice of Horse-Raddish given to drink, is held to be very effectual for the scurvy. It killeth the worms in children, being drank, and also laid upon the belly. The root bruised and laid to the place grieved with the sciatica, jointach, or the hard swellings of the liver and spleen, doth wonderfully help them all. The distilled water of the herb and root is more familiar to be taken with a little sugar for all the purposes aforesaid.

Garden Raddishes are in wantonness, by the gentry, eaten as a sallad, but they breed but scurvy humours in the ſtomach, and corrupt the blood, and then ſend for a phyſician as faſt as you can; this is one cauſe makes the owners of ſuch nice palates ſo unhealthful; yet for ſuch as are troubled with the gravel, ſtone, or ſtoppage of urine, they are good phyſick, if the body be ſtrong that takes them; you may make the juice of the roots into a ſyrup if you pleaſe, for that uſe: They purge by urine exceedingly.

RAGWORT.

IT is called alſo St James's-wort, and Stagger-wort, and Stammer-wort, and Segrum.

Deſcript.] The greater common Ragwort hath many large and long, dark green leaves lying on the ground, very much rent and torn on the ſides in many places; from among which riſe up ſometimes but one, and ſometimes two or three ſquare or creſted blackiſh or browniſh ſtalks, three or four feet high, ſometimes branched, bearing divers ſuch-like leaves upon them, at ſeveral diſtances unto the top, where it branches forth into many ſtalks bearing yellow flowers, conſiſting of divers leaves, ſet as a pale or border, with a dark yellow thrum in the middle, which do abide a great while, but at laſt are turned into down, and with the ſmall blackiſh grey ſeed, are carried away with the wind. The root is made of many fibres, whereby it is firmly faſtened into the ground, and abideth many years.

There is another ſort thereof different from the former only in this, that it riſeth not ſo high; the leaves are not ſo finely jagged, nor of ſo dark a green colour, but rather ſomewhat whithiſh, ſoft and woolly, and the flowers uſually paler.

Place.] They grow both of them wild in paſtures, and untilled grounds in many places, and oftentimes both in one field.

Time.] They flower in June and July, and the ſeed is ripe in Auguſt.

Government and Virtues.] Ragwort is under the command of Dame Venus, and cleanſeth, digeſteth, and diſcuſſeth. The decoction of the herb is good to waſh the mouth or throat that hath ulcers or ſores therein; and for

for ſwellings, hardneſs, or impoſthumations, for it thoroughly cleanſeth and healeth them; as alſo the quinſy, and the king's evil. It helpeth to ſtay catarrhs, thin rheums, and defluctions from the head into the eyes, noſe, or lungs. The juice is found by experience to be ſingular good to heal green wounds, and to cleanſe and heal all old and filthy ulcers in the privities, and in other parts of the body, as alſo inward wounds and ulcers; ſtayeth the malignity of fretting and running cankers, and hollow fiſtulas, not ſuffering them to ſpread farther. It is alſo much commended to help aches and pains either in the fleſhy part, or in the nerves and ſinews; as alſo the ſciatica, or pain of the hips or huckle-bone, to bathe the places with the decoction of the herb, or to anoint them with an ointment made of the herb, bruiſed and boiled in old hog's ſuet, with ſome maſtick and olibanum in powder added unto it after it is ſtrained forth. In Suſſex we call it Ragweed.

RATTLE GRASS.

OF this there are two kinds which I ſhall ſpeak of, *viz.* the red and yellow.

Deſcript.] The common Red Rattle hath ſundry reddiſh, hollow ſtalks, and ſometime green, riſing from the root lying for the moſt part on the ground, ſome growing more upright, with many ſmall reddiſh or green leaves ſet on both ſides of a middle rib, finely dented about the edges: The flowers ſtand at the tops of the ſtalks and branches, of a fine purpliſh red colour, like ſmall gaping hooks: after which come blackiſh ſeed in ſmall huſks, which lying looſe therein, will rattle with ſhaking. The root conſiſts of two or three ſmall whitiſh ſtrings wih ſome fibres thereat.

The common Yellow Rattle hath ſeldom above one round great ſtalk, riſing from the foot, about half a yard, or two feet high, and but few branches thereon, having two long, and ſomewhat broad leaves ſet at a joint, deeply cut in on the edges, reſembling the comb of a cock, broadeſt next to the ſtalk, and ſmaller to the end. The flowers grow at the tops of the ſtalks, with ſome ſhorter leaves with them, hooded after the ſame manner that the others are, but of a fair yellow colour, or in ſome paler,

and

and in some more white. The seed is contained in large husks, and being ripe, will rattle or make a noise with lying loose in them. The root is small and slender; perishing every year.

Place.] They grow in meadows and woods generally through this land.

Time.] They are in flower from Midsummer until August be past, sometimes.

Government and Virtues.] They are both of them under the dominion of the Moon. The Red Rattle is accounted profitable to heal up fistulas and hollow ulcers, and to stay the flux of humours in them, as also the abundance of womens courses, or any other flux of blood, being boiled in red wine, and drank.

The yellow Rattle, or Cock's Comb, is held to be good for those that are troubled with a cough, or dimness of sight, if the herb, being boiled with beans, and some honey put thereto, be drank or dropped into the eyes. The whole seed being put into the eyes, draweth forth any skin, dimness of film, from the sight, without trouble, or pain.

Rest Harrow, or Cammock.

Descript.] Common Rest Harrow riseth up with divers rough woody twigs half a yard or a yard high, set at the joints without order, with little roundish leaves, sometimes more than two or three at a place, of a dark green colour, without thorns while they are young; but afterwards armed in sundry places, with short and sharp thorns. The flowers come forth at the tops of the twigs and branches, whereof it is full fashioned like pease or broom blossoms, but lesser, flatter, and somewhat closer, of a faint purplish colour; after which come small pods containing small, flat, round seed: The root is blackish on the outside, and whitish within, very rough, and hard to break when it is fresh and green, and as hard as an horn when it is dried, thrusting down deep into the ground, and spreading likewise, every piece being apt to grow again if it be left in the ground.

Place.] It groweth in many places of this land, as well in the arable as waste ground.

Time.

Time.] It flowereth about the beginning or middle of July, and the ſeed is ripe in Auguſt.

Government and Virtues.] It is under the dominion of Mars. It is ſingular good to provoke urine when it is ſtopped, and to break and drive forth the ſtone, which the powder of the bark of the root taken in wine performeth effectually. Matthiolus ſaith, The ſame helpeth the diſeaſe called *Hernia Carnoſa* the fleſhy rupture, by taking the ſaid powder for ſome months together conſtantly, and that it hath cured ſome which ſeemed incurable by any other means than by cutting or burning. The decoction thereof made with ſome vinegar, gargled in the mouth, eaſeth the tooth-ach, eſpecially when it comes of rheum; and the ſaid decoction is very powerful to open obſtructions of the liver and ſpleen, and other parts. A diſtilled water in *Balneo Mariæ*, with four pounds of the root hereof firſt ſliced ſmall, and afterwards ſteeped in a gallon of Canary wine, is ſingular good for all the purpoſes aforeſaid, and to cleanſe the paſſages of the urine. The powder of the ſaid root made into an electuary, or lozenges, with ſugar, as alſo the bark of the freſh roots boiled tender, and afterwards beaten to a conſerve with ſugar, worketh the like effect. The powder of the roots ſtrewed upon the brims of ulcers, or mixed with any other convenient thing, and applied, conſumeth the hardneſs, and cauſeth them to heal the better.

ROCKET.

IN regard the Garden Rocket is rather uſed as a ſallad herb than to any phyſical purpoſes, I ſhall omit it, and only ſpeak of the common wild Rocket: The deſcription whereof take as followeth.

Deſcript.] The common wild Rocket hath longer and narrower leaves, much more divided into ſlender cuts and jags on both ſides the middle rib than the garden kinds have; of a ſad green colour, from among which riſe up divers ſtalks two or three feet high, ſometimes ſet with the like leaves, but ſmaller and ſmaller upwards, branched from the middle into divers ſtiff ſtalks, bearing ſundry yellow flowers on them, made of four leaves a-piece, as the others are, which afterwards yield them small reddish seed, in small long pods, of a more bitter and hot biting taste than the garden kinds, as the leaves are also.

Place.] It is found wild in divers places of this land.

Time.] It flowereth about June or July, and the seed is ripe in August.

Government and Virtues.] The wild Rockets are forbidden to be used alone, in regard their sharpness fumeth into the head, causing aches and pains therein, and are less hurtful to hot and cholerick persons, for fear of inflamming their blood, and therefore for such we may say a little doth but a little harm, for angry Mars rules them, and he sometimes will be rusty when he meets with fools. The wild Rocket is more strong and effectual to increase sperm and venerous qualities, whereunto all the seed is more effectual than the garden kind; it serveth also to help digestion, and provoketh urine exceedingly. The seed is used to cure the biting of serpents, the scorpion, and the shrew mouse, and other poisons, and expelleth worms, and other noisome creatures that breed in the bely. The herb boiled or stewed, and some sugar put thereto, helpeth the cough in children, being taken often. The seed also taken in drink, taketh away the ill scent of the arm-pits, increaseth milk in nurses, and wasteth the spleen. The seed mixed with honey, and used on the face, cleanseth the skin from morphew, and used with vinegar, taketh away freckles and redness in the face, or other parts; and with the gall of an ox, it mendeth foul scars, black and blue spots, and the marks of the small-pox.

WINTER-ROCKET, or CRESSES.

Descript.] WINTER Rocket, or Winter-Cresses, hath divers somewhat large sad green leaves lying upon the ground, torn or cut in divers parts, somewhat like unto Rocket or turnip leaves, with smaller pieces next the bottom, and broad at the ends, which so abide all the Winter, (if it spring up in Autumn, when it is used to be eaten) from among which rise up divers small round stalks, full of branches, bearing many small yellow flowers of four leaves a-piece, after which come small pods
with

with reddish seed in them. The root is somewhat stringy, and perisheth every year after the seed is ripe.

Place.] It groweth of its own accord in gardens and fields, by the way-sides, in divers places, and particularly in the next pasture to the conduit-head behind Gray's Inn, that brings water to Mr Lamb's conduit in Holborn.

Time.] It flowereth in May, seedeth in June, and then perisheth.

Government and Virtues.] This is profitable to provoke urine, to help strangury, and expel gravel and the stone. It is good for the scurvy, and found by experience to be a singular good wound herb to cleanse inward wounds; the juice or decoction being drank, or outwardly applied to wash foul ulcers and sores, cleansing them by sharpness, and hindering or abating the dead flesh from growing therein, and healing them by the drying quality.

ROSES.

I Hold it altogether needless to trouble the reader with a description of any of these, since both the garden Roses, and the Roses of the briars are so well known; take therefore the virtue of them as followeth: And first I shall begin with the garden kinds.

Government and Virtues.] What a pother have authors made with Roses! What a racket have they kept? I shall add, red roses are under Jupiter, Damask under Venus, white under the Moon, and provence under the King of France. The white and red roses are cooling and drying, and yet the white is taken to exceed the red in both the properties, but is seldom used inwardly in any medicine: The bitterness in the roses when they are fresh, especially the juice, purgeth choler, and watry humours; but being dried, and that heat which caused the bitterness being consumed, they have then a binding and astringent quality: Those also that are not full blown, do both cool and bind more than those that are full blown, and the white rose more than the red. The decoction of red roses made with wine and used, is very good for the head-ach, and pains in the eyes, ears, throat and gums; as also for the fundament, the lower parts of the belly and the matrix, being bathed or put into them. The

same

ſame decoction with the roſes remaining in it, is profitably applied to the region of the heart to eaſe the inflammation therein; as alſo St Anthony's fire, and other diſeaſes of the ſtomach. Being dried and beaten to powder, and taken in ſteeled wine or water, it helpeth to ſtay womens courſes. The yellow threads in the middle of the roſes (which are erroneouſly called the Roſe Seed) being powdered and drank in the diſtilled water of quinces, ſtayeth the overflowing of womens courſes, and doth wonderfully ſtay the defluctions of rheum upon the gums and teeth, preſerving them from corruption, and faſtening them if they be looſe, being waſhed and gargled therewith, and ſome vinegar of ſquills added thereto. The heads with the ſeed being uſed in powder, or in a decoction, ſtayeth the laſk and ſpitting of blood. Red Roſes do ſtrengthen the heart, the ſtomach and the liver, and the retentive faculty: They mitigate the pains that ariſe from heat, aſſuage inflammations, procure reſt and ſleep, ſtay both whites and reds in women, the gonorrhea, or running of the reins, and fluxes of the belly; the juice of them doth purge and cleanſe the body from choler and phlegm. The huſks of the roſes, with the beards and nails of the roſes, are binding and cooling, and the diſtilled water of either of them is good for the heat and redneſs in the eyes, and to ſtay and dry up the rheums and watering of them. Of the red roſes are uſually made many compoſitions, all ſerving to ſundry good uſes, viz. Electuary of Roſes, conſerve, both moiſt and dry, which is more uſually called ſugar of roſes, ſyrup of dry roſes, and honey of roſes. The cordial powder called *Diarrhodon Abbatis*, and *Aromatica Roſarum*. The diſtilled water of Roſes, vinegar of Roſes, ointment, and oil of Roſes, and the Roſe leaves dried, are of very great uſe and effect. To write at large of every one of theſe, would make my book ſwell too big, it being ſufficient for a volume of itſelf, to ſpeak fully of them. But briefly, the electuary is purging, whereof two or three drams taken by itſelf in ſome convenient liquor, is a purge ſufficient for a weak conſtitution, but may be increaſed to ſix drams, according to the ſtrength of the patient. It purgeth choler without trouble, and it is good in hot fevers, and pains

of

of the head arising from hot cholerick humours, and heat in the eyes, the jaundice also, and jont-achs proceeding of hot humours. The moist conserve is of much use, both binding and cordial, for until it be about two years old, it is more binding than cordial, and after that, more cordial than binding. Some of the younger conserve taken with mithridate mixed together, is good for those that are troubled with distillations of rheum from the brain to the nose, and defluction of rheum into the eyes; as also for fluxes and lasks of the belly; and being mixed with the powder of mastick, is very good for running of the reins, and for the looseness of humours in the body. The old conserve mixed with Aromaticum Rosarum, is a very good cordial against faintings, swoonings, weakness and tremblings of the heart, strengthens both it and a weak stomach helpeth digestion, stayeth casting, and is a very good preservative in the time of infection. The dry converse, which is called the Sugar of Roses, is a very good cordial to strengthen the heart and spirits; as also to stay defluctions. The syrup of dried red Roses strengthens a stomach given to casting, cooleth an over-heated liver, and the blood in agues, comforteth the heart, and resisteth putrefaction and infection, and helpeth to stay lasks and fluxes. Honey of Roses is much used in gargles and lotions to wash sores, either in the mouth, throat, or other parts, both to cleanse and heal them, and to stay the fluxes of humours falling upon them. It is also used in clysters both to cool and cleanse. The cordial powders, called Diarrhodon Abbatis and Aromatica Rosarum, do comfort and strengthen the heart and stomach, procure an appetite, help digestion, stay vomiting, and are very good for those that have slippery bowels, to strengthen them, and to dry up their moisture: Red Rose-water is well known, and of a familiar use on all occasions, and better than damask Rose-water, being cooling and cordial, refreshing, quickening the weak and faint spirits, used either in meats or broths, to wash the temples, to smell at the nose, or to smell the sweet vapours thereof out of a perfuming pot, or cast into a hot fire-shovel. It is also of much good use against the redness and inflammations of the eyes to bathe them therewith, and the temples of the head; as also against pain and ache, for which

Z purpose

purpose also vinegar of Roses is of much good use, and to procure rest and sleep, if some thereof and rose-water together, be used to smell unto, or the nose and temples moistened therewith, but more usually to moisten a piece of a red Rose-cake, cut for the purpose, and heated between a double folded cloth, with a little beaten nutmeg, and poppy-seed strewed on the side that must lie next to the forehead and temples, and bound so thereto all night. The ointment of Roses is much used against heat and inflammations in the head, to anoint the forehead and temples, and being mixed with *Unguentum Populneon*, to procure rest; it is also used for the heat of the liver, the back and reins, and to cool and heal pushes, wheals, and other red pimples rising in the face and other parts. Oil of roses is not only used by itself to cool any hot swellings or inflammations, and to bind and stay fluxes of humours unto sores, but is also put into ointments and plaisters that are cooling and binding, and restraining the flux of humours. The dried leaves of the red Roses are used both inwardly and outwardly, both cooling, binding, and cordial, for with them are made both *Aromaticum Rosarum*, *Diarrhodon Abbatis*, and *Saccharum Rosarum*, each of whose properties are before declared. Rose leaves and Mint, heated and applied outwardly to the stomach, stay castings, and very much strengthen a weak stomach; and applied as a fomentation to the region of the liver and heart, do much cool and temper them, and also serve instead of a Rose-cake (as is said before) to quiet the over-hot spirits, and cause rest and sleep. The syrup of damask roses, is both simple and compound, and made with agarick. The simple solutive syrup is a familiar, safe, gentle and easy medicine, purging choler, taken from one ounce to three or four, yet this is remarkable herein, that the distilled water of this syrup should notably bind the belly. The syrup with agarick is more strong and effectual, for one ounce thereof by itself will open the body more than the other, and worketh as much on phlegm as choler. The compound syrup is more forcible in working on melancholick humours; and available against the leprosy, itch, tetters, &c. and the French disease: Also honey of roses solutive is made of the same infusions that the syrup is made of, and there-

therefore worketh the same effect, both opening and purging but is oftener given to phlegmatick than cholerick persons, and is more used in clysters than in potions, as the syrup made with sugar is. The conserve and preserved leaves of those roses are also operative in gently opening the belly.

The simple water of the damask Roses is chiefly used for fumes to sweeten things, as the dried leaves thereof to make sweet powders, and fill sweet bags; and little use they are put to in physick, altho' they have some purging quality; the wild roses also are few or none of them used in physick, but are generally held to come near the nature of the manured roses. The fruit of the wild briar, which are called hips, being thoroughly ripe, and made into a conserve with sugar, besides the pleasantness of the taste, doth gently bind the belly, and stay defluctions from the head upon the stomach, drying up the moisture thereof, and helpeth digestion. The pulp of the hips dried into a hard consistence, like to the juice of liquorish, or so dried that it may be made into powder and taken in drink, stayeth speedily the whites in women. The briar ball is often used, being made into powder and drank, to break the stone, to provoke urine when it is stopped, and to ease and help the colick; some appoint it to be burnt, and then taken for the same purpose. In the middle of the balls are often found certain white worms, which being dried and made into powder, and some of it drank, is found by experience of many to kill and drive forth the worms of the belly.

Rosa Solis, or Sun Dew.

Descript.] IT hath divers small, round, hollow leaves somewhat greenish, but full of certain red hairs, which make them seem red, every one standing upon his own foot-stalk, reddish, hairy, likewise. The leaves are continually moist in the hottest day, yea, the hotter the sun shines on them, the moister they are, with a sliminess that will rope (as we say) the small hairs always holding this moisture. Among these leaves rise up slender stalks, reddish also, three or four fingers high, bearing divers small white knobs one above another, which are flowers;

after which in the heads are contained ſmall ſeeds. The root is a few ſmall hairs.

Place.] It groweth uſually in bogs and wet places, and ſometimes in moiſt woods.

Time.] It flowereth in June, and then the leaves are fitteſt to be gathered.

Government and Virtues.] The Sun rules it, and it is under the ſign Cancer. Roſa Solis is accounted good to help thoſe that have a ſalt rheum diſtilling on the lungs, which breedeth a conſumption, and therefore the diſtilled water thereof in wine is held fit and profitable for ſuch to drink, which water will be of a good yellow colour. The ſame water is held to be good for all other diſeaſes of the lungs, as phthiſicks, wheezings, ſhortneſs of breath, or the cough; as alſo to heal the ulcers that happen in the lungs; and it comforteth the heart and fainting ſpirits. The leaves outwardly applied to the ſkin, will raiſe bliſters, which has cauſed ſome to think it dangerous to be taken inwardly; but there are other things which will alſo draw bliſters, yet nothing dangerous to be taken inwardly. There is an uſual drink made thereof with aqua vitæ and ſpices frequently, and without any offence or danger, but to good purpoſe uſed in qualms and paſſions of the heart.

ROSEMARY.

OUR garden Roſemary is ſo well known, that I need not deſcribe it.

Time.] It flowereth in April and May with us, ſometimes again in Auguſt.

Government and Virtues.] The Sun claims privilege in it, and it is under the celeſtial Ram. It is an herb of as great uſe with us in theſe days as any whatſoever, not only for phyſicial but civil purpoſes. The phyſical uſe of it (being my preſent taſk) is very much both for inward and outward diſeaſes, for by the warming and comforting heat thereof it helpeth all cold diſeaſes, both of the head, ſtomach, liver, and belly. The decoction thereof in wine, helpeth the cold diſtillations of rheums into the eyes, and all other cold diſeaſes of the head and brain, as the giddineſs or ſwimmings therein, drowſineſs or dulneſs of the mind

mind and senses like a stupidness, the dumb palsy, or loss of speech, the lethargy, and falling-sickness, to be both drank, and the temples bathed therewith. It helpeth the pains in the gums and teeth, by rheum falling into them, not by putrefaction, causing an evil smell from them, or a stinking breath. It helpeth a weak memory, and quickeneth the senses. It is very comfortable to the stomach in all the cold griefs thereof, helpeth both retention of meat, and digestion, the decoction or powder being taken in wine. It is a remedy for the windiness in the stomach, bowels, and spleen, and expels it powerfully. It helpeth those that are liver-grown, by opening the obstructions thereof. It helpeth dim eyes, and procureth a clear sight, the flowers thereof being taken all the while it is flowering, every morning fasting, with bread and salt. Both Dioscorides and Galen say, That if a decoction be made thereof with water, and they that have the yellow jaundice exercise their bodies presently after the taking thereof, it will certainly cure them. The flowers, and conserve made of them, are singular good to comfort the heart, and to expel the contagion of the pestilence; to burn the herb in houses and chambers, correcteth the air in them. Both the flowers and leaves are very profitable for women that are troubled with the whites, if they be daily taken. The dried leaves shred small, and taken in a pipe, as tobacco is taken, helpeth those that have any cough, phthisick, or consumption, by warming and drying the thin distillations which cause those diseases. The leaves are very much used in bathings; and made into ointments or oil, are singular good to help cold benumbed joints, sinews, or members. The chymical oil drawn from the leaves and flowers, is a sovereign help for all the diseases aforesaid, to touch the temples and nostrils with two or three drops for all the diseases of the head and brain spoken of before; as also to take one drop, two, or three, as the case requireth, for the inward griefs: Yet must it be done with discretion, for it is very quick and piercing, and therefore but a very little must be taken at a time. There is also another oil made by insolation in this manner: Take what quantity you will of the flowers, and put them into a strong glass close stopped, tie a fine linen cloth over the mouth, and turn the mouth down into another ſtrong glaſs, which being ſet in the ſun, an oil will diſtil down into the lower glaſs, to be preſerved as precious for divers uſes, both inward and outward, as a ſovereign balm to heal the diſeaſes before mentioned, to clear dim ſights, and take away ſpots, marks, and ſcars in the ſkin.

RHUBARB, OR RAPHONTICK.

DO not ſtart, and ſay, This grows you know not how far off; and then aſk me, How it comes to paſs that I bring it among our Engliſh ſimples? For tho' the name may ſpeak it foreign, yet it grows with us in England, and that frequent enough in our gardens; and when you have thoroughly purſued its virtues, you will conclude it nothing inferior to that which is brought out of China, and by that time this hath been as much uſed as that hath been, the name which the other hath gotten will be eclipſed by the fame of this; take therefore a deſcription at large of it as followeth

Deſcript.] At the firſt appearing out of the ground, when the Winter is paſt, it hath a great round browniſh head, riſing from the middle or ſides of the root, which openeth itſelf into ſundry leaves one after another, very much crumpled or folded together at the firſt, and browniſh; but afterwards it ſpreadeth itſelf, and becometh ſmooth, very large and almoſt round, every one ſtanding on a browniſh ſtalk of the thickneſs of a man's thumb, when they are grown to their fulneſs, and moſt of them two feet and more in length, eſpecially when they grow in any moiſt or good ground; and the ſtalk of the leaf, from the bottom thereof to the leaf itſelf, being alſo two feet, the breadth thereof from edge to edge, in the broadeſt place, being alſo two feet, of a ſad or dark green colour, of a fine tart or ſouriſh taſte, much more pleaſant than the garden or wood ſorrel. From among theſe riſeth up ſome, but not every year, ſtrong thick ſtalks, not growing ſo high as the patience, or garden dock, with ſuch round leaves as grow below, but ſmaller at every joint up to the top, and among the flowers, which are white, ſpreading forth into many branches, conſiſting of five or ſix ſmall leaves a-piece, hardly to be diſcerned from the white threads

in

in the middle, and seeming to be all threads, after which come brownish three square seeds, like unto other docks, but larger, whereby it may be plainly known to be a dock. The root grows in time to be very great, with divers and sundry great spreading branches from it, of a dark brownish or reddish colour on the outside, with a pale yellow skin under it, which covereth the inner substance or root, which rind and skin being pared away, the root appears of so fresh and lively a colour, with fresh coloured veins running through it, that the choicest of that Rhubarb that is brought us from beyond the seas cannot excel it, which root, if it be dried carefully, and as it ought (which must be in our country by the gentle heat of a fire, in regard the sun is not hot enough here to do it, and every piece kept from touching one another) will hold its colour almost as well as when it is fresh, and hath been approved of, and commended by those who have oftentimes used them.

Place.] It groweth in gardens, and flowereth about the beginning or middle of June, and the seed is ripe in July.

Time.] The roots that are to be dried and kept all the year following, are not to be taken up before the stalk and leaves be quite withered and gone, and that is not until the middle or end of October, and if they be taken a little before the leaves do spring, or when they are sprung up, the roots will not have half so good a colour in them.

I have given the precedence unto this, because in virtues also it hath the pre-eminence, I come now to describe unto you that which is called Patience, or Monk's Rhubarb; and next unto that, the great round leaved Dock, or Bastard Rhubarb, for the one of these may happily supply in the absence of the other, being not much unlike in their virtues, only one more powerful and efficacious than the other. And lastly, shall shew you the virtues of all the three sorts.

GARDEN-PATIENCE, or MONK'S RHUBARB.

Descript.] THIS is a Dock bearing the name of Rhubarb for some purging quality therein, and groweth up with large tall stalks, set with somewhat broad and long fair green leaves, not dented at all. The

tops

tops of the ſtalks being divided into many ſmall branches, bear reddiſh or purpliſh flowers, and three-ſquare ſeed, like unto other docks. The root is long, great, and yellow, like unto the wild docks, but a little redder; and if it be a little dried, ſheweth leſs ſtore of diſcoloured veins than the next doth when it is dry.

Great round-leav'd Dock, or Baſtard Rhubarb.

Deſcript.] THIS hath divers large, round, thin, yellowiſh green leaves riſing from the root, a little waved about the edges, every one ſtanding upon a reaſonable thick and long browniſh foot-ſtalk, from among which riſeth up a pretty big ſtalk, about two feet high, with ſome ſuch like leaves growing thereon, but ſmaller; at the top whereof ſtand in a long ſpike many ſmall browniſh flowers, which turn into a hard three-ſquare ſhining brown ſeed, like the garden Patience before deſcribed. The root groweth greater than that, with many branches of great fibres thereat, yellow on the outſide, and ſomewhat pale; yellow within, with ſome diſcoloured veins like to the Rhubarb which is firſt deſcribed, but much leſs than it, eſpecially when it is dry.

Place and Time.] Theſe alſo grow in gardens, and flower and ſeed at or near the ſame time that our true Rhubarb doth, *viz.* they flower in June, and the ſeed is ripe in July.

Temperature and Virtues.] Mars claims predominancy over all theſe wholeſome herbs: You cry out upon him for an infortunate, when God created him for your good (only he is angry with fools.) What diſhonour is this, not to Mars, but to God himſelf? A dram of the dried root of Monk's Rhubarb, with a ſcruple of ginger made into powder, and taken faſting in a draught or meſs of warm broth, purgeth choler and phlegm downwards very gently and ſafely, without danger. The ſeed thereof contrary doth bind the belly, and helpeth to ſtay any ſort of laſks or bloody-flux. The diſtilled water thereof is very profitably uſed to heal ſcabs; alſo foul ulcerous ſores, and to lay the inflammation of them; the juice of the leaves or roots, or the decoction of them in vinegar, is uſed as a moſt effectual remedy to heal ſcabs and running ſores.

The Baſtard Rhubarb hath all the properties of the Monk's

Monk's Rhubarb, but more effectual for both inward and outward diseases. The decoction thereof without vinegar dropped into the ears, taketh away the pains; gargled in the mouth, taketh away the tooth-ach; and being drank, healeth the jaundice. The seed thereof taken, easeth the gnawing and griping pains of the stomach, and taketh away the loathing thereof unto meat. The root thereof helpeth the ruggedness of the nails, and being boiled in wine helpeth the swelling of the throat, commonly called the king's evil, as also the swellings of the kernels of the ears. It helpeth them that are troubled with the stone, provoketh urine, and helpeth the dimness of the sight. The roots of this Bastard Rhubarb are used in opening and purging diet-drinks, with other things, to open the liver, and to cleanse and cool the blood.

The properties of that which is called the English Rhubarb, are the same with the former, but much more effectual, and hath all the properties of the true Italian Rhubarbs, except the force in purging, wherein it is but of half the strength thereof, and therefore a double quantity must be used; it likewise hath not that bitterness and astriction; in other things it worketh almost in an equal quantity, which are these: It purgeth the body of choler and phlegm, being either taken of itself, made into powder, and drank in a draught of white wine, or steeped therein all night, and taken fasting, or put among other purges, as shall be thought convenient, cleansing the stomach, liver, and blood, opening obstructions, and helping those griefs that come thereof, as the jaundice, dropsy, swelling of the spleen, tertian and daily agues, and pricking pains of the sides; and also it stayeth spitting of blood. The powder taken with cassia dissolved, and washed Venice turpentine, cleanseth the reins, and strengtheneth them afterwards, and is very effectual to stay the running of the reins, or gonorrhea. It is also given for the pains and swellings in the head, for those that are troubled with melancholy, and helpeth the sciatica, gout, and the cramp. The powder of the Rhubarb taken with a little mummia and madder roots in some red wine, dissolveth clotted blood in the body, happening by any fall or bruise, and helpeth burstings and broken parts, as well inward as outward. The oil likewise

wherein

wherein it hath been boiled, worketh the like effects, being anointed. It is used to heal those ulcers that happen in the eyes or eyelids, being steeped and strained; as also to assuage the swellings and inflammations; and applied with honey, boiled in wine, it taketh away all blue spots or marks that happen therein. Whey or white wine are the best liquors to steep it in, and thereby it worketh more effectually in opening obstructions, and purging the stomach and liver. Many do use a little Indian spikenard as the best corrector thereof.

MEADOW-RUE.

Descript.] MEADOW-RUE riseth up with a yellow stringy root, much spreading in the ground, shooting forth new sprouts round about, with many herby green stalks, two feet high, crested all the length of them, set with joints here and there, and many large leaves on them, above as well as below, being divided into smaller leaves, nicked or dented in the forepart of them, of a red green colour on the upper side, and pale green underneath: Toward the top of the stalk there shooteth forth divers short branches, on every one whereof stand two, three, or four small heads, or buttons, which breaking the skin that incloseth them, shooteth forth a tuft of pale greenish yellow threads, which falling away, there come in their places small three cornered cods, wherein is contained small, long, and round seed. The whole plant hath a strong unpleasant scent.

Place.] It groweth in many places of this land, in the borders of moist meadows, and ditch-sides.

Time.] It flowereth about July, or beginning of August.

Government and Virtues.] Dioscorides saith, That this herb bruised and applied, perfectly healeth old sores, and the distilled water of the herb and flowers doth the like. It is used by some among other pot-herbs to open the body, and make it soluble; but the roots washed clean, and boiled in ale and drank, provoke to stool more than the leaves, but yet very gently. The root boiled in water, and the places of the body most troubled with vermin and lice washed therewith while it is warm, destroyeth them utterly.

terly,

terly. In Italy it is ufed againft the plague, and in Saxony againft the jaundice, as *Camerarius* faith.

GARDEN-RUE.

GARDEN-Rue is fo well known by this name, and the name Herb of Grace, that I fhall not need to write any further defcription of it, but fhall only fhew you the virtue of it, as followeth.

Government and Virtues.] It is an herb of the Sun, and under Leo. It provoketh urine and womens courfes, being taken either in meat or drink. The feed thereof taken in wine, is an antidote againft all dangerous medicines or deadly poifons. The leaves taken either by themfelves, or with figs and walnuts, is called Mithridate's counterpoifon againft the plague, and caufeth all venomous things to become harmlefs; being often taken in meat and drink, it abateth venery, and deftroyeth the ability to get children. A decoction made thereof with fome dried dill-leaves and flowers, eafeth all pains and torments, inwardly to be drank, and outwardly to be applied warm to the place grieved. The fame being drank, helpeth the pains both of the cheft and fides, as alfo coughs and hardnefs of breathing, the inflammations of the lungs, and the tormenting pains of the fciatica and the joints, being anointed, or laid to the places; as alfo the fhaking fits of agues, to take a draught before the fit comes; being boiled or infufed in oil, it is good to help the wind colick, the hardnefs and windinefs of the mother, and freeth women from the ftrangling or fuffocation thereof, if the fhare and the parts thereabouts be anointed therewith: It killeth and driveth forth the worms of the belly, if it be drank after it is boiled in wine to the half, with a little honey; it helpeth the gout or pains in the joints, hands, feet or knees, applied thereunto; and with figs it helpeth the dropfy, being bathed therewith: Being bruifed and put into the noftrils, it ftayeth the bleeding thereof; it helpeth the fwelling of the cods, if they be bathed with a decoction of Rue and bay leaves. It taketh away wheals and pimples, if being bruifed with a few myrtle leaves, it be made up with wax, and applied. It cureth the morphew, and taketh away all forts of warts, if boiled ed in wine with some pepper and nitre, and the place rubbed therewith, and with almond and honey, helpeth the dry scabs, or any tetter or ringworm. The juice thereof warmed in a pomegranate shell or rhind, and dropped into the ears, helpeth the pains of them. The juice of it and fennel, with a little honey, and the gall of a cock put thereunto, helpeth the dimness of the eye-sight. An ointment made of the juice thereof with oil of roses, ceruse, and a little vinegar, and anointed, cureth St Anthony's fire, and all running sores in the head; and the stinking ulcers of the nose, or other parts. The antidote used by Mithridates, every morning fasting, to secure himself from any poison or infection, was this: Take twenty leaves of rue, a little salt, a couple of walnuts, and a couple of figs, beaten together into a mess, with twenty juniper berries, which is the quantity appointed for every day. Another electuary is made thus: Take of nitre, pepper, and cummin seed, of equal parts; of the leaves of rue clean picked, as much in weight as all the other three weighed; beat them well together, and put as much honey as will make it up into an electuary (but you must first steep your cummin seed in vinegar twenty-four hours, and then dry it, or rather roast it in a hot fire-shovel, or in an oven) and is a remedy for the pains or griefs in the chest or stomach, of the spleen, belly, or sides, by wind or stitches; of the liver by obstructions; of the reins and bladder by the stopping of urine; and helpeth also to extenuate fat corpulent bodies. What an infamy is cast upon the ashes of Mithridates, or Methridates (as the Augustines read his name) by unworthy people. They that deserve no good report themselves, love to give none to others, *viz.* That renowned King of Pontus fortified his body by poison against poison. (*He cast out devils by* Beelzebub *Prince of the devils.*) What a sot is he that knows not if he had accustomed his body to cold poisons, hot poisons would have dispatched him? on the contrary, if not, corrosions would have done it. The whole world is at this present time beholden to him for his studies in physick, and he that useth the quantity but of an hazel-nut of that receipt every morning, to which his name is adjoined, shall to admiration preserve his body in health, if he do but consider that Rue is an herb of the

the Sun, and under Leo, and gather it and the rest accordingly.

RUPTURE-WORT.

Descript.] THIS spreads very many thready branches round about upon the ground, about a span long, divided into many other smaller parts full of small joints set very thick together, whereat come forth two very small leaves of a French yellow, green coloured branches and all, where groweth forth also a number of exceeding small yellowish flowers, scarce to be discerned from the stalks and leaves, which turn into seeds as small as the very dust. The root is very long and small, thrusting down deep into the ground. This hath neither smell nor taste at first, but afterwards hath a little astringent taste, without any manifest heat; yet a little bitter and sharp withal.

Place.] It groweth in dry sandy, and rocky places.

Time.] It is fresh and green all the Summer.

Government and Virtues.] They say Saturn causeth ruptures; if he do, he doth no more than he can cure; if you want wit, he will teach you, though to your cost. This herb is Saturn's own, and is a noble antivenerean. Rupture-wort hath not its name in vain; for it is found by experience to cure the rupture, not only in children, but also in elder persons, if the disease be not too inveterate, by taking a dram of the powder of the dried herb every day in wine, or a decoction made and drank for certain days together. The juice or distilled water of the green herb, taken in the same manner, helpeth all other fluxes either of man or woman; vomitings also, and the gonorrhea or running of the reins, being taken any of the ways aforesaid. It doth also most assuredly help those that have the strangury, or are troubled with the stone or gravel in the reins or bladder. The same also helpeth stiches in the sides, gripping pains of the stomach or belly, the obstructions of the liver, and cureth the yellow jaundice; likewise it kills also the worms in children. Being outwardly applied, it conglutinateth wounds notably, and helpeth much to stay defluctions of rheum from the head to the eyes, nose and teeth, being bruised green, and bound thereto;

 or

or the forehead, temples, or the nape of the neck behind, bathed with the decoction of the dried herb. It also drieth up the moisture of fistulous ulcers or any other that are foul and spreading.

RUSHES.

ALTHOUGH there are many kinds of Rushes, yet I shall only here insist upon those which are best known, and most medicinal; as the bulrushes, and other of the soft and smooth kinds, which grow so commonly in almost every part of this land, and are so generally noted, that I suppose it needless to trouble you with any description of them: Briefly then take the virtues of them as followeth.

Government and Virtues.] The seed of the soft Rushes, (saith Dioscorides and Galen, toasted, saith Pliny) being drank in wine and water, stayeth the lask and womens courses, when they come down too abundantly; but it causeth head-ach: It provoketh sleep likewise, but must be given with caution. The root boiled in water, to the consumption of one third, helpeth the cough.

Thus you see that conveniencies have their inconveniencies, and virtues are seldom unaccompanied with some vices. What I have written concerning Rushes, is to satisfy my countrymens questions: *Are our Rushes good for nothing?* Yes, and as good let them alone as take them. There are remedies enough without them for any disease, and therefore, as the proverb is, I care not a Rush for them; or rather, they will do you as much good as if one had given you a Rush.

RYE.

THIS is so well known in all the counties of this land, and especially to the country people, who feed much thereon, that if I did describe it, they would presently say, I might as well have spared that labour. Its virtues follow.

Government and Virtues.] Rye is more digesting than wheat; the bread and the leaven thereof ripeneth and breaketh imposthumes, boils, and other swellings: The meal of Rye put between a double cloth, and moistened with a little vinegar, and heated in a pewter dish, set over

ver a chafing dish of coals, and bound fast to the head while it is hot, doth much ease the continual pains of the head. Matthiolus saith, That the ashes of Rye straw put into water, and steeped therein a day and a night, and the chops of the hands or feet washed therewith, doth heal them.

SAFFRON.

THE herb needs no description, it being known generally where it grows.

Place.] It grows frequently at Walden in Essex, and in Cambridgeshire.

Government and Virtues.] It is an herb of the Sun, and under the Lion, and therefore you need not demand a reason why it strengthens the heart so exceedingly. Let not above ten grains be given at one time, for the Sun, which is the fountain of light, may dazzle the eyes, and make them blind; a cordial being taken in an immoderate quantity, hurts the heart instead of helping it. It quickeneth the brain, for the Sun is exalted in Aries, as well as he hath his house in Leo: It helps consumptions of the lungs, and difficulty of breathing: It is excellent in epidemical diseases, as pestilence, small-pox, and measles. It is a notable expulsive medicine, and a notable remedy for the yellow jaundice. My opinion is, (but I have no author for it) that hermodactyls are nothing else but the roots of Saffron dried; and my reason is, that the roots of all crocus, both white and yellow, purge phlegm as hermodactyls do; and if you please to dry the roots of any crocus, neither your eyes nor your taste shall distinguish them from hermodactyls.

SAGE.

OUR ordinary garden Sage needeth no description.

Time.] It flowereth in or about July.

Government and Virtues.] Jupiter claims this, and bids me tell you, it is good for the liver, and to breed blood. A decoction of the leaves and branches of Sage made and drank, saith Dioscorides, provoketh urine, bringeth down womens courses, helps to expel the dead child, and causeth the hair to become black. It stayeth the bleeding of wounds, and cleanseth foul ulcers or sores. The said decoction made in wine, taketh away the itching of the cods, if they be bathed therewith. Agrippa saith, that if women that cannot conceive by reason of the moist slipperiness of their wombs, shall take a quantity of the juice of Sage, with a little salt, for four days before they company with their husbands, it will help them not only to conceive, but also to retain the birth without miscarrying. Orpheus saith, Three spoonfuls of the juice of Sage taken fasting, with a little honey, doth presently stay the spitting or casting of blood of them that are in a consumption. These pills are much commended: Take of spikenard, ginger, of each two drams; of the seed of Sage toasted at the fire, eight drams; of long-pepper twelve drams; all these being brought into powder, put thereto so much juice of Sage as may make them into a mass of pills, taking a dram of them every morning fasting, and so likewise at night, drinking a little pure water after them. Matthiolus saith, it is very profitable for all manner of pains in the head coming of cold and rheumatick humours; as also for all pains of the joints, whether inwardly or outwardly, and therefore helpeth the falling-sickness, the lethargy, such as are dull and heavy of spirit, the palsy; and is of much use in all defluctions of rheum from the head, and for the diseases of the chest or breast. The leaves of Sage and nettles bruised together, and laid upon the imposthume that riseth behind the ears, doth assuage it much. The juice of Sage taken in warm water, helpeth a hoarseness and a cough. The leaves sodden in wine, and laid upon the place affected with the palsy, helpeth much, if the decoction be drank: Also, Sage taken with wormwood is good for the bloody-flux. Pliny saith, it procures womens courses, and stayeth them coming down too fast; helpeth the stinging and biting of serpents, and killeth the worms that breed in the ear, and in sores. Sage is of excellent use to help the memory, warming and quickening the senses; and the conserve made of the flowers is used to the same purpose, and also for all the former recited diseases. The juice of Sage drank with vinegar, hath been of good use in time of the plague at all times. Gargles likewise are made with Sage, rosemary,

rosemary, honey-suckles, and plantain, boiled in wine or water, with some honey or alum put thereto, to wash sore mouths and throats, cankers, or the secret parts of man or woman, as need requireth. And with other hot and comfortable herbs, Sage is boiled to bathe the body and the legs in the Summer time, especially to warm cold joints or sinews, troubled with the palsy and cramp, and to comfort and strengthen the parts. It is much commended against the stitch, or pains in the side coming of wind, if the place be fomented warm with the decoction thereof in wine, and the herb also after boiling be laid warm thereunto.

WOOD-SAGE.

Descript.] WOOD-Sage riseth up with square hoary stalks, two feet high at the least, with two leaves set at every joint, somewhat like other Sage leaves but smaller, softer, whiter, and rounder, and a little dented about the edges, and smelling somewhat stronger. At the tops of the stalks and branches stand the flowers, on a slender like spike, turning themselves all one way when they blow, and are of a pale and whitish colour, smaller than Sage, but hooded and gaping like unto them. The seed is blackish and round; four usually seem in a husk together; the root is long and stringy, with divers fibres thereat, and abideth many years.

Place.] It groweth in woods, and by wood-sides; as also in divers fields and bye-lanes in the land.

Time.] It flowereth in June, July and August.

Government and Virtues.] The herb is under Venus. The decoction of the Wood-Sage provoketh urine and womens courses: It also provoketh sweat, digesteth humours, and discusseth swellings and nodes in the flesh, and is therefore thought to be good against the French-pox. The decoction of the green herb, made with wine, is a safe and sure remedy for those who by falls, bruises, or blows, suspect some vein to be inwardly broken, to disperse and void the congealed blood, and to consolidate the veins. The drink used inwardly, and the herb used outwardly, is good for such as are inwardly or outwardly bursten, and is found to be a sure remedy for the palsy.

The juice of the herb, or the powder thereof dried, is good for moiſt ulcers and ſores in the legs, and other parts, to dry them, and cauſe them to heal more ſpeedily. It is no leſs effectual alſo in green wounds, to be uſed upon any occaſion.

SOLOMON'S SEAL.

Deſcript.] THE common Solomon's Seal riſeth up with a round ſtalk half a yard high, bowing or bending down to the ground, ſet with ſingle leaves one above another, ſomewhat large, and like the leaves of the lily-convally, or May-lily, with an eye of blueiſh upon the green, with ſome ribs therein, and more yellowiſh underneath. At the foot of every leaf, almoſt from the bottom up to the top of the ſtalk, come forth ſmall, long, white and hollow pendulous flowers, ſomewhat like the flowers of May-lily, but ending in five long points, for the moſt part two together, at the end of a long foot-ſtalk, and ſometimes but one, and ſometimes alſo two ſtalks, with flowers at the foot of a leaf, which are without any ſcent at all, and ſtand on one ſide of the ſtalk. After they are paſt, come in their places ſmall round berries, great at the firſt, and blackiſh green, tending to blueneſs when they are ripe, wherein lie ſmall, white, hard, and ſtoney ſeeds. The root is of the thickneſs of one's finger or thumb, white and knotted in ſome places, a flat round circle repreſenting a ſeal, whereof it took the name, lying along under the upper cruſt of the earth, and not growing downward, but with many fibres underneath.

Place.] It is frequent in divers places of this land; as, namely, in a wood two miles from Canterbury, by Fiſh-Pool Hill, as alſo in Buſhy Cloſe belonging to the parſonage of Alderbury, near Clarendon, two miles from Saliſbury; in Cheſſon-wood, on Cheſſon-hill, between Newington and Sittingbourn in Kent, and divers other places in Eſſex, and other counties.

Time.] It flowereth about May: The root abideth and ſhooteth a-new every year.

Government and Virtues.] Saturn owns the plant, for he loves his bones well. The root of Solomon's Seal is found by experience to be available in wounds, hurts, and outward

ward sores, to heal and close up the lips of those that are green, and to dry up and restrain the flux of humours to those that are old. It is singularly good to stay vomitings and bleeding wheresoever, as also all fluxes in man or woman, whether whites or reds in women, or the running of the reins in men; also, to knit any joint, which by weakness useth to be often out of place, or will not stay in long when it is set; also, to knit and join broken bones in any part of the body, the roots being bruised and applied to the places; yea, it hath been found by late experience, that the decoction of the root in wine, or the bruised root put into wine or other drink, and after a night's infusion, strained forth hard and drank, hath helped both man and beast, whose bones hath been broken by any occasion, which is the most assured refuge of help to people of divers counties of the land that they can have: It is no less effectual to help ruptures and burstings, the decoction in wine, or the powder in broth or drink, being inwardly taken, and outwardly applied to the place. The same is also available for inward or outward bruises, falls or blows, both to dispel the congealed blood, and to take away both the pains and the black and blue marks that abide after the hurt. The same also, or the distilled water of the whole plant, used to the face, or other parts of the skin, cleanseth it from morphew, freckles, spots, or marks whatsoever, leaving the place fresh, fair, and lovely; for which purpose it is much used by the Italian Dames.

SAMPHIRE.

Descript.] ROCK Samphire groweth up with a tender green stalk about half a yard, or two feet high at the most, branching forth almost from the very bottom, and stored with sundry thick and almost round (somewhat long) leaves, of a deep green colour, sometimes two together, and sometimes more on a stalk, and sappy, and of a pleasant, hot, and spicy taste. At the top of the stalks and branches stand umbels of white flowers, and after them come large seed bigger than fennel seed, yet somewhat like it. The root is great, white, and long, continuing many years, and is of an hot and spicy taste likewise.

Place.

Place.] It groweth on the rocks that are often moisten-ed at the least, if not overflowed with the sea water.

Time.] And it flowereth and seedeth in the end of July and August.

Government and Virtues.] It is an herb of Jupiter, and was in former times wont to be used more than now it is; the more is the pity. It is well known almost to every body, that ill digestions and obstructions are the cause of most of the diseases which the frail nature of man is subject to; both which might be remedied by a more frequent use of this herb. If people would have sauce to their meat, they may take some for profit as well as for pleasure. It is a safe herb, very pleasant both to taste and stomach, helping digestion, and in some sort opening obstructions of the liver and spleen; provoketh urine, and helpeth thereby to wash away the gravel and stone engendered in the kidneys or bladder.

SANICLE.

Descript.] ORDINARY Sanicle sendeth forth many great round leaves, standing upon long brownish stalks, every one somewhat deeply cut or divided into five or six parts, and some of these also cut in somewhat like the leaf of crow's-foot, or dove's-foot, and finely dented about the edges, smooth, and of a dark shining colour, and sometimes reddish about the brims; from among which arise up small, round green stalks, without any joint or leaf thereon, saving at the top, where it branches forth into flowers, having a leaf divided into three or four parts at that joint with the flowers, which are small and white, starting out of small round greenish yellow heads, many standing together in a tuft, in which afterwards are the seeds contained, which are small round burs, somewhat like the leaves of clevers, and stick in the same manner upon any thing that they touch. The root is composed of many blackish strings or fibres, set together at a little long head, which abideth with green leaves all the Winter, and perisheth not.

Place.] It is found in many shadowy woods, and other places of this land.

Time.

Time.] It flowereth in June, and the feed is ripe shortly after.

Government and Virtues.] This is one of Venus's herbs, to cure the wounds or mischiefs Mars inflicteth upon the body of man. It heals green wounds speedily, or any ulcers, imposthumes, or bleedings inward, also tumours in any part of the body; for the decoction or powder in drink taken, and the juice used outwardly, dissipateth the humours; and there is not found any herb that can give such present help either to man or beast, when the disease falleth upon the lungs or throat, and to heal up putrid malignant ulcers in the mouth, throat, and privities, by gargling or washing with the decoction of the leaves and roots made in water, and a little honey put thereto. It helpeth to stay womens courses, and all other fluxes of blood, either by the mouth, urine, or stool, and lasks of the belly; the ulcerations of the kidneys also, and the pains in the bowels, and gonorrhæa, or running of the reins, being boiled in wine or water, and drank. The same also is no less powerful to help any ruptures or burstings, used both inwardly and outwardly: And briefly, it is as effectual in binding, restraining, consolidating, heating, drying, and healing, as comfrey, bugle, self-heal, or any other of the vulnerary herbs whatsoever.

Saracens Confound, or Saracens Woundwort.

Descript.] THIS groweth high sometimes, with brownish stalks, and other whiles with green, to a man's height, having narrow green leaves snipped about the edges, somewhat like those of the peach-tree, or willow leaves, but not of such a white green colour. The tops of the stalks are furnished with many yellow star-like flowers, standing in green heads, which when they are fallen, and the seed ripe, which is somewhat long, small and of a brown colour, wrapped in down, is therewith carried away with the wind. The root is composed of fibres set together at a head, which perisheth not in Winter, altho' the stalks dry away, and no leaf appeareth in the winter. The taste hereof is strong and unpleasant; and so is the smell also.

Place.] It groweth in moist and wet grounds, by woodsides,

ſides, and ſometimes in the moiſt places of ſhadow groves, as alſo by the water ſide.

Time.] It flowereth in July, and the ſeed is ſoon ripe, and carried away with the wind.

Government and Virtues.] Saturn owns the herb, and it is of a ſober condition, like him. Among the Germans, this wound herb is preferred before all others of the ſame quality. Being boiled in wine, and drank, it helpeth the indiſpoſition of the liver, and freeth the gall from obſtructions; whereby it is good for the yellow jaundice, and for the dropſy in the beginning of it; for all inward ulcers of the reins, mouth or throat, and inward wounds and bruiſes, likewiſe for ſuch ſores as happen in the privy parts of men or women; being ſteeped in wine, and then diſtilled, the water thereof drank, is ſingular good to eaſe all gnawings in the ſtomach, or other pains of the body, as alſo the pains of the mother: And being boiled in water, it helpeth continual agues; and the ſaid water, or the ſimple water of the herb diſtilled, or the juice or decoction, are very effectual to heal any green wound, or old ſore or ulcer whatſoever, cleanſing them from corruption, and quickly healing them up: Briefly, whatſoever hath been ſaid of bugle or ſanicle, may be found herein.

Sauce-alone, or Jack by the Hedge-ſide.

Deſcript.] THE lower leaves of this are rounder than thoſe that grow towards the top of the ſtalks, and are ſet ſingly on a joint, being ſomewhat round and broad, pointed at the ends, dented alſo about the edges, ſomewhat reſembling nettle leaves for the form, but of a freſher green colour, not rough or pricking: The flowers are white, growing at the top of the ſtalks one above another, which being paſt, follow ſmall round pods, wherein are contained round ſeed ſomewhat blackiſh. The root ſtringy and thready, periſheth every year after it hath given ſeed, and raiſeth itſelf again of its own ſowing. The plant, or any part thereof, being bruiſed, ſmelleth of garlick, but more pleaſantly, and taſteth ſomewhat hot and ſharp, almoſt like unto rocket.

Place.] It groweth under walls, and by hedge-ſides, and path-ways in fields in many places.

Time.

Time.] It flowereth in June, July, and August.

Government and Virtues.] It is an herb of Mercury. This is eaten by many country people as sauce to their salt fish, and helpeth well to digest the crudities and other corrupt humours engendered thereby: It warmeth also the stomach, and causeth digestion: The juice thereof boiled with honey is accounted to be as good as hedge mustard for the cough, to cut and expectorate the tough phlegm. The seed bruised and boiled in wine, is a singular good remedy for the wind colick, or the stone, being drank warm: It is also given to women troubled with the mother, both to drink, and the seed put into a cloth, and applied while it is warm, is of singular good use. The leaves also, or the seed boiled, is good to be used in clysters to ease the pains of the stone. The green leaves are held to be good to heal the ulcers in the legs.

Winter and Summer SAVORY.

BOTH these are so well known (being entertained as constant inhabitants in our gardens) that they need no description.

Government and Virtues.] Mercury claims the dominion over this herb, neither is there a better remedy against the colick and iliac passion, than this herb; keep it dry by you all the year, if you love yourself and your ease, and it is a hundred pounds to a penny if you do not; keep it dry, make conserves and syrups of it for your use, and withal, take notice that the Summer kind is the best. They are both of them hot and dry, especially the Summer kind, which is both sharp and quick in taste, expelling wind in the stomach and bowels, and is a present help for the rising of the mother procured by wind; provoketh urine and womens courses, and is much commended for women with child to take inwardly, and to smell often unto. It cureth tough phlegm in the chest and lungs, and helpeth to expectorate it the more easily; quickens the dull spirits in the lethargy, the juice thereof being snuffed up into the nostrils. The juice dropped into the eyes, cleareth a dull sight, if it proceed of thin cold humours distilled from the brain. The juice heated with oil of Roses, and dropped into the ears, easeth them of the noise and singing in them,

and

and of deafneſs alſo: Outwardly applied with wheat flour, in manner of a poultice, it giveth eaſe to the ſciatica and palſied members, heating and warming them, and taketh away their pains. It alſo taketh away the pain that comes by ſtinging of bees, waſps, &c.

SAVINE.

TO deſcribe a plant ſo well known is needleſs, it being nurſed up almoſt in every garden, and abiding green all the winter.

Government and Virtues.] It is under the dominion of Mars, being hot and dry in the third degree, and being of exceeding clean parts, is of a very digeſting quality. If you dry the herb into powder, and mix it with honey, it is an excellent remedy to cleanſe old filthy ulcers and fiſtulas; but it hinders them from healing. The ſame is excellent good to break carbuncles and plague-ſores; alſo helpeth the king's evil, being applied to the place. Being ſpread over a piece of leather, and applied to the navel, kills the worms in the belly, helps ſcabs and itch, running ſores, cankers, tetters, and ringworms; and being applied to the place, may haply cure venereal ſores. This I thought good to ſpeak of, as it may be ſafely uſed outwardly, for inwardly it cannot be taken without manifeſt danger.

The common WHITE SAXIFRAGE.

Deſcript.] THIS hath a few ſmall reddiſh kernels of roots covered with ſome ſkins, lying among divers ſmall blackiſh fibres, which ſend forth divers round, faint or yellow green leaves, and greyiſh underneath, lying above the ground, unevenly dented about the edges, and ſomewhat hairy, every one upon a little foot-ſtalk, from whence riſeth up round, browniſh, hairy, green ſtalks, two or three feet high, with a few ſuch like round leaves as grow below, but ſmaller, and ſomewhat branched at the top, whereon ſtand pretty large white flowers of five leaves a-piece, with ſome yellow threads in the middle, ſtanding in a long creſted, browniſh, green huſk. After the flowers are paſt, there ariſeth ſometimes a round hard head, forked at the top, wherein is contained ſmall black ſeed,

ſeed, but uſually they fall away without any ſeed, and it is the kernels or grains of the root which are uſually called the White Saxifrage-ſeed, and ſo uſed.

Place.] It groweth in many places of our land, as well in the lowermoſt, as in the upper dry corners of meadows, and graſſy ſandy places. It uſed to grow near Lamb's conduit, on the backſide of Gray's Inn.

Time.] It flowereth in May, and then gathered, as well for that which is called the ſeed, as to diſtil, for it quickly periſheth down to the ground when any hot weather comes.

Government and Virtues.] It is very effectual to cleanſe the reins and bladder, and to diſſolve the ſtone engendered in them, and to expel it and the gravel by urine; to help the ſtrangury; for which purpoſe the decoction of the herb or roots in white wine, is moſt uſual, or the powder of the ſmall kernelly root, which is called the ſeed, taken in white wine, or in the ſame decoction made with white wine, is moſt uſual. The diſtilled water of the whole herb, root and flowers, is moſt familiar to be taken. It provoketh alſo womens courſes, and freeth and cleanſeth the ſtomach and lungs from thick and tough phlegm that trouble them. There are not many better medicines to break the ſtone than this.

BURNET SAXIFRAGE.

Deſcript.] THE greater ſort of our Engliſh Burnet Saxifrage groweth up with divers long ſtalks of winged leaves, ſet directly oppoſite one to another on both ſides, each being ſomewhat broad, and a little pointed and dented about the edges, of a ſad green colour. At the top of the ſtalks ſtand umbels of white flowers, after which come ſmall and blackiſh ſeed. The root is long and whitiſh, abiding long. Our leſſer Burnet Saxifrage hath much finer leaves than the former, and very ſmall, and ſet one againſt another, deeply jagged about the edges, and of the ſame colour as the former. The umbels of the flowers are white, and the ſeed very ſmall, and ſo is the root, being alſo ſomewhat hot and quick in taſte.

Place.] Theſe grow in moiſt meadows of this land, and

are easy to be found being well sought for among the grass, wherein many times they lie hid scarcely to be discerned.

Time.] They flower about July, and their seed is ripe in August.

Government and Virtues.] They are both of them herbs of the Moon. The Saxifrages are hot as pepper; and Tragus saith, by his experience, that they are wholesome. They have the same properties the parsleys have, but in provoking urine, and easing the pains thereof, and of the wind and colick, are much more effectual, the roots or seed being used either in powder, or in decoctions, or any other way; and likewise helpeth the windy pains of the mother, and to procure their courses, and to break and void the stone in the kidneys, to digest cold, viscous, and tough phlegm in the stomach, and is an especial remedy against all kind of venom. Castoreum being boiled in the distilled water thereof is singular good to be given to those that are troubled with cramps and convulsions. Some do use to make the seeds into comfits (as they do carraway seeds) which is effectual to all the purposes aforesaid. The juice of the herb dropped into the most grievous wounds of the head drieth up their moisture, and healeth them quickly. Some women use the distilled water to take away freckles or spots in the skin or face; and to drink the same sweetened with sugar for all the purposes aforesaid.

SCABIOUS, three Sorts.

Descript.] COMMON field Scabious groweth up with many hairy, soft, whitish green leaves, some whereof are very little, if at all jagged on the edges, others very much rent and torn on the sides, and have threads in them, which upon breaking may be plainly seen; from among which rise up divers hairy green stalks, three or four feet high, with such like hairy green leaves on them, but more deeply and finely divided, branched forth a little: At the tops thereof, which are naked and bare of leaves for a good space, stand round heads of flowers, of a pale blueish colour, set together in a head, the outermost whereof are larger than the inward, with many threads also in the middle, somewhat flat at the top, as the head with the seed is likewise; the root is great, white and thick, growing down deep into the ground, and abideth many years.

There

There is another ſort of Field Scabious different in nothing from the former, but only it is ſmaller in all reſpects.

The Corn Scabious differeth little from the firſt, but that it is greater in all reſpects, and the flowers more inclining to purple, and the root creepeth under the upper cruſt of the earth, and runneth not deep into the ground as the firſt doth.

Place.] The firſt groweth more uſually in meadows, eſpecially about London every where.

The ſecond in ſome of the dry fields about this city, but not ſo plentifully as the former.

The third in ſtanding corn, or fallow fields, and the borders of ſuch like fields.

Time.] They flower in June and July, and ſome abide flowering until it be late in Auguſt, and the ſeed is ripe in the mean time.

There are many other ſorts of Scabious, but I take theſe which I have here deſcribed to be moſt familiar with us: The virtues of both theſe and the reſt, being much alike, take them as followeth.

Government and Virtues.] Mercury owns the plant. Scabious is very effectual for all ſorts of coughs, ſhortneſs of breath, and all other diſeaſes of the breaſt and lungs, ripening and digeſting cold phlegm, and other tough humours, voideth them forth by coughing and ſpitting: It ripeneth alſo all ſorts of inward ulcers and impoſthumes; pleuriſy alſo, if the decoction of the herb dry or green be made in wine, and drank for ſome time together. Four ounces of the clarified juice of Scabious taken in the morning faſting, with a dram of mithridate, or Venice treacle, freeth the heart from any infection of peſtilence, if after the taking of it the party ſweat two hours in bed, and this medicine be again and again repeated, if need require. The green herb bruiſed and applied to any carbuncle or plague ſore, is found by certain experience to diſſolve and break it in three hours ſpace. The ſame decoction alſo drank, helpeth the pains and ſtitches in the ſide. The decoction of the roots taken for forty days together, or a dram of the powder of them taken at a time in whey, doth (as Matthiolus ſaith) wonderfully help thoſe that are troubled with running or ſpreading ſcabs, tetters, ringworms, yea, although they proceed from the French pox, which, he saith, he tried by experience. The juice or decoction drank, helpeth also scabs and breakings-out of the itch, and the like. The juice also made up into an ointment and used, is effectual for the same purpose. The same also healeth all inward wounds by the drying, cleansing, and healing quality therein: And a syrup made of the juice and sugar, is very effectual to all the purposes aforesaid, and so is the distilled water of the herb and flowers made in due season, especially to be used when the green herb is not in force to be taken. The decoction of the herb and roots outwardly applied, doth wonderfully help all sorts of hard or cold swellings in any part of the body, is effectual for shrunk sinews or veins, and healeth green wounds, old sores and ulcers. The juice of Scabious, made up with the powder of Borax and Samphire, cleanseth the skin of the face, or other parts of the body, not only from freckles and pimples, but also from morphew and leprosy; the head washed with the decoction, cleanseth it from dandriff, scurff, sores, itch, and the like, used warm. The herb bruised and applied, doth in a short time loosen, and draw forth any splinter, broken bone, arrow head, or other such like thing, lying in the flesh.

SCURVYGRASS.

Descript] OUR ordinary English Scurvygrass hath many thick flat leaves more long than broad, and sometimes longer and narrower; sometimes also smooth on the edges, and sometimes a little waved; sometimes plain, smooth and pointed, of a sad green, and sometimes a blueish colour, every one standing by itself upon a long foot-stalk, which is brownish or greenish also, from among which arise many slender stalks, bearing few leaves thereon like the other, but longer and lesser for the most part: At the tops whereof grow many whitish flowers, with yellow threads in the middle, standing about a green head, which becometh the seed vessel, which will be somewhat flat when it is ripe, wherein is contained reddish seed, tasting somewhat hot. The root is made of many white strings, which stick deeply into the mud, wherein it chiefly delights, yet it will well abide in the more upland

land and drier ground, and tasteth a little brackish and salt even there, but not so much as where it hath the salt water to feed upon.

Place.] It groweth all along the Thames side, both on the Essex and Kentish shores, from Woolwich round about the sea coasts to Dover, Portsmouth, and even to Bristol, where it is had in plenty; the other with round leaves groweth in the marshes in Holland, in Lincolnshire, and other places of Lincolnshire by the sea side.

Descript.] There is also another sort called Dutch Scurvygrass, which is most known, and frequent in gardens, which hath fresh, green, and almost round leaves rising from the root, not so thick as the former, yet in some rich ground, very large, even twice as big as in others, not dented about the edges, or hollow in the middle, standing on a long foot-stalk; from among these rise long slender stalks, higher than the former, with more white flowers at the tops of them, which turn into small pods, and smaller brownish seed than the former. The root is white, small, and thready. The taste is nothing salt at all; it hath a hot, aromatical, spicy taste.

Time.] It flowereth in April and May, and giveth seed ripe quickly after.

Government and Virtues.] It is an herb of Jupiter. The English Scurvygrass is more used for the salt taste it beareth, which doth somewhat open and cleanse; but the Dutch Scurvygrass is of better effect, and chiefly used (if it may be had) by those that have the scurvy, and is of singular good effect to cleanse the blood, liver, and spleen, taking the juice in the Spring every morning fasting in a cup of drink. The decoction is good for the same purpose, and openeth obstructions, evacuating cold, clammy and phlegmatick humours both from the liver and the spleen, and bringing the body to a more lively colour. The juice also helpeth all foul ulcers and sores in the mouth, gargled therewith; and used outwardly, cleanseth the skin from spots, marks, or scars that happen therein.

SELF-HEAL.

Called alſo Prunel, Carpenter's Herb, Hook-heal, and Sickle-wort.

Deſcript.] THE common Self-heal is a ſmall, low creeping herb, having many ſmall, roundiſh pointed leaves, like leaves of wild mints, of a dark green colour, without dents on the edges; from among which riſe ſquare hairy ſtalks, ſcarce a foot high, which ſpread ſometimes into branches with ſmall leaves ſet thereon, up to the tops, where ſtand brown ſpiked heads of ſmall browniſh leaves like ſcales and flowers ſet together, almoſt like the head of caſſidony, which flowers are gaping, and of a blueiſh purple, or more pale blue, in ſome places ſweet, but not ſo in others. The root conſiſts of many fibres downward, and ſpreadeth ſtrings alſo whereby it increaſeth. The ſmall ſtalks, with the leaves creeping on the ground, ſhoot forth fibres taking hold on the ground whereby it is made a great tuft in a ſhort time.

Place.] It is found in woods and fields every where.

Time.] It flowereth in May, and ſometimes in April.

Government and Virtues.] Here is another herb of Venus, Self-heal, whereby when you are hurt you may heal yourſelf: It is a ſpecial herb for inward and outward wounds. Take it inwardly in ſyrups for inward wounds: outwardly in unguents and plaiſters for outward. As Self-heal is like Bugle in form, ſo alſo in the qualities and virtues, ſerving for all the purpoſes whereto Bugle is applied with good ſucceſs, either inwardly or outwardly, for inward wounds or ulcers whatſoever within the body, for bruiſes or falls, and ſuch like hurts. If it be accompanied with Bugle, Sanicle, and other the like wound herbs, it will be more effectual to waſh or inject into ulcers in the parts outwardly. Where there is cauſe to repreſs the heat and ſharpneſs of humours flowing to any ſore, ulcers, inflammations, ſwellings, or the like, or to ſtay the flux of blood in any wound or part, this is uſed with ſome good ſucceſs; as alſo to cleanſe the the foulneſs of ſores, and cauſe them more ſpeedily to be healed. It is an eſpecial remedy for all green wounds, to ſolder the lips of them, and to keep the place from any further inconveniencies. The juice hereof

hereof used with oil of roses, to anoint the temples and forehead, is very effectual to remove the head-ach, and the same mixed with honey of roses, cleanseth and healeth all ulcers in the mouth and throat, and those also in the secret parts. And the proverb of the Germans, French, and others, is verified in this, *That he needeth neither physician nor surgeon that hath* Self-heal *and* Sanicle *to help himself.*

The SERVICE-TREE.

IT is so well known in the place where it grows, that it needeth no description.

Time.] It flowereth before the end of May, and the fruit is ripe in October.

Government and Virtues.] Services, when they are mellow, are fit to be taken to stay fluxes, scouring, and casting, yet less than medlars. If they be dried before they be mellow, and kept all the year, they may be used in decoctions for the said purpose, either to drink, or to bathe the parts requiring it; and are profitably used in that manner to stay the bleeding of wounds, and of the mouth or nose, to be applied to the forehead, and nape of the neck; and are under the dominion of Saturn.

SHEPHERD'S PURSE.

IT is called Whoreman's Permacety, Shepherd's Scrip, Shepherd's Pounce, Toywort, Pickpurse, and Casewort.

Descript.] The root is small, white, and perisheth every year. The leaves are small and long, of a pale green colour. and deeply cut in on both sides, among which spring up a stalk which is small and round, containing small leaves upon it even to the top. The flowers are white and very small; after which come the little cases which hold the seed, which are flat, almost in the form of a heart.

Place.] They are frequent in this nation, almost by every path-side.

Time.] They flower all the Summer long; nay, some of them are so fruitful, that they flower twice a year.

Government and Virtues.] It is under the dominion of Saturn, and of a cold, dry, and binding nature, like to him. It helps all fluxes of blood, either caused by inward

or

or outward wounds; as alſo flux of the belly, and bloody flux, ſpitting and piſſing of blood, ſtops the terms in women; being bound to the wriſts of the hands, and the ſoles of the feet, it helps the yellow jaundice. The herb being made into a poultice, helps inflammations and St Anthony's fire. The juice being dropped into the ears, heals the pains, noiſe, and matterings thereof. A good ointment may be made of it for all wounds, eſpecially wounds in the head.

SMALLAGE.

THIS is alſo very well known, and therefore I ſhall not trouble the reader with any deſcription thereof.

Place.] It groweth naturally in dry and marſhy ground; but if it be ſown in gardens, it there proſpereth very well.

Time.] It abideth green all the winter, and ſeedeth in Auguſt.

Government and Virtues.] It is an herb of Mercury. Smallage is hotter, drier, and much more medicinal than parſley, for it much more openeth obſtructions of the liver and ſpleen, rarefieth thick phlegm, and cleanſeth it and the blood withal. It provoketh urine and womens courſes, and is ſingular good againſt the yellow jaundice, tertian and quartan agues, if the juice thereof be taken, but eſpecially made up into a ſyrup. The juice alſo put to honey of roſes, and barley-water, is very good to gargle the mouth and throat of thoſe that have ſores and ulcers in them, and will quickly heal them. The ſame lotion alſo cleanſeth and healeth all other foul ulcers and cankers elſewhere, if they be waſhed therewith. The ſeed is eſpecially uſed to break and expel wind, to kill worms, and to help a ſtinking breath. The root is effectual to all the purpoſes aforeſaid, and is held to be ſtronger in operation than the herb, but eſpecially to open obſtructions, and to rid away any ague, if the juice thereof be taken in wine, or the decoction thereof in wine be uſed.

SOPEWORT, or BRUISEWORT.

Deſcript.] THE root creepeth under ground far and near, with many joints therein, of a brown colour on the outſide, and yellowiſh within, ſhooting forth in divers places weak round ſtalks, full of joints, ſet with two leaves a-piece at every one of them on the contrary ſide, which are ribbed ſomewhat like unto plaintain, and faſhioned like the common field white campion leaves, ſeldom having any branches from the ſides of the ſtalks, but ſet with flowers at the top, ſtanding in long huſks like the wild campions, made of five leaves a-piece, round at the ends, and dented in the middle, of a roſe colour, almoſt white, ſometimes deeper, ſometimes paler; of a reaſonable ſcent.

Place.] It groweth wild in many low and wet grounds of this land, by brooks and the ſides of running waters.

Time.] It flowereth uſually in July, and ſo continueth all Auguſt, and part of September, before they be quite ſpent.

Temperature and Virtues.] Venus owns it. The country people in divers places do uſe to bruiſe the leaves of Sopewort, and lay it to their fingers, hands or legs, when they are cut, to heal them up again. Some make great boaſt thereof, that it is diuretical to provoke urine, and thereby to expel gravel and the ſtone in the reins or kidneys, and do alſo account it ſingular good to void hydropical waters; and they no leſs extol it to perform an abſolute cure in the French-pox, more than either ſarſaparilla, guiacum, or China can do; which, how true it is, I leave others to judge.

SORREL.

OUR ordinary Sorrel, which grows in gardens, and alſo wild in the fields, is ſo well known, that it needeth no deſcription.

Government and Virtues.] It is under the dominion of Venus. Sorrel is prevalent in all hot diſeaſes, to cool any inflammation and heat of blood in agues, peſtilential or cholerick, or ſickneſs and fainting, ariſing from heat, and to refreſh the overſpent ſpirits with the violence of furious or fiery fits of agues; to quench thirſt, and procure an appetite in fainting or decaying ſtomachs: For it reſiſteth the putrefaction of the blood, killeth worms, and is a cordial to the heart, which the ſeed doth more effectually, being more drying and binding, and thereby ſtayeth

the

the hot fluxes of womens courses, or of humours in the bloody-flux, or flux of the stomach. The root also in a decoction, or in powder, is effectual for all the said purposes. Both roots and seeds, as well as the herb, are held powerful to resist the poison of the scorpion. The decoction of the roots is taken to help the jaundice, and to expel the gravel and the stone in the reins or kidneys. The decoction of the flowers made with wine and drank, helpeth the black jaundice, as also the inward ulcers of the body and bowels. A syrup made with the juice of Sorrel and fumitory, is a sovereign help to kill those sharp humours that cause the itch. The juice thereof, with a little vinegar, serveth well to be used outwardly for the same cause, and is also profitable for tetters, ringworms, &c. It helpeth also to discuss the kernels in the throat; and the juice gargled in the mouth, helpeth the sores therein.

The leaves wrapt in a colewort leaf and roasted in the embers, and applied to a hard imposthume, botch, boil, or plague sore, doth both ripen and break it. The distilled water of the herb is of much good use for all the purposes aforesaid.

WOOD SORREL.

Descript.] THIS groweth upon the ground, having a number of leaves coming from the root made of three leaves, like a trefoil, but broad at the ends, and cut in the middle, of a yellowish green colour, every one standing on a long foot-stalk, which at their first coming up are close folded together to the stalk, but opening themselves afterwards, and are of a fine sour relish, and yielding a juice which will turn red when it is clarified, and maketh a most dainty clear syrup, Among these leaves rise up divers slender, weak foot-stalks, with every one of them a flower at the top, consisting of five small pointed leaves, star-fashion, of a white colour, in most places, and in some dashed over with a small show of blueish, on the back-side only. After the flowers are past, follow small round heads, with small yellowish seed in them. The roots are nothing but small strings fastened to the end of a small long piece; all of them being of a yellowish colour.

Place.] It groweth in many places of our land, in woods and

and wood-ſides, where they be moiſt and ſhadowed, and in other places not too much open to the Sun.

Time.] It flowereth in April and May.

Government and Virtues.] Venus owns it. Wood Sorrel ſerveth to all the purpoſes that the other Sorrels do, and is more effectual in hindering putrefaction of blood, and ulcers in the mouth and body, and to quench thirſt, to ſtrengthen a weak ſtomach, to procure an appetite, to ſtay vomiting, and very excellent in any contagious ſickneſs or peſtilential fevers. The ſyrup made of the juice is effectual in all the caſes aforeſaid, and ſo is the diſtilled water of the herb. Spunges or linen cloths wet in the juice, and applied outwardly to any hot ſwelling or inflammations, doth much cool and help them. The ſame juice taken and gargled in the mouth, and after it is ſpit forth, taken afreſh, doth wonderfully help a foul ſtinking canker or ulcers therein. It is ſingular good to heal wounds, or to ſtay the bleeding of thruſts or ſtabs in the body.

SOW THISTLE.

SOW Thiſtles are generally ſo well known, that they need no deſcription.

Place.] They grow in gardens and manured grounds, ſometimes by old walls, path-ſides of fields and high-ways.

Government and Virtues.] This and the former are under the influence of Venus. Sow Thiſtles are cooling, and ſomewhat binding, and are very fit to cool a hot ſtomach, and eaſe the pains thereof. The herb boiled in wine, is very helpful to ſtay the diſſolution of the ſtomach, and the milk that is taken from the ſtalks when they are broken, given in drink, is beneficial to thoſe that are ſhort-winded, and have a wheezing. Pliny ſaith, That it hath cauſed the gravel and ſtone to be voided by urine, and that the eating thereof helpeth a ſtinking breath. The decoction of the leaves and ſtalks cauſeth abundance of milk in nurſes, and their children to be well coloured. The juice or diſtilled water is good for all hot inflammations, wheals, and eruptions or heat in the ſkin, itching of the hemorrhoids. The juice boiled or throughly heated in a little oil of bitter almonds in the peel of a pomegranate,

granate, and dropped into the ears, is a ſure remedy for deafneſs, ſingings, &c. Three ſpoonfuls of the juice taken warmed in white wine, and ſome wine put thereto, cauſeth women in travail to have ſo eaſy and ſpeedy delivery, that they may be able to walk preſently after. It is wonderfully good for women to waſh their faces with, to clear the ſkin, and give it a luſtre.

SOUTHERN WOOD.

SOUTHERN Wood is ſo well known to be an ordinary inhabitant in our gardens, that I ſhall not need to trouble you with any deſcription thereof.

Time.] It flowereth for the moſt part in July and Auguſt.

Government and Virtues.] It is a gallant mercurial plant, worthy of more eſteem than it hath. Dioſcorides ſaith, That the ſeed bruiſed, heated in warm water, and drank, helpeth thoſe that are burſten, or troubled with cramps or convulſions of the ſinews, the ſciatia, or difficulty in making water, and bringing down womens courſes. The ſame taken in wine is an antidote, or counter-poiſon againſt all deadly poiſon, and driveth away ſerpents and other venomous creatures; as alſo the ſmell of the herb, being burnt, doth the ſame. The oil thereof anointed on the back-bone before the fits of agues come, taketh them away: It taketh away inflammations in the eyes, if it be put with ſome part of a roaſted quince, and boiled with a few crumbs of bread, and applied. Boiled with barley-meal, it taketh away pimples, puſhes or wheals that ariſe in the face, or other parts of the body. The ſeed, as well as the dried herb, is often given to kill the worms in children: The herb bruiſed and laid to, helpeth to draw forth ſplinters and thorns out of the fleſh. The aſhes thereof drieth up and healeth old ulcers, that are without inflammation, although by the ſharpneſs thereof it biteth ſore, and putteth them to ſore pains; as alſo the ſores in the privy parts of man or woman. The aſhes mingled with old ſallad oil, helpeth thoſe that have hair fallen, and are bald, cauſing the hair to grow again either on the head or beard. Daranters ſaith, That the oil made of Southernwood, and put among the ointments that are uſed againſt the French diſeaſe, is very effectual, and likewiſe killeth

lice

lice in the head. The diſtilled water of the herb is ſaid to help them much that are troubled with the ſtone, as alſo for the diſeaſes of the ſpleen and mother. The Germans commend it for a ſingular wound herb, and therefore call it Stabwort. It is held by all writers, ancient and modern, to be more offenſive to the ſtomach than wormwood.

SPIGNEL.

Deſcript.] THE roots of common Spignel do ſpread much and deep in the ground, many ſtrings or branches growing from one head, which is hairy at the top, of a blackiſh brown colour on the outſide, and white within, ſmelling well, and of an aromatical taſte, from whence riſe ſundry long ſtalks of moſt fine cut leaves like hair, ſmaller than dill, ſet thick on both ſides of the ſtalks, and of a good ſcent. Among theſe leaves riſe up round ſtiff ſtalks, with a few joints and leaves on them, and at the tops an umbel of fine pure white flowers; at the edges whereof ſometimes will be ſeen a ſhew of the reddiſh blueiſh colour, eſpecially before they be full blown, and are ſucceeded by ſmall ſomewhat round ſeeds, bigger than the ordinary fennel, and of a brown colour, divided into two parts, and cruſted on the back, as moſt of the umbelliferous ſeeds are.

Place.] It groweth wild in Lancaſhire, Yorkſhire, and other northern counties, and is alſo planted in gardens.

Government and Virtues.] It is an herb of Venus. Galen ſaith, The roots of Spignel are available to provoke urine, and womens courſes; but if too much thereof be taken it cauſeth head-ach. The roots boiled in wine or water, and drank, helpeth the ſtrangury and ſtoppings of the urine, the wind, ſwellings and pains in the ſtomach, pains of the mother, and all joint-achs. If the powder of the root be mixed with honey, and the ſame taken as a licking medicine, it breaketh tough phlegm, and drieth up the rheum that falleth on the lungs. The roots are accounted very effectual againſt the ſtinging or biting of any venomous creature, and is one of the ingredients in Mithridate and other antidotes of the ſame.

SPLEENWORT, or CETERACH.

Descript.] THE smooth Spleenwort, from a black, thready and bushy root, sendeth forth many long single leaves, cut in on both sides into round dents almost to the middle, which is not so hard as that of polypody, each division being not always set opposite unto the other, cut between each, smooth, and of a light green on the upper side, and a dark yellowish roughness on the back, folding or rolling itself inward at the first springing up.

Place.] It groweth as well upon stone walls, as moist and shadowy places, about Bristol, and other the west parts plentifully; as also on Framlingham Castle, on Beaconsfield church in Berkshire, at Stroude in Kent, and elsewhere, and abideth green all the winter.

Government and Virtues.] Saturn owns it. It is generally used against infirmities of the spleen: It helpeth the strangury, and wasteth the stone in the bladder, and is good against the yellow jaundice, and the hiccough; but the juice of it in women hindereth conception. Matthiolus saith, That if a dram of the dust that is on the backside of the leaves be mixed with half a dram of amber in powder, and taken with the juice of the purslain or plantain, it helps the running of the reins speedily, and that the herb and root being boiled and taken, helpeth all melancholy diseases, and those especially that arise from the French disease. Camerarius saith, That the distilled water thereof being drank, is very effectual against the stone in the reins and bladder; and that the lee that is made of the ashes thereof being drank for some time together, helpeth splenetick persons. It is used in outward remedies for the same purpose.

STAR THISTLE.

Descript.] A Common Star Thistle hath divers narrow leaves lying next the ground, cut on the edges somewhat deeply into many parts, soft a little woolly all over green, among which rise up divers weak stalks parted into many branches, all lying down to the ground, that it seemeth a pretty bush, set with divers the like divided

vided leaves up to the tops, where ſeverally do ſtand ſmall whitiſh green heads, ſet with ſharp white pricks, (no part of the plant elſe being prickly) which are ſomewhat yellowiſh; out of the middle whereof riſeth the flowers, compoſed of many ſmall reddiſh purple threads; and in the heads, after the flowers are paſt, come ſmall whitiſh round ſeed lying down as others do. The root is ſmall, long and woody, periſhing every year, and riſing again of their own ſowing.

Place.] It groweth wild in the fields about London in many places, as at Mile-End green, in Finſbury fields, beyond the Windmills, and many other places.

Time.] It flowereth early, and ſeedeth in July, and ſometimes in Auguſt.

Government and Virtues.] This, as almoſt all Thiſtles are, is under Mars. The ſeed of this Star Thiſtle made into powder, and drank in wine, provoketh urine, and helpeth to break the ſtone, and driveth it forth. The root in powder, and given in wine and drank, is good againſt the plague and peſtilence; and drank in the morning faſting for ſome time together, it is very profitable for a fiſtula in any part of the body. Baptiſta Sardas doth much commend the diſtilled water hereof, being drank, to help the French diſeaſe, to open the obſtructions of the liver, and cleanſe the blood from corrupted humours, and is profitable againſt the quotidian or tertian ague.

STRAWBERRIES.

THESE are ſo well known through this land, that they need no deſcription.

Time] They flower in May ordinarily, and the fruit is ripe ſhortly after.

Government and Virtues.] Venus owns the herb. Strawberries, when they are green, are cool and dry; but when they are ripe they are cool and moiſt: The berries are excellent good to cool the liver, the blood, and the ſpleen, or an hot cholerick ſtomach; to refreſh and comfort the fainting ſpirits, and quench thirſt: They are good alſo for other inflammations; yet it is not amiſs to refrain from them in a fever, leſt by their putrefying in the ſtomach they increaſe the fits. The leaves and roots boiled in wine and water, and drank, do likewise cool the liver and blood, and assuage all inflammations in the reins and bladder, provoke urine, and allay the heat and sharpness thereof. The same also being drank stayeth the bloody-flux and womens courses, and helps the swelling of the spleen. The water of the berries carefully distilled, is a sovereign remedy and cordial in the panting and beating of the heart, and is good for the yellow jaundice. The juice dropped into foul ulcers, or they washed therewith, or the decoction of the herb and root, doth wonderfully cleanse and help to cure them. Lotions and gargles for sore mouths, or ulcers therein, or in the privy parts or elsewhere, are made with the leaves and roots thereof; which is also good to fasten loose teeth, and to heal spungy foul gums. It helpeth also to stay catarrhs, or defluxions of rheum in the mouth, throat, teeth, or eyes. The juice or water is singular good for hot and red inflamed eyes, if dropped into them, or they bathed therewith. It is also of excellent property for all pushes, wheals, and other breakings forth of hot and sharp humours in the face and hands, and other parts of the body, to bathe them therewith, and to take away any redness in the face, or spots, or other deformities in the skin, and to make it clear and smooth. Some use this medicine: Take so many Strawberries as you shall think fitting, and put them into a distillatory, or body of glass fit for them, which being well closed, set it in a bed of horse dung for your use. It is an excellent water for hot inflamed eyes, and to take away a film or skin that beginneth to grow over them, and for such other defects in them as may be helped by any outward medicine.

SUCCORY.

Descript.] THE garden Succory hath longer and narrower leaves than the Endive, and more cut in or torn on the edges, and the root abideth many years. It beareth also blue flowers like Endive, and the seed is hardly distinguished from the seed of the smooth or ordinary Endive.

The wild Succory hath divers long leaves lying on the ground, very much cut in or torn on the edges, on both sides,

ſides, even to the middle rib, ending in a point; ſometimes it hath a rib down to the middle of the leaves, from among which riſeth up a hard, round, woody ſtalk, ſpreading into many branches, ſet with ſmaller and leſſer divided leaves on them up to the tops, where ſtand the flowers, which are like the garden kind, and the ſeed is alſo (only take notice that the flowers of the garden kind are gone in on a ſunny day, they being ſo cold, that they are not able to endure the beams of the ſun, and therefore more delight in the ſhade) the root is white, but more hard and woody than the garden kind. The whole plant is exceeding bitter.

Place.] This groweth in many places of our land in waſte untilled and barren fields. The other only in gardens.

Government and Virtues.] It is an herb of Jupiter. Garden Succory, as it is more dry and leſs cold than Endive, ſo it openeth more. An handful of the leaves, or roots boiled in wine or water, and a draught thereof drank faſting, driveth forth cholerick and phlegmatick humours, openeth obſtructions of the liver, gall and ſpleen; helpeth the yellow jaundice, the heat of the reins, and of the urine; the dropſy alſo; and thoſe that have an evil diſpoſition in their bodies, by reaſon of long ſickneſs, evil diet, &c. which the Greeks call Cachexia. A decoction thereof made with wine, and drank, is very effectual againſt long lingering agues; and a dram of the ſeed in powder, drank in wine, before the fit of the ague, helpeth to drive it away. The diſtilled water of the herb and flowers (if you can take them in time) hath the like properties, and is eſpecially good for hot ſtomachs, and in agues, either peſtilential or of long continuance; for ſwoonings and paſſions of the heart, for the heat and head-ach in children, and for the blood and liver. The ſaid water, or the juice, or the bruiſed leaves applied outwardly, allays ſwellings, inflammations, St Anthony's fire, puſhes, wheals and pimples, eſpecially uſed with a little vinegar; as alſo to waſh peſtiferous ſores. The ſaid water is very effectual for ſore eyes that are inflamed with redneſs, for nurſes breaſts that are pained by the abundance of milk.

The wild Succory, as it is more bitter, ſo it is more ſtrengthening to the ſtomach and liver.

Stone-Crop, Prick-Madam, or Small-Houseleek.

Descript.] IT groweth with divers trailing branches upon the ground, set with many thick, flat, roundish, whitish green leaves, pointed at the ends. The flowers stand many of them together, somewhat loosely. The roots are small, and run creeping under ground.

Place.] It groweth upon the stone-walls and mud-walls, upon the tiles of houses, and pent-houses, and amongst rubbish, and in other gravelly places.

Time.] It flowereth in June and July, and the leaves are green all the winter.

Government and Virtues.] It is under the dominion of the Moon, cold in quality, and something binding, and therefore very good to stay defluctions, especially such as fall upon the eyes. It stops bleeding, both inward and outward, helps cankers, and all fretting sores and ulcers: It abates the heat of choler, thereby preventing diseases arising from cholerick humours. It expels poison much, resisteth pestilential fevers, being exceeding good also for tertian agues: You may drink the decoction of it, if you please, for all the foregoing infirmities. It is so harmless an herb, you can scarce use it amiss: Being bruised and applied to the place, it helps the king's evil, and any other knots or kernels in the flesh; as also the piles.

ENGLISH TOBACCO.

Descript.] THIS riseth up with a round thick stalk, about two feet high, whereon do grow thick, flat green leaves, nothing so large as the other Indian kind, somewhat round pointed also, and nothing dented about the edges. The stalk branches forth, and beareth at the tops divers flowers set on great husks like the other, but nothing so large; scarce standing above the brims of the husks, round pointed also, and of a greenish yellow colour. The seed that followeth is not so bright, but larger, contained in the like great heads. The roots are neither so great nor woody; it perisheth every year with the hard frosts in winter, but riseth generally of its own sowing.

Place.] This came from some parts of Brasil, as it is thought,

thought, and is more familiar in our country than any of the other sorts; early giving ripe seed, which the others seldom do.

Time.] It flowereth from June, sometimes to the end of August, or later, and the seed ripeneth in the mean time.

Government and Virtues.] It is a martial plant. It is found by good experience to be available to expectorate tough phlegm from the stomach, chest and lungs. The juice thereof made into a syrup, or the distilled water of the herb drank with some sugar, or without, if you will, or the smoke taken by a pipe, as is usual, but fasting, helpeth to expel worms in the stomach and belly, and to ease the pains in the head, or megrim and the gripping pains in the bowels. It is profitable for those that are troubled with the stone in the kidneys, both to ease the pains by provoking urine, and also to expel gravel and the stone engendered therein, and hath been found very effectual to expel windiness, and other humours, which cause the strangling of the mother. The seed hereof is very effectual to expel the tooth-ach, and the ashes of the burnt herb to cleanse the gums, and make the teeth white. The herb bruised and applied to the place grieved with the king's evil, helpeth it in nine or ten days effectually. Monardus saith, it is a counter-poison against the biting of any venomous creature, the herb also being outwardly applied to the hurt place. The distilled water is often given with some sugar before the fit of an ague, to lessen it, and take it away in three or four times using. If the distilled fæces of the herb, having been bruised before the distillation, and not distilled dry, be set in warm dung for fourteen days, and afterwards be hung up in a bag in a wine cellar, the liquor that distilleth therefrom is singularly good to use for cramps, aches, the gout and sciatica, and to heal itches, scabs, and running ulcers, cankers, and all foul sores whatsoever. The juice is also good for all the said griefs, and likewise to kill lice in children's heads. The green herb bruised and applied to any green wounds, cureth any fresh wound or cut whatsoever; and the juice put into old sores, both cleanseth and healeth them. There is also made hereof a singular good salve to help imposthumes, hard tumours, and other swellings by blows and falls.

The

The TAMARISK TREE.

IT is so well known in the places where it grows, that it needeth no description.

Time.] It flowereth about the end of May, or in June, and the seed is ripe and blown away in the beginning of September.

Government and Virtues.] A gallant Saturnine herb it is. The root, leaves, young branches, or bark boiled in wine, and drank, stays the bleeding of the hæmorrhodical veins, the spitting of blood, the too abounding of womens courses, the jaundice, the colick, and the biting of all venomous serpents, except the asp; and outwardly applied, is very powerful against the hardness of the spleen, and the tooth-ach, pains in the ears, red and watering eyes. The decoction, with some honey put thereto, is good to stay gangrenes and fretting ulcers, and to wash those that are subject to nits and lice. Alpinus and Veslingius affirm, That the Egyptians do with good success use the wood of it to cure the French disease, as others do with lignum vitæ or guiacum; and give it also to those who have the leprosy, scabs, ulcers, or the like. Its ashes doth quickly heal blisters raised by burnings or scaldings. It helps the dropsy, arising from the hardness of the spleen, and therefore to drink out of cups made of the wood is good for splenetic persons. It is also helpful for melancholy, and the black jaundice that ariseth thereof.

GARDEN TANSY.

GARDEN Tansy is so well known, that it needeth no description.

Time.] It flowereth in June and July.

Government and Virtues.] Dame Venus was minded to pleasure women with child by this herb, for there grows not an herb fitter for their use than this is; it is just as tho' it were cut out for the purpose. This herb bruised and applied to the navel, stays miscarriages; I know no herb like it for that use: Boiled in ordinary beer, and the decoction drank, doth the like; and if her womb be not as she would have it, this decoction will make it so. Let those women that desire children love this herb, it is their best

beſt companion, their huſband excepted. Alſo it conſumes the phlegmatick humours, the cold and moiſt conſtitution of Winter moſt uſually affects the body of man with, and that was the firſt reaſon of eating Tanſies in the Spring. At laſt the world being over-run with Popery, a monſter called ſuperſtition perks up his head; and, as a judgment of God, obſcures the bright beams of knowledge by his diſmal looks; (phyſicians ſeeing the Pope and his imps ſelfiſh, they began to do ſo too) and now forſooth Tanſies muſt be eaten only on Palm and Eaſter Sundays, and their neighbour days: At laſt ſuperſtition being too hot to hold, and the ſelfiſhneſs of phyſicians walking in the clouds; after the friars and monks had made the people ignorant, the ſuperſtition of the time was found out, by the virtue of the herb hidden, and now it is almoſt, if not altogether, left off. Surely our phyſicians are beholden to none ſo much as they are to monks and friars: For want of eating this herb in Spring, maketh people ſickly in Summer; and that makes work for the phyſician. If it be againſt any man or woman's conſcience to eat Tanſy in the Spring, I am as unwilling to burthen their conſcience, as I am that they ſhould burthen mine; they may boil it in wine and drink the decoction, it will work the ſame effect. The decoction of the common Tanſy, or the juice drank in wine, is a ſingular remedy for all the griefs that come by ſtopping of the urine, helpeth the ſtrangury, and thoſe that have weak reins and kidneys. It is alſo very profitable to diſſolve and expel wind in the ſtomach, belly or bowels, to procure womens courſes, and expel windineſs in the matrix, if it be bruiſed and often ſmelled unto, as alſo applied to the lower part of the belly. It is alſo very profitable for ſuch women as are given to miſcarry in child-bearing, to cauſe them to go out their full time: It is uſed alſo againſt the ſtone in the reins, eſpecially to men. The herb fried with eggs (as it is accuſtomed in the Spring-time) which is called a Tanſy, helpeth to digeſt and carry downward thoſe bad humours that trouble the ſtomach. The ſeed is very profitable given to children for the worms, and the juice in drink is as effectual. Being boiled in oil, it is good for the ſinews ſhrunk by cramps, or pained with colds, if thereto applied.

WILD TANSY, or SILVER WEED.

THIS is alſo ſo well known, that it needed no deſcription.

Place.] It groweth almoſt in every place.

Time.] It flowereth in June and July.

Government and Virtues.] Now Dame Venus hath fitted women with two herbs of one name, one to help conception, the other to maintain beauty, and what more can be expected of her? What now remains for you, but to love your huſbands, and not to be wanting to your poor neighbours? Wild Tanſy ſtayeth the laſk, and all the fluxes of blood in men and women, which ſome ſay it will do, if the green herb be worn in the ſhoes, ſo it be next the ſkin; and it is true enough, that it will ſtop the terms, if worn ſo, and the whites too, for ought I know. It ſtayeth alſo ſpitting or vomiting of blood. The powder of the herb taken in ſome of the diſtilled water, helpeth the whites in women, but more eſpecially if a little coral and ivory in powder be put to it. It is alſo commended to help children that are burſten, and have a rupture, being boiled in water and ſalt. Being boiled in water and drank, it eaſeth the gripping pains of the bowels, and is good for the ſciatica and joint-achs. The ſame boiled in vinegar, with honey and alum, and gargled in the mouth, eaſeth the pains of the tooth-ach, faſteneth looſe teeth, helpeth the gums that are ſore, and ſettleth the palate of the mouth in its place, when it is fallen down. It cleanſeth and healeth ulcers in the mouth or ſecret parts, and is very good for inward wounds, and to cloſe the lips of green wounds, and to heal old, moiſt, and corrupt running ſores in the legs or elſewhere. Being bruiſed and applied to the ſoles of the feet and hand wriſts, it wonderfully cooleth the hot fits of agues, be they never ſo violent. The diſtilled water cleanſeth the ſkin of all diſcolourings therein, as morphew, ſun-burnings, &c. as alſo pimples, freckles, and the like; and dropped into the eyes, or cloths wet therein and applied, taketh away the heat and inflammations in them..

THISTLES.

OF these are many kinds growing here in England, which are so well known, that they need no description: Their difference are easily known by the places where they grow, *viz.*

Place.] Some grow in fields, some in meadows, and some among the corn; others on heaths, greens, and waste grounds in many places.

Time.] They flower in June and August, and their seed is ripe quickly after.

Government and Virtues.] Surely Mars rules it, it is such a prickly business. All these Thistles are good to provoke urine, and to mend the stinking smell thereof; as also the rank smell of the arm-pits, or the whole body, being boiled in wine and drank, and are said also to help a stinking breath, and to strengthen the stomach. Pliny saith, That the juice bathed on the place that wanteth hair, it being fallen off, will cause it to grow again speedily.

The MELANCHOLY THISTLE.

Descript.] IT riseth up with tender single hoary green stalks, bearing thereon four or five green leaves, dented about the edges; the points thereof are little or nothing prickly, and at the top usually but one head, yet sometimes from the bosom of the uppermost leaves there shooteth forth another small head, scaly and prickly, with many reddish thrumbs or threads in the middle, which being gathered fresh, will keep the colour a long time, and fadeth not from the stalk a long time, while it perfects the seed, which is of a mean bigness, lying in the down. The root hath many strings fastened to the head or upper part, which is blackish, and perisheth not.

There is another sort, little differing from the former, but that the leaves are more green above, and more hoary underneath, and the stalk being about two feet high, beareth but one scaly head, with threads and seeds as the former.

Place.] They grow in many moist meadows of this land, as well in the southern, as in the northern parts.

Time.] They flower about July or August, and their seed ripeneth quickly after.

Government

Government and Virtues.] It is under Capricorn, and therefore under both Saturn and Mars; one rids melancholy by sympathy, the other by antipathy. Their virtues are but few, but those not to be despised; for the decoction of the thistle in wine being drank, expels superfluous melancholy out of the body, and makes a man as merry as a cricket: superfluous melancholy causeth care, fear, sadness despair, envy, and many evils more besides; but religion teacheth to wait upon God's providence, and cast our care upon him who careth for us. What a fine thing were it if men and women could live so? And yet seven years care and fear makes a man never the wiser, nor a farthing richer. Dioscorides saith, the root borne about one doth the like, and removes all diseases of melancholy. Modern writers laugh at him: *Let them laugh that win,* my opinion is, that it is the best remedy against all melancholy diseases that grows; they that please may use it.

Our LADY'S THISTLE.

Descript.] OUR Lady's Thistle hath divers very large and broad leaves lying on the ground cut in, and as it were crumpled, but somewhat hairy on the edges, of a white green shining colour, wherein are many lines and streaks of a milk-white colour running all over, and set with many sharp and stiff prickles all about, among which riseth up one or more strong, round and prickly stalks, set full of the like leaves up to the top, where, at the end of every branch, comes forth a great prickly thistle-like head, strongly armed with prickles, and with bright purple thrumbs rising out of the middle: After they are past, the seed groweth in the said heads, lying in soft white down, which is somewhat flattish in the ground, and many strings and fibres fastened thereunto. All the whole plant is bitter in taste.

Place.] It is frequent on the banks of almost every ditch.

Time.] It flowereth and seedeth in June, July, and August.

Government and Virtues.] Our Lady's Thistle is under Jupiter, and thought to be as effectual as Carduus Benedictus for agues, and to prevent and cure the infection of the plague; as also to open the obstructions of the liver and spleen, and thereby is good against the jaundice. It provoketh

voketh urine, breaketh and expelleth the ſtone, and is good for the dropſy. It is effectual alſo for the pains in the ſides, and many other inward pains and gripings. The ſeed and diſtilled water are held powerful to all the purpoſes aforeſaid, and beſides, it is often applied both outwardly with cloths or ſpunges, to the region of the liver, to cool the diſtemper thereof, and to the region of the heart, againſt ſwoonings and paſſions of it. It cleanſeth the blood exceedingly; and in Spring, if you pleaſe to boil the tender plant (but cut off the prickles, unleſs you have a mind to choak yourſelf) it will change your blood as the ſeaſon changeth, and that is the way to be ſafe.

The WOOLLEN, OR COTTON THISTLE.

Deſcript.] THIS hath many large leaves lying upon the ground, ſomewhat cut in, and as it were crumpled on the edges, of a green colour on the upper ſide, but covered over with a long hairy wool or cotton down, ſet with moſt ſharp and cruel pricks; from the middle of whoſe heads of flowers come forth many purpliſh crimſon threads, and ſometimes white, although but ſeldom. The ſeed that followeth in thoſe white downy heads, is ſomewhat large and round, reſembling the ſeed of Lady's Thiſtle, but paler: The root is great and thick, ſpreading much, yet uſually dieth after ſeed-time.

Place.] It groweth on divers ditch-banks, and in the corn fields and highways, generally throughout the land, and is often growing in gardens.

Government and Virtues.] It is a plant of Mars. Dioſcorides and Pliny write, That the leaves and roots hereof taken in drink, help thoſe that have a crick in their neck, that they cannot turn it, unleſs they turn their whole body. Galen ſaith, That the roots and leaves hereof are good for ſuch perſons that have their bodies drawn together by ſome ſpaſm or convulſion, or other infirmities; as the rickets (or as the college of phyſicians would have it, rachites, about which name they have quarrelled ſufficiently) in children, being a diſeaſe that hindereth their growth, by binding their nerves, ligaments, and whole ſtructure of their body.

The Fuller's Thistle, or Teasle.

IT is so well known, that it needs no description, being used with the cloth-workers.

The wild Teasle is in all things like the former, but that the prickles are small, soft, and upright, not hooked or stiff, and the flowers of this are of a fine blueish, or pale carnation colour, but of the manured kind, whitish.

Place.] The first groweth, being sown, in gardens or fields for the use of cloth-workers: The other near ditches and rills of water in many places of this land.

Time.] They flower in July, and are ripe in the end of August.

Government and Virtues.] It is an herb of Venus. Dioscorides saith, That the root bruised and boiled in wine, till it be thick, and kept in a brazen vessel, and after spread as a salve, and applied to the fundament, doth heal the cleft thereof, cankers and fistulas therein, also taketh away warts and wens. The juice of the leaves dropped into the ears, killeth worms in them. The distilled water of the leaves dropped into the eyes, taketh away redness and mists in them that hinder the sight, and is often used by women to preserve their beauty, and to take away redness and inflammations, and all other heat or discolourings.

Treacle Mustard.

Descript.] IT riseth with a hard round stalk, about a foot high, parted into some branches, having divers soft green leaves, long and narrow, set thereon, waved, but not cut into the edges, broadest towards the ends, somewhat round pointed; the flowers are white that grow at the tops of the branches, spike-fashion, one above another; after which come round pouches, parted in the middle with a furrow, having one blackish brown seed on either side, somewhat sharp in taste, and smelling of garlick, especially in the fields where it is natural, but not so much in gardens: The roots are small and thready, perishing every year.

Give me leave here to add Mithridate Mustard, altho' it may seem more properly by the name to belong to M, in the alphabet.

MITH-

MITHRIDATE MUSTARD.

Descript.] THIS groweth higher than the former, spreading more and higher branches, whose leaves are smaller and narrower, sometimes unevenly dented about the edges. The flowers are small and white, growing on long branches, with much smaller and rounder vessels after them, and parted in the same manner, having smaller brown seeds than the former, and much sharper in taste. The root perisheth after seed time, but abideth the first winter after springing.

Place.] They grow in sundry places in this land, as half a mile from Hatfield, by the river-side, under a hedge as you go to Hatfield, and in the street of Peckham on Surry-side.

Time.] They flower and seed from May to August.

Government and Virtues.] Both of them are herbs of Mars. The Mustards are said to purge the body both upwards and downwards, and procureth womens courses so abundantly, that it suffocateth the birth. It breaketh inward imposthumes, being taken inwardly; and used in clysters, helpeth the sciatica. The seed applied, doth the same. It is an especial ingredient unto mithridate and treacle, being of itself an antidote resisting poison, venom, and putrefaction. It is also available in many cases for which the common Mustard is used, but somewhat weaker.

The BLACK THORN, or SLOE-BUSH.

IT is so well known, that it needeth no description.

Place.] It groweth in every county, in the hedges and borders of fields.

Time.] It flowereth in April, and sometimes in March, but the fruit ripeneth after all other plumbs whatsoever, and is not fit to be eaten until the Autumn frost mellow them.

Government and Virtues.] All the parts of the Sloe Bush are binding, cooling and dry, and all effectual to stay bleeding at the nose and mouth, or any other place; the lask of the belly or stomach, or the bloody-flux, the too much abounding of womens courses, and helpeth to ease the pains of the sides, bowels, and guts, that come by over-much ſcouring, to drink the decoction of the bark of the roots, or more uſually the decoction of the berries, either freſh or dried. The conſerve alſo is of very much uſe, and more familiarly taken for the purpoſe aforeſaid. But the diſtilled water of the flowers firſt ſteeped in ſack for a night, and drawn therefrom by the heat of Balneum, Anglice, a bath, is a moſt certain remedy, tried and approved, to eaſe all manner of gnawings in the ſtomach, the ſides and bowels, or any griping pains in any of them, to drink a ſmall quantity when the extremity of pain is upon them. The leaves alſo are good to make lotions to gargle and waſh the mouth and throat wherein are ſwellings, ſores, or kernels; and to ſtay the defluctions of rheum to the eyes, or other parts; as alſo to cool the heat and inflammations of them, and eaſe hot pains of the head, to bathe the forehead and temples therewith. The ſimple diſtilled water of the flowers is very effectual for the ſaid purpoſes, and the condenſate juice of the Sloes. The diſtilled water of the green berries is uſed alſo for the ſaid effects.

THOROUGH WAX, or THOROUGH LEAF.

Deſcript.] COMMON Thorough-Wax ſendeth forth a ſtrait round ſtalk, two feet high, or better, whoſe lower leaves being of a blueiſh colour, are ſmaller and narrower than thoſe up higher, and ſtand cloſe thereto, not compaſſing it; but as they grow higher, they do more encompaſs the ſtalks, until it wholly paſs through them, branching toward the top into many parts, where the leaves grow ſmaller again, every one ſtanding ſingly, and never two at a joint. The flowers are ſmall and yellow, ſtanding in tufts at the heads of the branches, where afterwards grow the ſeed, being blackiſh, many thick thruſt together. The root is ſmall, long and woody, periſhing every year, after ſeed-time, and riſing again plentifully of its own ſowing.

Place.] It is found growing in many corn-fields and paſture-grounds in this land.

Time.] It flowereth in July, and the ſeed is ripe in Auguſt.

Temperature and Virtues.] Both this and the former are under the influence of Saturn. Thorough-Wax is of ſingular

gular good uſe for all ſorts of bruiſes and wounds either inward or outward; and old ulcers and ſores likewiſe, if the decoction of the herb with water and wine be drank, and the place waſhed therewith, or the juice of the green herb bruiſed, or boiled, either by itſelf, or with other herbs, in oil or hog's greaſe, to be made into an ointment to ſerve all the year. The decoction of the herb, or powder of the dried herb, taken inwardly, and the ſame, or the leaves bruiſed, and applied outwardly, is ſingular good for all ruptures and burſtings, eſpecially in children before they be too old. Being applied with a little flour and wax to childrens navels that ſtick forth, it helpeth them.

THYME.

IT is in vain to deſcribe an herb ſo commonly known.

Government and Virtues.] It is a noble ſtrengthener of the lungs, as notable a one as grows; neither is there ſcarce a better remedy growing for that diſeaſe in children which they commonly call the Chin-cough, than it is. It purgeth the body of phlegm, and is an excellent remedy for ſhortneſs of breath. It kills worms in the belly, and being a notable herb of Venus, provokes the terms, gives ſafe and ſpeedy delivery to women in travail, and brings away the after-birth. It is ſo harmleſs you need not fear the uſe of it. An ointment made of it takes away hot ſwellings and warts, helps the ſciatica and dulneſs of ſight, and takes away pains and hardneſs of the ſpleen: 'Tis excellent for thoſe that are troubled with the gout; as alſo, to anoint the cods that are ſwelled. It eaſeth pains in the loins and hips. The herb taken any way inwardly, comforts the ſtomach much, and expels wind.

WILD THYME, or MOTHER of THYME.

WILD Thyme alſo is ſo well known, that it needeth no deſcription.

Place.] It may be found commonly in commons, and other barren places throughout the nation.

Government and Virtues.] It is under the dominion of Venus, and under the ſign Aries, and therefore chiefly appropriated to the head. It provoketh urine and the terms, and eaſeth the griping pain of the belly, cramps, ruptures, and inflammation of the liver. If you make a vinegar of the herb, as vinegar of roses is made (you may find out the way in my translation of the London Dispensatory) and anoint the head with it, it presently stops the pains thereof. It is excellent good to be given either in phrenzy or lethargy, although they are two contrary diseases: It helps spitting and pissing of blood, coughing, and vomiting; it comforts and strengthens the head, stomach, reins, and womb, expels wind, and breaks the stone.

TORMENTIL, OR SEPTFOIL.

Descript.] THIS hath reddish, slender, weak branches rising from the root, lying on the ground, rather leaning than standing upright, with many short leaves that stand closer to the stalks than cinquefoil (to which this is very like) with the foot-stalk compassing the branches in several places; but those that grow to the ground are set upon long foot-stalks, each whereof are like the leaves of cinquefoil, but somewhat long and lesser, dented about the edges, many of them divided but into five leaves, but most of them into seven, whence it is also called Septfoil; yet some may have six, and some eight, according to the fertility of the soil. At the tops of the branches stand divers small yellow flowers, consisting of five leaves, like those of cinquefoil, but smaller. The root is smaller than bistort, somewhat thick, but blacker without, and not so red within, yet sometimes a little crooked, having blackish fibres thereat.

Place.] It groweth as well in woods and shadowy places, as in the open champain country, about the borders of fields in many places of this land, and almost in every broom field in Essex.

Time.] It flowereth all the Summer long.

Government and Virtues.] This is a gallant herb of the Sun. Tormentil is most excellent to stay all kind of fluxes of blood or humours in man or woman, whether at nose, mouth, or belly. The juice of the herb and root, or the decoction thereof, taken with some Venice treacle, and the person laid to sweat, expels any venom or poison, or the plague, fever, or other contagious diseases, as pox, measles, &c. for it is an ingredient in all antidotes or counter-

counter-poisons. Andreas Valesius is of opinion, that the decoction of this root is no less effectual to cure the French pox than Guiacum or China; and it is not unlikely, because it so mightily resisteth putrefaction. The root taken inwardly is most effectual to help any flux of the belly, stomach, spleen, or blood; and the juice wonderfully opens obstructions of the liver and lungs, and thereby helpeth the yellow jaundice. The powder or decoction drank, or to sit thereon as a bath, is an assured remedy against abortion in women, if it proceed from the over flexibility or weakness of the inward retentive faculty; as also a plaister made therewith, and vinegar applied to the reins of the back, doth much help not only this, but also those that cannot hold their water, the powder being taken in the juice of plantain, and is also commended against the worms in children. It is very powerful in ruptures and burstings, as also for bruises or falls, to be used as well outwardly as inwardly. The root hereof made up with pellitory of Spain and alum, and put into a hollow tooth, not only assuageth the pain, but stayeth the flux of humours which causeth it. Tormentil is no less effectual and powerful a remedy against outward wounds, sores and hurts, than for inward, and is therefore a special ingredient to be used in wound drinks, lotions and injections, for foul corrupt rotten sores and ulcers of the mouth, secrets, or other parts of the body. The juice or powder of the root put in ointments, plaisters, and such things, that are to be applied to wounds or sores, is very effectual, as the juice of the leaves and the root bruised and applied to the throat, or jaws, healeth the king's evil, and easeth the pain of the sciatica; the same used with a little vinegar, is a special remedy against the running sores of the head or other parts; scabs also, and the itch, or any such eruptions in the skin, proceeding of salt and sharp humours. The same is also effectual for the piles or hæmorrhoids, if they be washed or bathed therewith, or with the distilled water of the herb and roots. It is found also helpful to dry up any sharp rheum that distilleth from the head into the eyes, causing redness, pain, waterings, itching, or the like, if a little prepared tutia, or white amber, be used with the distilled water thereof.

Many

Many women use this water as a secret to help themselves and others, when they are troubled with too much flowing of the whites or reds, both to drink it, or inject it with a syringe. And here is enough, only remember the Sun challengeth this herb.

TURNSOLE, OR HELIOTROPIUM.

Descript.] THE greater Turnsole riseth with one upright stalk, about a foot high, or more, dividing itself almost from the bottom, into divers small branches, of a hoary colour; at each joint of the stalk and branches grow small broad leaves, somewhat white and hoary. At the tops of the stalks and branches stand small white flowers, consisting of four, and sometimes five small leaves, set in order one above another, upon a small crooked spike, which turneth inwards like a bowed finger, opening by degrees as the flowers blow open; after which in their place come forth cornered seed, four for the most part standing together; the root is small and thready, perishing every year, and the seed shedding every year, raiseth it again the next spring.

Place.] It groweth in gardens, and flowereth and seedeth with us, notwithstanding it is not natural to this land, but to Italy, Spain, and France, where it grows plentifully.

Government and Virtues.] It is an herb of the Sun, and a good one too. Dioscorides saith, That a good handful of this, which is called the Great Turnsole, boiled in water, and drank, purgeth both choler and phlegm; and boiled with cummin, helpeth the stone in the reins, kidneys, or bladder, provoketh urine and womens courses, and causeth an easy and speedy delivery in child-birth. The leaves bruised and applied to places pained with the gout, or that have been out of joint, and newly set, and full of pain, do give much ease: the seed and juice of the leaves also being rubbed with a little salt upon warts or wens, and other kernels in the face, eye-lids, or any other part of the body, will, by often using, take them away.

MEADOW TREFOIL, OR HONEYSUCKLES.

IT is so well known, especially by the name of Honeysuckles, white and red, that I need not describe them.

Place.

Place.] They grow almoſt every place in this land.

Government and Virtues.] Mercury hath dominion over the common ſorts. Dodoneus ſaith, The leaves and flowers are good to eaſe the griping pains of the gout, the herb being boiled and uſed in a clyſter. If the herb be made into a poultice, and applied to inflammations, it will eaſe them. The juice dropped in the eyes, is a familiar medicine, with many country people, to take away the pin and web (as they call it) in the eyes; it alſo allayeth the heat and blood-ſhooting of them. Country people do alſo in many places drink the juice thereof againſt the biting of an adder; and having boiled the herb in water, they firſt waſh the place with the decoction, and then lay ſome of the herb alſo to the hurt place. The herb alſo boiled in ſwine's greaſe, and ſo made into an ointment, is good to apply to the biting of any venomous creatures. The herb alſo bruiſed and heated between tiles, and applied hot to the ſhare, cauſeth them to make water who had it ſtopt before. It is held likewiſe to be good for wounds, and to take away ſeed. The decoction of the herb and flowers, with the ſeed and root, taken for ſome time, helpeth women that are troubled with the whites. The ſeed and flowers boiled in water, and after made into a poultice with ſome oil, and applied, helpeth hard ſwellings and impoſthumes.

HEART TREFOIL.

BESIDES the ordinary ſort of Trefoil, here are two more remarkable, and one of which may be probably called Heart Trefoil, not only becauſe the leaf is triangular, like the heart of a man, but alſo becauſe each leaf contains the perfect icon of a heart, and that in its proper colour, viz. a fleſh colour.

Place.] It groweth between Longford and Bow, and beyond Southwark, by the highway and parts adjacent.

Government and Virtues.] It is under the dominion of the Sun, and if it were uſed, it would be found as great a ſtrengthener of the heart, and cheriſher of the vital ſpirits as grows, relieving the body againſt fainting and ſwoonings, fortifying it againſt poiſon and peſtilence, defending the heart againſt the noiſome vapours of the ſpleen.

PEARL

PEARL TREFOIL.

IT differs not from the common ſort, ſave only in this one particular, it hath a white ſpot in the leaf like a pearl. It is particularly under the dominion of the Moon, and its icon ſheweth that it is of a ſingular virtue againſt the pearl, or pin and web in the eyes.

TUTSAN, or PARK LEAVES.

Deſcript.] IT hath browniſh ſhining round ſtalks, creſted the length thereof, riſing two by two, and ſometimes three feet high, branching forth even from the bottom, having divers joints, and at each of them two fair large leaves ſtanding, of a dark blueiſh green colour on the upper ſide, and of a yellowiſh green underneath; turning reddiſh toward Autumn. At the top of the ſtalks ſtand large yellow flowers, and heads with ſeed, which, being greeniſh at the firſt, and afterwards reddiſh, turn to be of a blackiſh purple colour when they are ripe, with ſmall browniſh ſeed within them, and they yield a reddiſh juice or liquor, ſomewhat reſinous, and of a harſh and ſtypick taſte, as the leaves alſo and the flowers be, altho' much leſs, but do not yield ſuch a clear claret wine colour, as ſome ſay it doth; the root is browniſh, ſomewhat great, hard, and woody, ſpreading well in the ground.

Place.] It groweth in many woods, groves, and woody grounds, as parks and foreſts, and by hedge-ſides in many places in this land, as in Hampſtead wood, by Ratley in Eſſex, in the wilds of Kent, and in many other places needleſs to recite.

Time.] It flowereth later than St John's or St Peter's wort.

Government and Virtues.] It is an herb of Saturn, and a moſt noble antivenerean. Tutſan purgeth cholerick humours, as St Peter's-wort is ſaid to do, for therein it worketh the ſame effects, both to help the ſciatica and gout, and to heal burning by fire; it ſtayeth all the bleedings of wounds, if either the green herb be bruiſed, or the powder of the dry be applied thereto. It hath been accounted, and certainly it is, a ſovereign herb to heal either wound or ſore, either outwardly or inwardly, and therefore always uſed in drinks, lotions, balms, oils, ointments

ments, or any other sorts of green wounds, old ulcers, or sores, in all which the continual experience of former ages hath confirmed the use thereof to be admirable good, though it be not so much in use now, as when physicians and surgeons were so wise as to use herbs more than now they do.

GARDEN VALERIAN.

Descript.] THIS hath a thick short greyish root, lying for the most part above ground, shooting forth on all other sides such like small pieces of roots, which have all of them many long green strings and fibres under them in the ground, whereby it draweth nourishment. From the head of these roots spring up many green leaves, which at first are somewhat broad and long, without any divisions at all in them, or denting on the edges; but those that rise up after are more and more divided on each side, some to the middle rib, being winged, as made of many leaves together on a stalk, and those upon a stalk, in like manner more divided, but smaller towards the top than below; the stalk riseth to be a yard high or more, sometimes branched at the top, with many small whitish flowers, sometimes dashed over at the edges with a pale purplish colour, of a little scent, which passing away, there followeth small brownish white seed, that is easily carried away with the wind. The root smelleth more strong than either leaf or flower, and is of more use in medicines.

Place.] It is generally kept with us in gardens.

Time.] It flowereth in June and July, and continueth flowering until the frost pull it down.

Government and Virtues.] This is under the influence of Mercury. Dioscorides saith, That the Garden Valerian hath a warming faculty, and that being dried and given to drink it provoketh urine, and helpeth the strangury. The decoction thereof taken, doth the like also, and taketh away pains of the sides, provoketh womens courses, and is used in antidotes. Pliny saith, That the powder of the root given in drink, or the decoction thereof taken, helpeth all stoppings and stranglings in any part of the body, whether they proceed of pains in the chest or sides, and

taketh

taketh them away. The root of Valerian boiled with liquorice, raisins, and anniseed, is singular good for those that are short-winded, and for those that are troubled with the cough, and helpeth to open the passages, and to expectorate phlegm easily. It is given to those who are bitten or stung by any venomous creature, being boiled in wine. It is of a special virtue against the plague, the decoction thereof being drank, and the root being used to smell to. It helpeth to expel the wind in the belly. The green herb with the root taken fresh, being bruised and applied to the head, taketh away the pains and prickings there, stayeth rheum and thin distillations, and being boiled in white wine, and a drop thereof put into the eyes, taketh away the dimness of the sight, or any pin or web therein: It is of excellent property to heal any inward sores or wounds, and also for outward hurts or wounds, and drawing away splinters or thorns out of the flesh.

VERVAIN.

Descript.] THE common Vervain hath somewhat long broad leaves next the ground deeply gashed about the edges, and some only deeply dented, or cut all alike, of a blackish green colour on the upper side, somewhat grey underneath. The stalk is square, branched into several parts, rising about two feet high, especially if you reckon the long spike of flowers at the tops of them, which are set on all sides one above another, and sometimes two or three together, being small and gaping, of a blue colour and white intermixed, after which come small round seed, in small and somewhat long heads: The root is small and long but of no use.

Place.] It groweth generally throughout this land in divers places of the hedges and way-sides, and other waste grounds.

Time.] It flowereth in July, and the seed is ripe soon after.

Government and Virtues.] This is an herb of Venus, and excellent for the womb to strengthen and remedy all the cold griefs of it, as Plantain doth the hot. Vervain is hot and dry, opening obstructions, cleansing and healing: It helpeth the yellow jaundice, the dropsy and the

gout;

gout; it killeth and expelleth worms in the belly, and causeth a good colour in the face and body, strengtheneth as well as correcteth the diseases of the stomach, liver, and spleen; helps the cough, wheezings, and shortness of breath, and all the defects of the reins and bladder, expelling the gravel and stone. It is held to be good against the biting of serpents, and other venomous beasts, against the plague, and both tertian and quartan agues. It consolidateth and healeth also all wounds, both inward and outward, stayeth bleedings, and used with some honey, healeth all old ulcers and fistulas in the legs or other parts of the body; as also those ulcers that happen in the mouth; or used with hog's grease, it helpeth the swellings and pains of the secret parts in man or woman, also for the piles or hæmorrhoids; applied with some oil of roses and vinegar unto the forehead and temples, it easeth the inveterate pains and ache of the head, and is good for those that are frantick. The leaves bruised, or the juice of them mixed with some vinegar, doth wonderfully cleanse the skin, and taketh away morphew, freckles, fistulas, and other such like inflammations and deformities of the skin in any part of the body. The distilled water of the herb when it is in full strength, dropped into the eyes, cleanseth them from films, clouds, or mists, that darken the sight, and wonderfully strengthens the optick nerves: The said water is very powerful in all the diseases aforesaid, either inward or outward, whether they be old corroding sores, or green wounds.

The VINE.

THE leaves of the English Vine (I do not mean to send you to the Canaries for a medicine) being boiled, make a good lotion for sore mouths; being boiled with barley-meal into a poultice, it cools inflammations of wounds; the dropping of the Vine, when it is cut in the Spring, which country people call Tears, being boiled in a syrup, with sugar, and taken inwardly, is excellent to stay womens longings after every thing they see, which is a disease many women with child are subject to. The decoction of Vine leaves in white wine doth the like: Also the tears of the Vine, drank two or three spoonfuls at a time, breaks the ſtone in the bladder. This is a very good remedy, and it is diſcreetly done, to kill a vine to cure a man, but the ſalt of the leaves are held to be better. The aſhes of the burnt branches will make teeth that are as black as coal, to be as white as ſnow, if you but every morning rub them with it. It is a moſt gallant Tree of the Sun, very ſympathetical with the body of man, and that is the reaſon ſpirit of wine is the greateſt cordial among all vegetables.

VIOLETS.

BOTH the tame and the wild are ſo well known, that they need no deſcription.

Time.] They flower until the end of July, but are beſt in March, and the beginning of April.

Government and Virtues.] They are a fine, pleaſing plant of Venus, of a mild nature, no way harmful. All the Violets are cold and moiſt while they are freſh and green, and are uſed to cool any heat, or diſtemperature of the body, either inwardly or outwardly, as inflammations in the eyes, in the matrix or fundament, in impoſthumes alſo, and hot ſwellings, to drink the decoction of the leaves and flowers made with water in wine, or to apply them poultice-wiſe to the grieved places: It likewiſe eaſeth pains in the head, cauſed through want of ſleep; or any other pains ariſing of heat, being applied in the ſame manner, or with oil of roſes. A dram weight of the dried leaves or flowers of Violets, but the leaves more ſtrongly, doth purge the body of cholerick humours, and aſſuageth the heat, being taken in a draught of wine, or any other drink; the powder of the purple leaves of the flowers, only picked and dried and drank in water, is ſaid to help the quinſy, and the falling-ſickneſs in children, eſpecially in the beginning of the diſeaſe. The flowers of the white Violets ripen and diſſolve ſwellings. The herb or flowers, while they are freſh, or the flowers when they are dry, are effectual in the pleuriſy, and all diſeaſes of the lungs, to lenify the ſharpneſs of hot rheums, and the hoarſeneſs of the throat, the heat alſo and ſharpneſs of urine, and all the pains of the back or reins, and bladder. It is good alſo for the liver and the jaundice, and all hot agues, to cool the heat, and quench the thirst; but the syrup of Violets is of most use, and of better effect, being taken in some convenient liquor; and if a little of the juice or syrup of lemons be put to it, or a few drops of the oil of vitriol, it is made thereby the more powerful to cool the heat, and quench the thirst, and giveth to the drink a claret wine colour, and a fine tart relish, pleasing the taste. Violets taken, or made up with honey, do more cleanse and cool, and with sugar contrary-wise. The dried flowers of Violets are accounted amongst the cordial drinks, powders, and other medicines, especially where cooling cordials are necessary. The green leaves are used with other herbs to make plaisters and poultices for inflammations and swellings, and to ease all pains whatsoever, arising of heat, and for the piles also, being fried with yolks of eggs, and applied thereto.

VIPER'S BUGLOSS.

Descript.] THIS hath many long rough leaves lying on the ground, from among which arise up divers hard round stalks, very rough, as if they were thick set with prickles or hairs, whereon are set such like rough, hairy, or prickly sad green leaves, somewhat narrow; the middle rib for the most part being white. The flowers stand at the top of the stalk, branched forth in many long spiked leaves of flowers, bowing or turning like the turnsole, all opening for the most part on the one side, which are long and hollow, turning up the brims a little, of a purplish violet colour in them that are fully blown, but more reddish while they are in the bud, as also upon their decay and withering; but in some places of a paler purple colour with a long pointel in the middle, feathered or parted at the top. After the flowers are fallen, the seeds growing to be ripe, are blackish, cornered and pointed somewhat like the head of a viper. The root is somewhat great and blackish, and woolly, when it groweth toward seed-time, and perisheth in the winter.

There is another sort, little differing from the former, only in this, that it beareth white flowers.

Place.] The first groweth wild almost every where.

That with white flowers about the castle-walls in Lewes in Sussex.

Time.] They flower in Summer, and their seed is ripe quickly after.

Government and Virtues.] It is a most gallant herb of the Sun; it is a pity it is no more in use than it is. It is an especial remedy against the biting of the Viper, and all other venomous beasts, or serpents; as also against poison, or poisonable herbs. Dioscorides and others say, That whosoever shall take of the herb or root before they be bitten, shall not be hurt by the poison of any serpent. The root or seed is thought to be most effectual to comfort the heart, and expel sadness, or causeless melancholy; it tempers the blood, and allayeth hot fits of agues. The seed drank in wine, procureth abundance of milk in womens breasts. The same also being taken, easeth the pain in the loins, back, and kidneys. The distilled water of the herb when it is in flower, or its chief strength, is excellent, to be applied either inwardly or outwardly, for all the griefs aforesaid. There is a syrup made hereof very effectual for the comforting the heart, and expelling sadness and melancholy.

WALL-FLOWERS, or Winter-Gilliflowers.

THE garden kind are so well known, that they need no description.

Descript.] The common single Wall-flowers, which grow wild abroad, have sundry small, long, narrow, dark green leaves, set without order upon small, round, whitish woody stalks, which bear at the tops divers single yellow flowers one above another, every one bearing four leaves a-piece, and of a very sweet scent; after which come long pods, containing a reddish seed. The roots are white, hard and thready.

Place.] It groweth upon church-walls, and old walls of many houses, and other stone-walls in divers places: The other sort in gardens only.

Time.] All the single kinds do flower many times in the end of Autumn; and if the Winter be mild, all the winter long, but especially in the months of February, March, and April, and until the heat of the Spring do spend them.

But

But thè double kinds continue not flowering in that manner all the year long, although they flower very early ſometimes, and in ſome places very late.

Government and Virtues.] The Moon rules them. Galen, in his ſeventh book of ſimple medicines, ſaith, That the yellow Wall-flowers work more powerfully than any of the other kinds, and are therefore of more uſe in phyſick. It cleanſeth the blood, and freeth the liver and reins from obſtructions, provoketh womens courſes, expelleth the ſecundine, and the dead-child; helpeth the hardneſs and pains of the mother, and of the ſpleen alſo; ſtayeth inflammations and ſwellings, comforteth and ſtrengtheneth any weak part, or out of joint; helpeth to cleanſe the eyes from miſtineſs and films on them, and to cleanſe the filthy ulcers in the mouth, or any other part, and is a ſingular remedy for the gout, and all achs and pains in the joints and ſinews. A conſerve made of the flowers, is uſed for a remedy both for the apoplexy and palſy.

The WALNUT TREE.

IT is ſo well known, that it needeth no deſcription.

Time.] It bloſſometh early before the leaves come forth, and the fruit is ripe in September.

Government and Virtues.] This is alſo a plant of the Sun. Let the fruit of it be gathered accordingly, which you ſhall find to be of moſt virtues whilſt they are green, before they have ſhells. The bark of the Tree doth bind and dry very much, and the leaves are much of the ſame temperature; but the leaves, when they are older, are heating and drying in the ſecond degree, and harder of digeſtion than when they are freſh, which, by reaſon of their ſweetneſs, are more pleaſing, and better digeſting in the ſtomach; and taken with ſweet wine, they move the belly downwards, but being old, they grieve the ſtomach; and in hot bodies cauſe the choler to abound, and the head-ach, and are an enemy to thoſe that have the cough; but are leſs hurtful to thoſe that have a colder ſtomach, and are ſaid to kill the broad worms in the belly or ſtomach. If they be taken with onions, ſalt and honey, they help the biting of a mad dog, or the venom, or infectious poiſon of any beaſt, &c. Caius Pompeius found in the treasury of Mithridates, king of Pontus, when he was overthrown, a scroll of his own hand writing, containing a medicine against any poison or infection; which is this: Take two dry Walnuts, and as many good figs, and twenty leaves of rue, bruised and beaten together with two or three corns of salt and twenty juniper berries, which take every morning fasting, preserveth from danger of poison and infection that day it is taken. The juice of the other green husks boiled with honey, is an excellent gargle for sore mouths, or the heat and inflammations in the throat and stomach. The kernels, when they grow old, are more oily, and therefore not fit to be eaten, but are then used to heal the wounds of the sinews, gangrenes and carbuncles. The said kernels being burned, are then very astringent, and will stay lasks and womens courses, being taken in red wine, and stay the falling of the hair, and make it fair, being anointed with oil and wine. The green husks will do the like, being used in the same manner. The kernels beaten with rue and wine, being applied, helpeth the quinsy; and bruised with some honey, and applied to the ears, easeth the pains and inflammations of them. A piece of the green husks put into a hollow tooth, easeth the pain. The catkins hereof, taken before they fall off, dried, and given a dram thereof in powder with white wine, wonderfully helpeth those that are troubled with the rising of the mother. The oil that is pressed out of the kernels, is very profitable taken inwardly like oil of almonds, to help the colick, and to expel wind very effectually; an ounce or two thereof may be taken at any time. The young green nuts taken before they be half ripe, and preserved with sugar, are of good use for those that have weak stomachs, or defluctions thereon. The distilled water of the green husks, before they be half ripe, is of excellent use to cool the heat of agues, being drank an ounce or two at a time; as also to resist the infection of the plague, if some of the same be also applied to the sores thereof. The same also cooleth the heat of green wounds and old ulcers, and healeth them, being bathed therewith. The distilled water of the green husks being ripe, when they are shelled from the nuts, and drank with a little vinegar, is good for the plague,

so

ſo as before the taking thereof a vein be opened. The ſaid water is very good againſt the quinſy, being gargled and bathed therewith, and wonderfully helpeth deafneſs, the noiſe, and other pains in the ears. The diſtilled water of the young green leaves in the end of May, performeth a ſingular cure on foul running ulcers and ſores, to be bathed, with wet cloths or ſponges applied to them every morning.

WOLD, WELD, or DYER'S WEED.

THE common kind groweth buſhing with many leaves, long, narrow, and flat upon the ground; of a dark blueiſh green colour, ſomewhat like unto Woad, but nothing ſo large, a little crumpled, and as it were round-pointed, which do ſo abide the firſt year; and the next Spring from among them, riſe up divers round ſtalks, two or three feet high, beſet with many ſuch like leaves thereon, but ſmaller, and ſhooting forth ſmall branches, which with the ſtalks carry many ſmall yellow flowers, in a long ſpiked head at the top of them, where afterwards come the ſeed, which is ſmall and black, incloſed in heads that are divided at the tops into four parts. The root is long, white, and thick, abiding the Winter. The whole herb changeth to be yellow, after it hath been in flower a while.

Place.] It groweth every where by the way ſides, in moiſt grounds, as well as dry, in corners of fields and bye-lanes, and ſometimes all over the field. In Suſſex and Kent they call it Green Weed.

Time.] It flowereth about June.

Government and Virtues.] Matthiolus ſaith, that the root hereof cureth tough phlegm, digeſteth raw phlegm, thinneth groſs humours, diſſolveth hard tumours, and openeth obſtructions. Some do highly commend it againſt the biting of venomous creatures, to be taken inwardly and applied outwardly to the hurt place; as alſo for the plague or peſtilence. The people in ſome counties of this land, do uſe to bruiſe the herb, and lay it to cuts or wounds in the hands or legs, to heal them.

WHEAT.

ALL the several kinds hereof are so well known unto almost all people, that it is altogether needless to write a description thereof.

Government and Virtues.] It is under Venus. Dioscorides saith, That to eat the corn of green Wheat is hurtful to the stomach, and breedeth worms. Pliny saith, That the corn of Wheat roasted upon an iron pan, and eaten, are a present remedy for those that are child with cold. The oil pressed from Wheat, between two thick plates of iron, or copper heated, healeth all tetters and ringworms, being used warm; and hereby Galen saith, he hath known many to be cured. Matthiolus commendeth the same to be put into hollow ulcers to heal them up, and it is good for chops in the hands and feet, and to make rugged skin smooth. The green corns of Wheat being chewed, and applied to the place bitten by a mad dog, heals it; slices of Wheat bread soaked in red rose water, and applied to the eyes that are hot, red and inflamed, or blood-shotten, helpeth them. Hot bread applied for an hour, at times, for three days together, perfectly healeth the kernels in the throat, commonly called the king's evil. The flour of Wheat mixed with the juice of henbane, stay the flux of humours to the joints, being laid thereon. The said meal boiled in vinegar, helpeth the shrinking of the sinews, saith Pliny; and mixed with vinegar, and boiled together, healeth all freckles, spots and pimples on the face. Wheat flower, mixed with the yolk of an egg, honey and turpentine, doth draw, cleanse and heal any boil, plague sore, or foul ulcer. The bran of Wheat meal steeped in sharp vinegar, and then bound in a linen cloth, and rubbed on those places that have the scurf, morphew, scabs or leprosy, will take them away, the body being first well purged and prepared. The decoction of the bran of Wheat or barley, is of good use to bathe those places that are bursten by a rupture; and the said bran boiled in good vinegar, and applied to swollen breasts, helpeth them, and stayeth all inflammations. It helpeth also the biting of vipers (which I take to be no other than our English adder) and all other venomous creatures. The leaves of Wheat meal, applied

applied with ſome ſalt, take away hardneſs of the ſkin, warts and hard knots in the fleſh. Starch moiſtened with roſe water, and laid to the cods, taketh away their itching. Wafters put in water, and drank, ſtayeth the laſks and bloody-flux, and are profitably uſed both inwardly and outwardly for the ruptures in children. Boiled in water unto a thick jelly, and taken, it ſtayeth ſpitting of blood; and boiled with mint and butter, it helpeth the hoarſeneſs of the throat.

The WILLOW TREE.

THESE are ſo well known that they need no deſcription; I ſhall therefore only ſhew you the virtues thereof.

Government and Virtues.] The Moon owns it. Both the leaves, bark, and the ſeed, are uſed to ſtanch bleeding of wounds, and at mouth and noſe, ſpitting of blood, and other fluxes of blood in man or woman, and to ſtay vomiting, and provocation thereunto, if the decoction of them in wine be drank. It helpeth alſo to ſtay thin, hot, ſharp, ſalt diſtillations from the head upon the lungs, cauſing a conſumption. The leaves bruiſed with ſome pepper, and drank in wine, helps much the wind colick. The leaves bruiſed and boiled in wine, and drank, ſtayeth the heat of luſt in man or woman, and quite extinguiſheth it, if it be long uſed: The ſeed is alſo of the ſame effect. Water that is gathered from the Willow, when it flowereth, the bark being ſlit, and a veſſel fitting to receive it, is very good for redneſs and dimneſs of ſight, or films that grow over the eyes, and ſtay the rheums that fall into them; to provoke urine, being ſtopped, if it be drank; to clear the face and ſkin from ſpots and diſcolourings. Galen ſaith, The flowers have an admirable faculty in drying up humours, being a medicine without any ſharpneſs or corroſion; you may boil them in white wine, and drink as much as you will, ſo you drink not yourſelf drunk. The bark works the ſame effect, if uſed in the ſame manner, and the Tree hath always a bark upon it, though not always flowers; the burnt aſhes of the bark being mixed with vinegar, taketh away warts, corns, and ſuperfluous fleſh, being applied to the place. The decoction of the leaves or

bark

bark in wine, takes away ſcurff and dandriff by waſhing the place with it. It is a fine cool tree, the boughs of which are very convenient to be placed in the chamber of one ſick of a fever.

WOAD.

Deſcript.] IT hath divers large leaves, long, and ſomewhat broad withal, like thoſe of the greater plantain, but larger, thicker, of a greeniſh colour, ſomewhat blue withal. From among which leaves riſeth up a luſty ſtalk, three or four feet high, with divers leaves ſet thereon; the higher the ſtalk riſeth, the ſmaller are the leaves; at the top it ſpreadeth divers branches, at the end of which appear very pretty, little yellow flowers, and after they paſs away like other flowers of the field, come huſks, long and ſomewhat flat withal; in form they reſemble a tongue, in colour they are black, and they hang bobbing downwards. The ſeed contained within theſe huſks (if it be a little chewed) give an azure colour. The root is white and long.

Place.] It is ſowed in fields for the benefit of it, where thoſe that ſow it, cut it three times a-year.

Time.] It flowers in June, but it is long after before the ſeed is ripe.

Government and Virtues.] It is a cold and dry plant of Saturn. Some people affirm the plant to be deſtructive to bees, and fluxes them, which, if it be, I cannot help it. I ſhould rather think, unleſs bees be contrary to other creatures, it poſſeſſeth them with the contrary diſeaſe, the herb being exceeding dry and binding. However, if any bees be diſeaſed thereby, the cure is, to ſet urine by them, but ſet it in a veſſel, that they cannot drown themſelves, which may be remedied, if you put pieces of cork in it. The herb is ſo drying and binding, that it is not fit to be given inwardly. An ointment made thereof, ſtancheth bleeding. A plaiſter made thereof, and applied to the region of the ſpleen which lies on the left ſide, takes away the hardneſs and pains thereof. The ointment is excellent good in ſuch ulcers as abound with moiſture, and takes away the corroding and fretting humours: It cools inflammations,

flammations, quencheth St Anthony's fire, and ſtayeth defluction of the blood to any part of the body.

WOODBINE, or HONEY-SUCKLES.

IT is a plant ſo common, that every one that hath eyes knows it, and he that hath none, cannot read a deſcription, if I ſhould write it.

Time.] They flower in June, and the fruit is ripe in Auguſt.

Government and Virtues.] Doctor Tradition, that grand introducer of errors, that hater of truth, that lover of folly, and that mortal foe to Dr Reaſon, hath taught the common people to uſe the leaves or flowers of this plant in mouth-water, and by long continuance of time, hath ſo grounded it in the brains of the vulgar, that you cannot beat it out with a beetle: All mouth-waters ought to be cooling and drying, but Honey-Suckles are cleanſing, conſuming and digeſting, and therefore no way fit for inflammations; thus Dr Reaſon. Again if you pleaſe, we will leave Dr Reaſon a while, and come to Dr Experience, a learned gentleman, and his brother: Take a leaf and chew it in your mouth, and you will quickly find it likelier to cauſe a ſore mouth and throat than to cure it. Well then, if it be not good for this, What is it good for? It is good for ſomething, for God and nature made nothing in vain. It is an herb of Mercury, and appropriated to the lungs; the celeſtial Crab claims dominion over it; neither is it a foe to the lion; if the lungs be afflicted by Jupiter, this is your cure: It is fitting a conſerve made of the flowers of it were kept in every gentlewoman's houſe; I know no better cure for an aſthma than this: beſides, it takes away the evil of the ſpleen, provokes urine, procures ſpeedy delivery of women in travail, helps cramps, convulſions, and palſies, and whatſoever griefs come of cold or ſtopping: if you pleaſe to make uſe of it as an ointment, it will clear your ſkin of morphew, freckles, and ſun-burnings, or whatever elſe diſcolours it, and then the maids will love it. Authors ſay, The flowers are of more effect than the leaves, and that is true; but they ſay the ſeeds are leaſt effectual of all. But Dr Reaſon told me, That there was a vital ſpirit in every ſeed to beget its like; and Dr Experience told me, That there was a greater heat in the ſeed than there was in any other part of the plant; and withal, That heat was the mother of action, and then judge if old Dr Tradition (who may well be honoured for his age, but not for his goodneſs) hath not ſo poiſoned the world with errors before I was born, that it was never well in its wits ſince, and there is great fear it will die mad.

WORMWOOD.

THREE Wormwoods are familiar with us; one I ſhall not deſcribe, another I ſhall deſcribe, and the third be critical at: and I care not greatly if I begin with the laſt firſt.

Sea Wormwood hath gotten as many names as virtues, (and perhaps one more) Seriphian, Santonieon, Belchion, Narbinenſe, Hantonicon, Miſneule, and a matter of twenty more which I ſhall not blot paper withal. A Papiſt got the toy by the end, and he called it Holy Wormwood; and in truth, I am of opinion, their giving ſo much holineſs to herbs, is the reaſon there remains ſo little in themſelves. The ſeed of this Wormwood is that which uſually women give their children for the worms. Of all Wormwoods that grow here, this is the weakeſt, but doctors commend it, and apothecaries ſell it; the one muſt keep his credit, and the other get money, and that is the key of the work. The herb is good for ſomething, becauſe God made nothing in vain: Will you give me leave to weigh things in the balance of reaſon; Then thus; The ſeeds of the common Wormwood are far more prevalent than the ſeed of this, to expel worms in children, or people of ripe age; of both, ſome are weak, ſome are ſtrong. The Seriphian Wormwood is the weakeſt, and haply may prove to be fitteſt for the weak bodies, (for it is weak enough of all conſcience.) Let ſuch as are ſtrong take the common Wormwood, for the others will do but little good. Again near the ſea many people live, and Seriphian grows near them, and therefore is more fitting for their bodies, becauſe nouriſhed by the ſame air; and this I had from Dr Reaſon. In whoſe body Dr Reaſon dwells not, dwells Dr Madneſs, and he brings in his brethren, Dr Ignorance, Dr

Dr Folly, and Dr Sickneſs, and theſe together make way for Death, and the latter end of that man is worſe than the beginning. Pride was the cauſe of Adam's fall; pride begat a daughter, I do not know the father of it, unleſs the devil, but ſhe chriſtened it, and called it Appetite, and ſent her daughter to taſte theſe Wormwoods, who finding this the leaſt bitter, made the ſqueamiſh wench extol it to the ſkies, though the virtues of it never reached to the middle region of the air. Its due praiſe is this: It is weakeſt, therefore fitteſt for weak bodies, and fitter for thoſe bodies that dwell near it, than thoſe that live far from it; my reaſon is, the ſea (thoſe that live far from it, know when they come near it) caſteth not ſuch a ſmell as the land doth. The tender mercies of God being over all his works, hath by his eternal Providence, planted Seriphian by the ſea ſide, as a fit medicine for the bodies of thoſe that live near it. Laſtly, It is known to all that know any thing in the courſe of nature, that the liver delights in ſweet things, if ſo, it abhors bitter; then if your liver be weak, it is none of the wiſeſt courſes to plague it with an enemy. If the liver be weak, a conſumption follows; would you know the reaſon? It is this, A man's fleſh is repaired by blood, by a third concoction, which tranſmutes the blood into fleſh, it is well I ſaid, (concoction) ſay I, if I had ſaid (boiling) every cook would have underſtood me. The liver makes blood, and if it be weakended that it makes not enough, the fleſh waſteth; and why muſt fleſh always be renewed? Becauſe the eternal God, when he made the creation, made one part of it in continual dependency upon another: And why did he ſo? Becauſe himſelf only is permanent; to teach us, That we ſhould not fix our affections upon what is tranſitory, but upon what endures for ever. The reſult of this is, if the liver be weak, and cannot make blood enough, (I would have ſaid Sanguify, if I had written only to ſcholars) the Seriphian, which is the weakeſt of Wormwoods, is better than the beſt. I have been critical enough, if not too much.

Place.] It grows familiarly in England, by the ſea ſide.

Deſcript.] It ſtarts up out of the earth, with many round, woody, hairy ſtalks from one root. Its height is four feet, or three at leaſt. The leaves in longitude are long, in latitude narrow, in colour white, in form hoary, in ſimilitude like Southernwood, only broader and longer; in taſte rather ſalt than bitter, becauſe it grows ſo near the ſalt-water: At the joints, with the leaves toward the tops it bears little yellow flowers; the root lies deep, and is woody.

Common Wormwood I ſhall not deſcribe, for every boy that can eat an egg knows it.

Roman Wormwood; and why Roman, ſeeing it grows familiarly in England? It may be ſo called, becauſe it is good for a ſtinking breath which the Romans cannot be very free from, maintaining ſo many bawdy-houſes by authority of his holineſs.

Deſcript.] The ſtalks are ſlender, and ſhorter than the common Wormwood by one foot at leaſt; the leaves are more finely cut and divided than they are, but ſomething ſmaller; both leaves and ſtalks are hoary, the flowers of a pale yellow colour; it is altogether like the common Wormwood, ſave only in bigneſs, for it is ſmaller; in taſte, for it is not ſo bitter; in ſmell, for it is ſpicy.

Place.] It groweth upon the tops of the mountains (it ſeems 'tis aſpiring) there 'tis natural, but uſually nurſed up in gardens for the uſe of the apothecaries in London.

Time.] All Wormwoods uſually flower in Auguſt, a little ſooner or later.

Government and Virtues.] Will you give me leave to be critical a little? I muſt take leave: Wormwood is an herb of Mars, and if Pontanus ſay otherwiſe, he is beſide the bridge; I prove it thus: What delights in martial places, is a martial herb; but Wormwood delights in martial places (for about forges and iron works you may gather a cart-load of it) *ergo*, it is a martial herb. It is hot and dry in the firſt degree, viz. juſt as hot as your blood, and no hotter. It remedies the evils choler can inflict on the body of man by ſympathy. It helps the evils Venus and the wanton Boy produce, by antipathy: and it doth ſomething elſe beſides. It cleanſeth the body of choler (who dares ſay Mars doth no good?) It provokes urine, helps ſurfeits, or ſwellings in the belly; it cauſeth appetite to meat, becauſe Mars rules the

the attractive faculty in man: The ſun never ſhone upon a better herb for the yellow jaundice than this: Why ſhould men cry out ſo much upon Mars for an infortunate, (or Saturn either?) Did God make creatures to do the creation a miſchief? This herb teſtifies, that Mars is willing to cure all diſeaſes he cauſes; the truth is, Mars loves no cowards, nor Saturn fools, nor I neither. Take of the flowers of Wormwood, Roſemary, and Black Thorn, of each a like quantity, half that quantity of ſaffron; boil this in Rheniſh wine, but put it not in ſaffron till it is almoſt boiled: This is the way to keep a man's body in health, appointed by Camerarius, in his book intitled, *Hortus Medicus*, and it is a good one too. Beſides all this, Wormwood provokes the terms. I would willingly teach aſtrologers, and make them phyſicians (if I knew how) for they are moſt fitting for the calling; if you will not believe me, aſk Dr Hippocrates, and Dr Galen, a couple of gentlemen that our college of phyſicians keep to vapour with not to follow. In this our herb, I ſhall give the pattern of a ruler, the ſons of art rough caſt, yet as near the truth as the men of Benjamin could throw a ſtone: Whereby, my brethren, the aſtrologers may know by a penny how a ſhilling is coined: As for the college of phyſicians, they are too ſtately to learn, and too proud to continue. They ſay a mouſe is under the dominion of the Moon, and that is the reaſon they feed in the night; the houſe of the Moon is Cancer; rats are of the ſame nature with mice, but they are a little bigger; Mars receives his fall in Cancer, *ergo*, Wormwood being an herb of Mars, is a preſent remedy for the biting of rats and mice. Muſhrooms (I cannot give them the title of Herba, Frutex or Arbor) are under the dominion of Saturn, (and take one time with another, they do as much harm as good); if any have poiſoned himſelf by eating them, Wormwood, an herb of Mars, cures him, becauſe Mars is exalted in Capricorn, the houſe of Saturn, and this it doth by ſympathy, as it did the other by antipathy. Wheals, puſhes, black and blue ſpots, coming either by bruiſes or beatings, Wormwood, an herb of Mars, helps, becauſe Mars, (as bad as you love him, and as you hate him) will not break your head, but he will give you a plaister. If he do but teach you to know yourselves, his courtesy is greater than his discourtesy. The greatest antipathy between the planets, is between Mars and Venus; one is hot the other cold; one diurnal, the other nocturnal; one dry, the other moist; their houses is opposite, one masculine, the other feminine; one public, the other private; one is valiant, the other effeminate; one loves the light, the other hates it; one loves the field, the other sheets; then the throat is under Venus, the quinsy lies in the throat, and is an inflammation there: Venus rules the throat (it being under Taurus her sign). Mars eradicates all diseases in the throat by his herbs (of which wormwood is one) and sends them to Egypt on an errand never to return more, this done by antipathy. The eyes are under the Luminaries; the right eye of a man, and the left eye of a woman the Sun claims dominion over; the left eye of a man, and the right eye of a woman, are privileges of the Moon, Wormwood, an herb of Mars, cures both; what belongs to the Sun by sympathy, because he is exalted in his house; but what belongs to the Moon by antipathy, because he hath his fall in her's. Suppose a man be bitten or stung by a martial creature, imagine a wasp, a hornet, a scorpion, Wormwood, an herb of Mars, giveth you a present cure; then Mars, cholerick as he is, hath learned that patience, to pass by your evil speeches of him, and tells you by my pen, That he gives you no affliction, but he gives you a cure; you need not run to Apollo, nor Æsculapius; and if he was so cholerick as you make him to be, he would have drawn his sword for anger, to see the ill conditions of those people that can spy his vices, and not his virtues. The eternal God, when he made Mars, made him for public good, and the sons of men shall know it in the latter end of the world. *E. cœlum Mars solus habet.* You say Mars is a destroyer; mix a little Wormwood, an herb of Mars, with your ink, neither rats nor mice touch the paper written with it, and then Mars is a preserver. Astrologers think Mars causeth scabs and itch, and the virgins are angry with him, because wanton Venus told them he deforms their skins; but, quoth Mars, My only desire is, they should know themselves; my herb worm-

wormwood will reſtore them to the beauty they formerly had, and in that I will not come an inch behind my oppoſite, Venus; for which doth the greateſt evil, he that takes away an innate beauty, and when he has done, knows how to reſtore it again? or ſhe that teaches a company of wanton laſſes to paint their faces? If Mars be in a Virgin, in the nativity, they ſay he cauſeth the colick (it is well God hath ſet ſomebody to pull down the pride of man). He in the Virgin troubles none with the colick, but them that know not themſelves (for who knows himſelf, may eaſily know all the world.) Wormwood, an herb of Mars, is a preſent cure for it; and whether it be moſt like a Chriſtian to love him for his good, or hate him for his evil, judge ye. I had almoſt forgotten, that charity thinks no evil. I was once in the tower and viewed the wardrobe, and there was a great many fine cloaths: (I can give them no other title, for I was never either linen or woollen draper) yet as brave as they looked, my opinion was that the moths might conſume them; moths are under the dominion of Mars; this herb Wormwood being laid among cloaths, will make a moth ſcorn to meddle with the cloaths, as much as a lion ſcorns to meddle with a mouſe, or an eagle with a fly. You ſay Mars is angry, and it is true enough he is angry with many countrymen, for being ſuch fools to be led by the noſe by the college of phyſicians, as they lead bears to Paris garden. Melancholy men cannot endure to be wronged in point of good fame, and that doth ſorely trouble old Saturn, becauſe they call him the greateſt infortunate; in the body of man he rules the ſpleen, (and that makes covetous men ſo ſplenetick) the poor old man lies crying out of his left ſide. Father Saturn's angry, Mars comes to him; Come, brother, I confeſs thou art evil ſpoken of, and ſo am I; thou knoweſt I have my exaltation in thy houſe, I give him an herb of mine, Wormwood to cure the poor man; Saturn conſented, but ſpoke little, and ſo Mars cured him by ſympathy. When Mars was free from war, (for he loves to be fighting, and is the beſt friend a ſoldier hath) I ſay, when Mars was free from war, he called a council of war in his own brain, to know how he ſhould do poor ſinful man good, deſiring to forget his abuſes in being called an infortunate. He musters up his own forces, and places them in battalia. Oh! quoth he, why do I hurt a poor silly man or woman? His angel answers him, It is because they have offended their God. (Look back to Adam:) Well, says Mars, tho' they speak evil of me, I will do good to them; Death's cold, my herb shall heat them; they are full of ill humours (else they would never have spoken ill of me;) my herb shall cleanse them, and dry them; they are poor weak creatures, my herb shall strengthen them; they are dull witted, my herb shall fortify their apprehensions; and yet among astrologers all this does not deserve a good word: Oh the patience of Mars!

Felix qui potuit rerum cognoscere causas,
Inque domus superum scandere cura facit.
Oh happy he that can the knowledge gain,
To know th' eternal God made nought in vain.

To this I add,

I know the reason causeth such a dearth
Of knowledge; 'tis because men love the earth.

The other day Mars told me he met with Venus, and he asked her, What was the reason that she accused him for abusing women? He never gave them the pox. In the dispute they fell out, and in anger parted, and Mars told me that his brother Saturn told him, that an antivenerean medicine was the best against the pox. Once a-month he meets with the Moon. Mars is quick enough of speech, and the Moon not much behind hand, (neither are most women.) The Moon looks much after children, and children are much troubled with the worms; she desired a medicine of him, he bid her take his own herb, Wormwood. He had no sooner parted with the Moon, but he met with Venus, and she was drunk as a bitch: Alas! poor Venus, quoth he; What! thou a fortune, and be drunk? I'll give thee an antipathetical cure: Take my herb Wormwood, and thou shalt never get a surfeit by drinking. A poor silly countryman hath got an ague, and cannot go about his business; he wishes he had it not, and so do I; but I will tell him a remedy, whereby he shall prevent it: Take the herb of Mars, Wormwood, and if infortunes will do do good, what will fortunes do? Some think the lungs are under Jupiter; and if the lungs then the breath; and tho' ſometimes a man gets a ſtinking breath, and yet Jupiter is a fortune, forſooth; up comes Mars to him: Come, brother Jupiter, thou knoweſt I ſent thee a couple of trines to thy houſe laſt night, the one from Aries, and the other from Scorpio; give me thy leave by ſympathy to cure this poor man with drinking a draught of Wormwood beer every morning. The Moon was weak the other day, and ſhe gave a man two terrible miſchiefs, a dull brain and a weak ſight; Mars laid by his ſword, and comes to her: Siſter Moon, ſaid he, this man hath angered thee, but I beſeech thee take notice he is but a fool; prithee be patient, I will with my herb Wormwood cure him of both infirmities by antipathy, for thou knoweſt thou and I cannot agree; with that the Moon began to quarrel; Mars (not delighting much in womens tongues) went away, and did it whether ſhe would or no.

He that reads this, and underſtands what he reads, hath a jewel of more worth than a diamond; he that underſtands it not, is as little fit to give phyſic. There lies a key in theſe words which will unlock (if it be turned by a wiſe hand) the cabinet of phyſic: I have delivered it as plain as I durſt; it is not only upon Wormwood as I wrote, but upon all plants, trees, and herbs; he that underſtands it not, is unfit (in my opinion) to give phyſic. This ſhall live when I am dead. And thus I leave it to the world not careing a farthing whether they like or diſlike it. The grave equals all men, and therefore ſhall equal me with all princes; until which time the eternal Providence is over me: Then the ill tongue of a prating fellow, or one that hath more tongue than wit, or more proud than honeſt, ſhall never trouble me. *Wiſdom is juſtified by her children.* And ſo much for Wormwood.

YARROW, *called* Noſe-bleed, Milfoil, *and* Thouſand-leaf.

Deſcript.] IT hath many long leaves ſpread upon the ground, finely cut, and divided into many ſmall parts: Its flowers are white, but not all of a whiteneſs,

neſs, and ſtayed in knots, upon divers green ſtalks which riſe from among the leaves.

Place.] It is frequent in all paſtures.

Time.] It flowereth late, even in the latter end of Auguſt.

Government and Virtues.] It is under the influence of Venus. An ointment of them cures wounds, and is moſt fit for ſuch as have inflammations, it being an herb of Dame Venus; it ſtops the terms in women, being boiled in white wine, and the decoction drank; as alſo the bloody-flux; the ointment of it is not only good for green wounds, but alſo for ulcers and fiſtulas, eſpecially ſuch as abound with moiſture. It ſtays the ſhedding of hair, the head being bathed with the decoction of it; inwardly taken it helps the retentive faculty of the ſtomach; it helps the running of the reins in men, and the whites in women, and helps ſuch as cannot hold their water; and the leaves chewed in the mouth eaſeth the tooth-ach; and theſe virtues being put together, ſhew the herb to be drying and binding. Achilles is ſuppoſed to be the firſt that left the virtues of this herb to poſterity, having learned them of his maſter Chiron, the Centaur; and certainly a very profitable herb it is in cramps, and therefore called Militaris.

DIRECTIONS.

DIRECTIONS.

HAVING in divers places of this Treatiſe promiſed you the way of making Syrups, Conſerves, Oils, Ointments, *&c.* of herbs, roots, flowers, *&c.* whereby you may have them ready for your uſe at ſuch times when they cannot be had otherwiſe; I come now to perform what I promiſed, and you ſhall find me rather better than worſe than my word.

That this may be done methodically, I ſhall divide my directions into two grand ſections, and each ſection into ſeveral chapters, and then you ſhall ſee it look with ſuch a countenance as this is.

SECT. I.

Of gathering, drying, and keeping Simples, and their Juices.

Chap. 1. *Of leaves of Herbs*, &c.
Chap. 2. *Of Flowers.*
Chap. 3. *Of Seeds.*
Chap. 4. *Of Roots.*
Chap. 5. *Of Barks.*
Chap. 6. *Of Juices.*

SECT. II.

Of making and keeping Compounds.

Chap. 1. *Of diſtilled Waters.*
Chap. 2. *Of Syrups.*
Chap. 3. *Of Juleps.*
Chap. 4. *Of Decoctions.*
Chap. 5. *Of Oils.*
Chap. 6. *Of Electuaries.*
Chap. 7. *Of Conſerves.*
Chap. 8. *Of Preſerves.*
Chap. 9. *Of Lohochs.*
Chap. 10. *Of Ointments.*
Chap. 11. *Of Plaiſters.*
Chap. 12. *Of Poultices.*
Chap. 13. *Of Troches.*
Chap. 14. *Of Pills.*
Chap. 15. *The way of fitting Medicines to Compound Diſeaſes.*

Of all theſe in order.

CHAP. I.

Of Leaves of Herbs, or Trees.

1. OF leaves, chooſe only ſuch as are green, and full of juice; pick them carefully, and caſt away ſuch as are any way declining, for they will putrefy the reſt:

So ſhall one handful be worth ten of thoſe you buy in Cheapſide.

2. Note what places they moſt delight to grow in, and gather them there; for Betony that grows in the ſhade, is far better than that which grows in the Sun, becauſe it delights in the ſhade; ſo alſo ſuch herbs as delight to grow near the water, ſhould be gathered near it, though happily you may find ſome of them upon dry ground: The Treatiſe will inform you where every herb delights to grow.

3. The leaves of ſuch herbs as run up to ſeed, are not ſo good when they are in flower as before, (ſome few excepted, the leaves of which are ſeldom or never uſed) in ſuch caſes, if through ignorance they were not known, or through negligence ſorgotten, you had better take the top and the flowers, than the leaf.

4. Dry them well in the Sun, and not in the ſhade, as the ſaying of phyſicians is; for if the Sun draw away the virtues of the herb, it muſt needs do the like by hay, by the ſame rule, which the experience of every country farmer will explode for a notable piece of nonſenſe.

5. Such as are artiſts in aſtrology, (and indeed none elſe are fit to make phyſicians) ſuch I adviſe; let the planet that governs the herb be angular, and the ſtronger the better; if they can in herbs of Saturn, let Saturn be in the aſcendant; in the herbs of Mars, let Mars be in the mid heaven, for in thoſe houſes they delight; let the Moon apply to them by good aſpect, and let her not be in the houſes of her enemies; if you cannot well ſtay till ſhe apply to them, let her apply to a planet of the ſame triplicity; if you cannot wait that time neither, let her be with a fixed ſtar of their nature.

6. Having well dried them, put them up in brown paper, ſewing the paper up like a ſack, and preſs them not too hard together, and keep them in a dry place near the fire.

7. As for the duration of dried herbs, a juſt time cannot be given, let authors prate their pleaſure; for,

1ſt, Such as grow upon dry grounds will keep better than ſuch as grow on moiſt.

2dly, Such herbs as are full of juice, will not keep ſo long as ſuch as are drier.

3dly,

3dly, Such herbs as are well dried, will keep longer than ſuch as are ſlack dried. Yet you may know when they are corrupted, by their loſs of colour, or ſmell, or both; and, if they be corrupted, reaſon will tell you that they muſt needs corrupt the bodies of thoſe people that take them.

8. Gather all leaves in the hour of that planet that governs them.

CHAP. II. *Of Flowers.*

THE flower, which is the beauty of the plant, and of none of the leaſt uſe in phyſick, groweth yearly, and is to be gathered when it is in its prime.

2. As for the time of gathering them, let the planetary hour, and the plant they come of, be obſerved, as we ſhewed you in the foregoing chapter; as for the time of the day, let it be when the ſun ſhines upon them, that ſo they may be dry; for, if you gather either flowers or herbs when they are wet or dewy, they will not keep.

3. Dry them well in the ſun, and keep them in papers near the fire, as I ſhewed you in the foregoing chapter.

4. So long as they retain the colour and ſmell, they are good; either of them being gone, ſo is their virtue alſo.

CHAP. III. *Of Seeds.*

THE ſeed is that part of the plant which is endowed with a vital faculty to bring forth its like, and it contains potentially the whole plant in it.

2. As for place, let them be gathered from the place where they delight to grow.

3. Let them be full ripe when they are gathered; and forget not the celeſtial harmony before-mentioned, for I have found by experience that their virtues are twice as great at ſuch times as others: "There is an appointed "time for every thing under the ſun."

4. When you have gathered them, dry them a little, and but a little in the ſun before you lay them up.

5. You need not be ſo careful of keeping them ſo near the fire, as the other before-mentioned, becauſe they are fuller of ſpirit, and therefore not ſo ſubject to corrupt.

6. As for the time of their duration, it is palpable they will

will keep a good many years; yet, they are beſt the firſt year, and this I make appear by a good argument. They will grow ſooneſt the firſt year they be ſet, therefore then they are in their prime; and it is an eaſy matter to renew them yearly.

CHAP. IV. *Of Roots.*

1. OF roots, chuſe ſuch as are neither rotten nor wormeaten, but proper in their taſte, colour and ſmell; ſuch as exceed neither in ſoftneſs nor hardneſs.

2. Give me leave to be a little critical againſt the vulgar received opinion, which is, That the ſap falls down into the roots in the Autumn, and riſes again in the Spring, as men go to bed at night, and riſe in the morning; and this idle talk of untruth is ſo grounded in the heads, not only of the vulgar, but alſo of the learned, that a man cannot drive it out by reaſon. I pray let ſuch ſapmongers anſwer me this argument: If the ſap falls into the roots in the fall of the leaf, and lies there all the Winter, then muſt the root grow only in the Winter. But the root grows not at all in the Winter, as experience teacheth, but only in the Summer: Therefore, If you ſet an apple-kernel in the Spring, you ſhall find the root to grow to a pretty bigneſs in that Summer, and be not a whit bigger next Spring. What doth the ſap do in the root all that while? Pick ſtraws! 'Tis as rotten as a rotten poſt.

The truth is, when the ſun declines from the tropic of Cancer, the ſap begins to congeal both in root and branch; when he touches the tropic of Capricorn, and aſcends to us-ward, it begins to wax thin again, and by degrees, as it congealed. But to proceed,

3. The drier time you gather the roots in, the better they are; for they have the leſs excrementitious moiſture in them.

4. Such roots as are ſoft, your beſt way is to dry in the ſun, or elſe hang them in the chimney corner upon a ſtring; as for ſuch as are hard, you may dry them any where.

5. Such roots as are great, will keep longer than ſuch as are ſmall; yet moſt of them will keep a year.

6. Such roots as are ſoft, it is your beſt way to keep them always near the fire, and to take this general rule for

for it: If in Winter-time you find any of your roots, herbs or flowers begin to be moiſt, as many times you ſhall (for it is your beſt way to look to them once a-month) dry them by a very gentle fire; or, if you can with conveniency keep them near the fire, you may ſave yourſelf the labour.

7. It is in vain to dry roots that may commonly be had, as Parſley, Fennel, Plantain, &c. but gather them only for preſent need.

CHAP. V. *Of Barks.*

1. BArks, which Phyſicians uſe in medicine, are of theſe ſorts: Of fruits, of roots, of boughs.

2. The barks of fruits are to be taken when the fruit is full ripe, as Oranges, Lemons, &c. but becauſe I have nothing to do with exotics here, I paſs them without any more words.

3. The barks of trees are beſt gathered in the Spring, if of oaks, or ſuch great trees; becauſe then they come eaſier off, and ſo you may dry them if you pleaſe; but indeed the beſt way is to gather all barks only for preſent uſe.

4. As for the barks of roots, 'tis thus to be gotten. Take the roots of ſuch herbs as have a pith in them, as parſley, fennel, &c. ſlit them in the middle, and when you have taken out the pith (which you may eaſily do) that which remains is called (tho' improperly) the bark, and indeed is only to be uſed.

CHAP. VI. *Of Juices.*

1. JUices are to be preſſed out of herbs when they are young and tender, out of ſome ſtalks and tender tops of herbs and plants, and alſo out of ſome flowers.

2. Having gathered the herb, you would preſerve the juice of it, when it is very dry (for otherwiſe the juice will not be worth a button) bruiſe it very well in a ſtone mortar with a wooden peſtle, then having put it into a canvas bag, the herb I mean, not the mortar, for that will give but little juice, preſs it hard in a preſs, then take the juice and clarify it.

3. The manner of clarifying it is this: Put it into a pipkin or ſkillet, or ſome ſuch thing, and ſet it over the

 fire;

fire; and when the ſcum ariſeth, take it off; let it ſtand over the fire till no more ſcum ariſe; when you have your juice clarified, caſt away the ſcum as a thing of no uſe.

4. When you have thus clarified it, you have two ways to preſerve it all the year.

(1.) When it is cold, put it into a glaſs, and put ſo much oil on it as will cover it to the thickneſs of two fingers; the oil will ſwim at the top, and ſo keep the air from coming to putrify it: When you intend to uſe it, pour it into a porringer, and if any oil come out with it, you may eaſily ſcum it off with a ſpoon, and put the juice you uſe not into the glaſs again, it will quickly ſink under the oil. This is the firſt way.

(2.) The ſecond way is a little more difficult, and the juice of fruits is uſually preſerved this way. When you have clarified it, boil it over the fire, till (being cold) it be of the thickneſs of honey: This is moſt commonly uſed for diſeaſes of the mouth, and is called Roba and Saba. And thus much for the firſt ſection, the ſecond follows.

SECT. II.

The way of making and keeping all neceſſary Compounds.

CHAP. I. *Of Diſtilled Waters.*

Hitherto we have ſpoke of medicines which conſiſt in in their own nature, which authors vulgarly call Simples, though ſomething improperly; for in truth, nothing is ſimple but pure elements; all things elſe are compounded of them. We come now to treat of the artificial medicines, in the form of which (becauſe we muſt begin ſomewhere) we ſhall place diſtilled waters; in which conſider.

1. Waters are diſtilled of herbs, flowers, fruits, and roots.

2. We treat not of ſtrong waters, but of cold, as being to act Galen's part, and not Paracelſus's.

3. The herbs ought to be diſtilled when they are in the greateſt vigour, and ſo ought the flowers alſo.

4. The vulgar way of diſtillations which people uſe, becauſe

because they know no better, is in a pewter ſtill; and altho' diſtilled waters are the weakeſt of artificial medicines, and good for little but mixtures of other medicines, yet they are weaker by many degrees, than they would be were they diſtilled in ſand. If I thought it not impoſſible, to teach you the way of diſtilling in ſand, I would attempt it.

5. When you have diſtilled your water, put it into a glaſs, covered over with a paper pricked full of holes, ſo that the excrementitious and fiery vapours may exhale, which cauſe that ſettling in diſtilled waters called the Mother, which corrupt them, then cover it cloſe, and keep it for your uſe.

6. Stopping diſtilled waters with a cork, makes them muſty, and ſo does paper, if it but touch the water; it is beſt to ſtop them with a bladder, being firſt put in water, and bound over the top of the glaſs.

Such cold waters as are diſtilled in a pewter ſtill (if well kept) will endure a year; ſuch as are diſtilled in ſand, as they are twice as ſtrong, ſo they endure twice as long.

CHAP. II. *Of Syrups.*

1. A Syrup is a medicine of a liquid form, compoſed of infuſion, decoction and juice. And, 1. For the more grateful taſte. 2. For the better keeping of it; with a certain quantity of honey or ſugar, hereafter mentioned, boiled to the thickneſs of new honey.

2. You ſee at the firſt view, That this aphoriſm divides itſelf into three branches, which deſerve ſeverally to be treated of, viz.

1. Syrups made by infuſion.
2. Syrups made by decoction.
3. Syrups made by juice.

Of each of theſe, (for your inſtruction-ſake, kind countrymen and women) I ſpeak a word, or two apart.

1ſt, Syrups made by infuſion, are uſually made of flowers, and of ſuch flowers as ſoon loſe their colour and ſtrength by boiling, as roſes, violets, peach-flowers, &c. My tranſlation of the London Diſpenſatory will inſtruct you in the reſt. They are thus made: Having picked your flowers clean, to every pound of them add three pounds or three pints, which you will (for it is all one) of ſpring water, made boiling hot; firſt put your flowers into a pewter pot, with a cover, and pour the water on them; then ſhutting the pot, let it ſtand by the fire, to keep hot twelve hours, and ſtrain it out; (in ſuch ſyrups as purge) as damaſk roſes, peach flowers, &c. the uſual, and indeed the beſt way, is to repeat this infuſion, adding freſh flowers to the ſame liquor divers times, (that ſo it may be the ſtronger) having ſtrained it out, put the infuſion into a pewter baſon, or an earthen one well glazed, and to every pint of it add two pounds of ſugar, which being only melted over the fire, without boiling, and ſcummed, will produce you the ſyrup you deſire.

2dly, Syrups made by decoction are uſually made of compounds, yet may any ſimple herb be thus converted into ſyrup: Take the herb, root, or flowers you would make into a ſyrup, and bruiſe it a little; then boil it in a convenient quantity of ſpring water; the more water you boil it in, the weaker it will be; a handful of the herb or root is a convenient quantity for a pint of water; boil it till half the water be conſumed, then let it ſtand till it be almoſt cold, and ſtrain it thro' a woollen cloth, letting it run out at leiſure; without preſſing: To every pint of this decoction add one pound of ſugar, and boil it over the fire till it come to a ſyrup, which you may know, if you now and then cool a little of it with a ſpoon: Scum it all the while it boils, and when it is ſufficiently boiled, whilſt it is hot, ſtrain it again through a woollen cloth, but preſs it not. Thus you have the ſyrup perfected.

3dly, Syrups made of juice, are uſually made of ſuch herbs as are full of juice, and indeed they are better made into a ſyrup this way than any other; the operation is thus: Having beaten the herb in a ſtone mortar, with a wooden peſtle, preſs out the juice, and clarify it, as you are taught before in the juices; then let the juice boil away till about a quarter of it be conſumed: To a pint of this add a pound of ſugar, and boil it to a ſyrup

ſyrup, always ſcumming it, and when it is boiled enough, ſtrain it through a woollen cloth, as we taught you before, and keep it for your uſe.

3. If you make a ſyrup of roots that are any thing hard, as parſley, fennel, and graſs roots, *&c.* when you have bruiſed them, lay them in ſteep ſome time in that water which you intend to boil them in, hot, ſo will the virtue the better come out.

4. Keep your ſyrups either in glaſſes or ſtone pots, and ſtop them not with cork nor bladder, unleſs you would have the glaſs break, and the ſyrup loſt, only bind paper about the mouth.

5. All ſyrups, if well made, continue a year with ſome advantage; yet ſuch as are made by infuſion, keep ſhorteſt.

CHAP. II. *Of Juleps.*

JULEPS were firſt invented, as I ſuppoſe, in Arabia; and my reaſon is, becauſe the word Julep is an Arabick word.

2. It ſignifies only a pleaſant potion, as is vulgarly uſed by ſuch as are ſick, and want help, or ſuch as are in health, and want no money to quench thirſt.

3. Now-a-days it is commonly uſed,

1. To prepare the body for purgation.
2. To open obſtructions and the pores.
3. To digeſt tough humours.
4. To qualify hot diſtempers, *&c.*

4. Simple Juleps (for I have nothing to ſay to compounds here) are thus made: Take a pint of ſuch diſtilled water, as conduces to the cure of your diſtemper, which this treatiſe will plentifully furniſh you with, to which add two ounces of ſyrup, conducing to the ſame effect; (I ſhall give you rules for it in the next chapter) mix them together, and drink a draught of it at your pleaſure. If you love tart things, add ten drops of oil of vitriol to your pint, and ſhake it together, and it will have a fine grateful taſte.

5. All juleps are made for preſent uſe; and therefore it is in vain to ſpeak of their duration.

CHAP. IV. *Of Decoctions.*

1. ALL the difference between decoctions, and ſyrup made by decoction, is this: Syrups are made to keep, decoctions only for preſent uſe; for you can hardly keep a decoction a week at any time; if the weather be hot, not half ſo long.

2. Decoctions are made of leaves, roots, flowers, ſeeds, fruits or barks, conducing to the cure of the diſeaſe you make them for; are made in the ſame manner as we ſhewed you in ſyrups.

3. Decoctions made with wine laſt longer than ſuch as are made with water; and if you take your decoction to cleanſe the paſſages of the urine, or open obſtructions, your beſt way is to make it with white wine inſtead of water, becauſe this is penetrating.

4. Decoctions are of moſt uſe in ſuch diſeaſes as lie in the paſſages of the body, as the ſtomach, bowels, kidneys, paſſages of urine and bladder, becauſe decoctions paſs quicker to thoſe places than any other form of medicines.

5. If you will ſweeten your decoction with ſugar, or any ſyrup fit for the occaſion you take it for, which is better, you may, and no harm.

6. If in a decoction, you boil both roots, herbs, flowers, and ſeed together, let the roots boil a good while firſt, becauſe they retain their virtue longeſt; then the next in order by the ſame rule, *viz.* 1. Barks. 2. The herbs. 3. The ſeeds. 4. The flowers. 5. The ſpices, if you put any in, becauſe their virtues come ſooneſt out.

7. Such things as by boiling cauſe ſlimineſs to a decoction, as figs, quince-ſeed, linſeed, *&c.* your beſt way is, after you have bruiſed them, to tie them up in a linen rag, as you tie up calf's brains, and ſo boil them.

8. Keep all decoctions in a glaſs cloſe ſtopped, and in the cooler place you keep them, the longer they will laſt ere they be ſour.

Laſtly, The uſual doſe to be given at one time, is uſually two, three, four, or five ounces, according to the age and ſtrength of the patient, the ſeaſon of the year, the ſtrength of the medicine, and the quality of the diſeaſe.

CHAP.

CHAP. V. *Of Oils.*

OIL Olive, which is commonly known by the name of Sallad Oil, I ſuppoſe, becauſe it is uſually eaten with ſallads by them that love it, if it be preſſed out of ripe olives, according to Galen, is temperate, and exceeds in no one quality.

2. Of oils, ſome are ſimple, and ſome are compound.

3. Simple oils are ſuch as are made of fruits or ſeeds by expreſſion, as oil of ſweet and bitter almonds, linſeed and rape-ſeed oil, &c. of which ſee in my Diſpenſatory.

4. Compound oils, are made of oil of olives, and other ſimples, imagine herbs, flowers, roots, &c.

5. The way of making them is this: Having bruiſed the herbs or flowers you would make your oil of, put them into an earthen pot, and to two or three handfuls of them pour a pint of oil, cover the pot with a paper, ſet it in the ſun about a fortnight or ſo, according as the ſun is in hotneſs; then, having warmed it very well by the fire, preſs out the herb, &c. very hard in a preſs, and add as many more herbs to the ſame oil; bruiſe the herbs (I mean not the oil) in like manner, ſet them in the ſun as before; the oftner you repeat this, the ſtronger your oil will be: At laſt when you conceive it ſtrong enough, boil both herbs and oil together, till the juice be conſumed, which you may know by its leaving its bubbling, and the herbs will be criſp; then ſtrain it while it is hot, and keep it in a ſtone or glaſs veſſel for your uſe.

6. As for chymical oils, I have nothing to ſay here.

7. The general uſe of theſe oils, is for pains in the limbs, roughneſs of the ſkin, the itch, &c. as alſo for ointments and plaiſters.

8. If you have occaſion to uſe it for wounds or ulcers, in two ounces of oil, diſſolve half an ounce of turpentine, the heat of the fire will quickly do it; for oil itſelf is offenſive to wounds, and the turpentine qualifies it.

CHAP. VI. *Of Electuaries.*

PHyſicians make more a quoil than needs by half, about electuaries. I ſhall preſcribe but one general way of making them up; as for ingredients, you may vary

vary them as you pleaſe, and as you find occaſion, by the laſt chapter.

1. That you may make electuaries when you need them, it is requiſite that you keep always herbs, roots, flowers, ſeeds, &c. ready dried in your houſe, that ſo you may be in a readineſs to beat them into powder when you need them.

2. It is better to keep them whole than beaten; for being beaten, they are more ſubject to loſe their ſtrength, becauſe the air ſoon penetrates them.

3. If they be not dry enough to beat into powder when you need them, dry them by a gentle fire till they are ſo.

4. Having beaten them, ſift them through a fine tiffany ſearce, that no great pieces may be found in your electuary.

5. To one ounce of your powder add three ounces of clarified honey; this quantity I hold to be ſufficient. If you would make more or leſs electuary, vary your proportion accordingly.

6. Mix them well together in a mortar, and take this for a truth, you cannot mix them too much.

7. The way to clarify honey, is to ſet it over the fire in a convenient veſſel, till the ſcum riſe, and when the ſcum is taken off, it is clarified.

8. The uſual doſe of cordial electuaries, is from half a dram to two drams; of purging electuaries, from half an ounce to an ounce.

9. The manner of keeping them is in a pot.

10. The time of taking them, is either in a morning faſting, and faſting an hour after them; or at night going to bed, three or four hours after ſupper.

CHAP. VII. *Of Conſerves.*

THE way of making conſerves is twofold, one of herbs and flowers, and the other of fruits.

2. Conſerves of herbs and flowers, are thus made: If you make your conſerve of herbs, as of ſcury-graſs, wormwood, rue, and the like, take only the leaves and tender tops (for you may beat your heart out, before you can beat the ſtalks ſmall) and having beaten them, weigh them,

and

and to every pound of them add three pounds of ſugar, you cannot beat them too much.

3. Conſerves of fruits, as of barberries, ſloes and the like, is thus made: Firſt, Scald the fruit, then rub the pulp through a thick hair ſieve made for the purpoſe, called a pulping ſieve; you may do it for a need with the back of a ſpoon; then take this pulp thus drawn, and add to it its weight of ſugar, and no more; put it into a pewter veſſel, and over a charcoal fire; ſtir it up and down till the ſugar be melted, and your conſerve is made.

4. Thus you have the way of making conſerves; the way of keeping them is in earthen pots.

5. The doſe is uſually the quantity of a nutmeg at a time, morning and evening, or, (unleſs they are purging) when you pleaſe.

6. Of conſerves, ſome keep many years, as conſerves of roſes; others but a year, as conſerves of borage, bugloſs, cowſlips, and the like.

7. Have a care of the working of ſome conſerves preſently after they are made; look to them once a day, and ſtir them about: Conſerves of borage, bugloſs, wormwood, have gotten an excellent faculty at that ſport.

8. You may know when your conſerves are almoſt ſpoiled by this; you ſhall find a hard cruſt at top with little holes in it, as though worms had been eating there.

CHAP. VIII. *Of Preſerves.*

OF Preſerves are ſundry ſorts, and the operations of all being ſomewhat different, we will handle them all apart. Theſe are preſerved with ſugar:

1. Flowers.	3. Roots.
2. Fruits.	4. Barks.

1. Flowers are very ſeldom preſerved; I never ſaw any that I remember, ſave only cowſlip flowers, and that was a great faſhion in Suſſex when I was a boy. It is thus done: Take a flat glaſs, we call them jat glaſſes; ſtrew in a laying of fine ſugar, on that a laying of flowers, on that another laying of ſugar, on that another laying of flowers, ſo do till your glaſs be full; then tie it over with a paper, and in a little time you ſhall have very excellent and pleaſant preſerves, it,

Thend

There is another way of preſerving flowers; namely, with vinegar and ſalt, as they pickle capers and broom buds; but as I have little ſkill in it myſelf, I cannot teach you.

2. Fruits, as quinces, and the like, are preſerved two ways:

(1.) Boil them well in water, and then pulp them thro' a ſieve, as we ſhewed you before; then with the like quantity of ſugar, boil the water they were boiled in into a ſyrup, *viz.* a pound of ſugar to a pint of liquor; to every pound of this ſyrup, add four ounces of the pulp; then boil it with a very gentle fire to their right conſiſtence, which you may eaſily know, if you drop a drop of it upon a trencher; if it be enough, it will not ſtick to to your fingers when it is cold.

(2.) Another way to preſerve fruits is this: Firſt, Pare off the rind; then cut them in halves, and take out the core; then boil them in water till they are ſoft; if you know when beef is boiled enough, you may eaſily know when they are: Then boil the water with its like weight of ſugar into a ſyrup; put the ſyrup into a pot, and put the boiled fruit as whole as you left it when you cut it into it, and let it remain till you have occaſion to uſe it.

3. Roots are thus preſerved: Firſt, Scrape them very clean, and cleanſe them from the pith, if they have any, for ſome roots have not, as Eringo and the like: Boil them in water till they be ſoft, as we ſhewed you before in the fruits; then boil the water you boiled the root in into a ſyrup, as we ſhewed you before; then keep the root whole in the ſyrup till you uſe them.

4. As for barks, we have but few come to our hands to be done, and of thoſe the few that I can remember, are oranges, lemons, citrons, and the outer bark of walnuts, which grow without-ſide the ſhell, for the ſhells themſelves would make but ſcurvy preſerves; theſe be they I can remember; if there be any more, put them into the number.

The way of preſerving theſe, is not all one in authors, for ſome are bitter, ſome are hot; ſuch as are bitter, ſay authors, muſt be ſoaked in warm water, oftentimes chang-

ing

ing till their bitter taſte be fled: But I like not this way, and my reaſon is this: Becauſe I doubt when their bitterneſs is gone, ſo is their virtue alſo; I ſhall then preſcribe one common way, namely, the ſame with the former, *viz.* Firſt boil them whole till they be ſoft, then make a ſyrup with ſugar and the liquor you boiled them in, and keep the barks in the ſyrup.

5. They are kept in glaſſes, or in glaz'd pots.

6. The preſerved flowers will keep a year, if you can forbear eating of them; the roots and barks much longer.

7. This art was plainly and firſt invented for delicacy, yet came afterwards to be of excellent uſe in phyſick: For,

(1.) Hereby medicines are made pleaſant for ſick and ſqueamiſh ſtomachs; which elſe would loath them.

(2.) Hereby they are preſerved from decaying a long time.

CHAP. IX. *Of Lohocks.*

1. THAT which the Arabians call Lohocks, and the Greeks Eclegma, the Latins call Linctus, and in plain Engliſh ſignifies nothing elſe but a thing to be lick'd up.

2. They are in body thicker than a ſyrup, and not ſo thick as an electuary.

3. The manner of taking them is, often to take a little with a liquoriſh ſtick, and let it go down at leiſure.

4. They are eaſily thus made: Make a decoction of pectoral herbs, and the treatiſe will furniſh you with enough; and when you have ſtrained it, with twice its weight of honey or ſugar, boil it to a lohock; if you are moleſted with much phlegm, honey is better than ſugar; and if you add a little vinegar to it, you will do well; if not, I hold ſugar to be better than honey.

5. It is kept in pots, and may be kept a year and longer.

6. It is excellent for roughneſs of the wind-pipe, inflammations and ulcers of the lungs, difficulty of breathing, aſthmas, coughs, and diſtillations of humours.

CHAP. X. *Of Ointments.*

1. VArious are the ways of making ointments, which authors have left to poſterity, which I ſhall omit, and

and quote one which is easiest to be made, and therefore most beneficial to people that are ignorant in physick, for whose sake I write this. It is thus done:

Bruise those herbs, flowers, or roots, you will make an ointment of, and to two handfuls of your bruised herbs add a pound of hog's grease dried, or cleansed from the skins, beat them very well together in a stone mortar with a wooden pestle, then put it into a stone pot, (the herb and grease I mean, not the mortar) cover it with a paper, and set it either in the sun, or some other warm place, three, four, or five days, that it may melt; then take it out and boil it a little; then whilst it is hot, strain it out, pressing it out very hard in a press; to this grease add as many more herbs bruised as before; let them stand in like manner as long, then boil them as you did the former: If you think your ointment not strong enough, you may do it the third and fourth time; yet this I will tell you, the fuller of juice the herbs are, the sooner will your ointment be strong; the last time you boil it, boil it so long till your herbs be crisp, and the juice consumed, then strain it, pressing it hard in a press, and to every pound of ointment add two ounces of turpentine, and as much wax, because grease is offensive to wounds as well as oil.

2. Ointments are vulgarly known to be kept in pots, and will last above a year, some above two years.

CHAP. XI. *Of Plaisters.*

1. THE Greeks made their plaisters of divers simples, and put metals into most of them, if not all; for, having reduced their metals into powder, they mixed them with that fatty substance whereof the rest of the plaister consisted, whilst it was yet hot, continually stirring it up and down, lest it should sink to the bottom; so they continually stirr'd it till it was stiff; then they made it up in rolls, which when they needed for use, they could melt by fire again.

2. The Arabians made up theirs with oil and fat, which needeth not so long boiling.

3. The Greeks emplaisters consisted of these ingredients, metals, stones, divers sorts of earth, feces, juices, liquors,

liquors, ſeeds, roots, herbs, excrements of creatures, wax, roſin, gums.

CHAP. XII. *Of Poultices.*

POultices are thoſe kind of things which the Latins call *Cataplaſmata*, and our learned fellows, that if they can read Engliſh, that's all, call them Cataplaſms, becauſe 'tis a crabbed word few underſtand; it is indeed a very fine kind of medicine to ripen ſores.

2. They are made of herbs and roots, fitted for the diſeaſe and members afflicted, being chopped ſmall, and boiled in water almoſt to a jelly; then by adding a little barley-meal, or meal of lupins, and a little oil, or rough ſweet ſuet, which I hold to be better, ſpread upon a cloth and apply to the grieved place.

3. Their uſe is to eaſe pain, to break ſores, to cool inflammations, to diſſolve hardneſs, to eaſe the ſpleen, to concoct humours, and diſſipate ſwellings.

4. I beſeech you take this caution along with you; Uſe no poultices (if you can help it) that are of an healing nature, before you have firſt cleanſed the body, becauſe they are ſubject to draw the humours to them from every part of the body.

CHAP. XIII. *Of Troches.*

1. THE Latins call them *Placentula*, or little cakes, and the Greeks, *Prochikois*, *Kukliſcoi*, and *Artiſcoi*; they are uſually little round flat cakes, or you may make them ſquare if you will.

2. Their firſt invention was, that powders being ſo kept, might reſiſt the intermiſſion of air, and ſo endure pure the longer.

3. Beſides, they are eaſier carried in the pockets of ſuch as travel; as many a man (for example) is forced to travel whoſe ſtomach is too cold, or at leaſt not ſo hot as it ſhould be, which is moſt proper, for the ſtomach is never cold till a man be dead; in ſuch a caſe, it is better to carry troches of wormwood, or galangal, in a paper in his pocket, than to lay a gallipot, along with him.

4. They are made thus: At night when you go to bed, take two drams of fine gum tragacanth; put it into a

 gallipot,

gallipot, and put half a quarter of a pint of any diſtilled water fitting for the purpoſe you would make your troches for, to cover it, and the next morning you ſhall find it in ſuch a jelly as the phyſicians call mueilage: With this you may (with a little pains taking) make a powder into a paſte, and that paſte into cakes called troches.

5. Having made them, dry them in the ſhade, and keep them in a pot for your uſe.

CHAP. XIV. *Of Pills.*

1. THEY are called *Pilulæ*, becauſe they reſemble little balls; the Greeks call them *Catapotia*.

2. It is the opinion of modern phyſicians, that this way of making medicines, was invented only to deceive the palate, that ſo, by ſwallowing them down whole, the bitterneſs of the medicine might not be perceived, or at leaſt it might not be unſufferable; and indeed moſt of their pills, tho' not all, are very bitter.

3. I am of a clean contrary opinion to this. I rather think they were done up in this hard form, that ſo they might be the longer in digeſting; and my opinion is grounded upon reaſon too, not upon fancy, or hearſay. The firſt invention of pills was to purge the head; now, as I told you before, ſuch infirmities as lie near the paſſages, were beſt removed by decoctions, becauſe they paſs to the grieved part ſooneſt; ſo here, if the infirmity lies in the head, or any other remote part, the beſt way is to uſe pills, becauſe they are longer in digeſtion, and therefore the better able to call the offending humour to them.

4. If I ſhould tell you here a long tale of medicines working by ſympathy and antipathy, you would not underſtand a word of it: They that are ſet to make phyſicians, may find it in the treatiſe. All modern phyſicians know not what belongs to a ſympathetical cure, no more than a cuckow what belongs to flats and ſharps in muſic, but follow the vulgar road, and call it a hidden quality, becauſe 'tis hidden from the eyes of dunces, and indeed none but aſtrologers can give a reaſon for it; and phyſic without reaſon, is like a pudding without fat.

5. The way to make pills is very eaſy, for with the

help of a peſtle and mortar, and a little diligence, you may make any powder into pills, either with ſyrup, or the jelly I told you before.

CHAP. XV. *The way of mixing medicines, according to the cauſe of the diſeaſe, and part of the body afflicted.*

THIS being indeed the key of the work, I ſhall be ſomewhat the more diligent in it. I ſhall deliver myſelf thus:

1. To the vulgar.

2. To ſuch as ſtudy Aſtrology; or ſuch as ſtudy phyſic aſtrologically.

1ſt, To the Vulgar. Kind ſouls, I am ſorry it hath been your hard miſhap to have been ſo long trained in ſuch Egyptian darkneſs, even darkneſs which to your ſorrow may be felt: The vulgar road of phyſic is not my practice, and I am therefore the more unfit to give you advice. I have now publiſhed a little book, (*Galen's Art of Phyſic*) which will fully inſtruct you, not only in the knowledge of your own bodies, but alſo in fit medicines to remedy each part of it when afflicted; in the mean ſeaſon take theſe few rules to ſtay your ſtomachs.

1. With the diſeaſe, regard the cauſe, and the part of the body afflicted; for example, ſuppoſe a woman be ſubject to miſcarry, thro' wind; thus do:

(1.) Look Abortion in the table of diſeaſes, and you ſhall be directed by that, how many herbs prevent miſcarriage.

(2.) Look Wind in the ſame table, and you ſhall ſee how many of theſe herbs expel wind.

Theſe are the herbs medicinal for your grief.

2. In all diſeaſes ſtrengthen the part of the body afflicted.

3. In mix'd diſeaſes there lies ſome difficulty, for ſometimes two parts of the body are afflicted with contrary humours, as ſometimes the liver is afflicted with choler and water, as when a man hath both the dropſy and the yellow jaundice; and this is uſually mortal.

In the former, Suppoſe the brain be too cold and moiſt, and the liver be too hot and dry; thus do:

1. Keep your head outwardly warm.

2. Accuſtom yourſelf to the ſmell of hot herbs.

3. Take a pill that heats the head at night going to bed.

4. In the morning take a decoction that cools the liver, for that quickly passeth the stomach, and is at the liver immediately.

You must not think, courteous people, that I can spend time to give you examples of all diseases: These are enough to let you see so much light as you without art are able to receive: If I should set you to look at the sun, I should dazzle your eyes, and make you blind.

2dly, To such as study Astrology, (who are the only men I know that are fit to study physic, physic without astrology, being like a lamp without oil); you are the men I exceedingly respect, and such documents as my brain can give you at present (being absent from my study) I shall give you.

1. Fortify the body with herbs of the nature of the Lord of the Ascendant, 'tis no matter whether he be a fortune or infortune in this case.

2. Let your medicine be something antipathetical to the Lord of the Sixth.

3. Let your medicine be something of the nature of the sign ascending.

4. If the Lord of the Tenth be strong, make use of his medicines.

5. If this cannot well be, make use of the medicines of the Light of Time.

6. Be sure always to fortify the grieved part of the body by sympathetical remedies.

7. Regard the Heart, keep that upon the wheels, because the Sun is the foundation of life, and therefore those universal remedies, *Aurum Potabile*, and the Philosopher's Stone, cure all diseases by fortifying the heart.

TABLE OF DISEASES.

D

Pox

F I N I S.

www.ingramcontent.com/pod-product-compliance
Lightning Source LLC
Chambersburg PA
CBHW021357210326
41599CB00011B/912
9783742840349